Pedicled Flaps in Partial Breast Reconstruction

Moustapha Hamdi • Raghavan Vidya
Amit Agrawal
Editors

Pedicled Flaps in Partial Breast Reconstruction

Springer

Editors
Moustapha Hamdi
Plastic Surgery Department
Brussels University Hospital
Vrije Universiteit Brussel
Brussels, Belgium

Raghavan Vidya
Department of Breast Surgery
The Royal Wolverhampton NHS Trust
Wolverhampton, UK

Amit Agrawal
Oncoplastic Breast Surgery
Cambridge University Hospitals
Cambridge, UK

This work contains media enhancements, which are displayed with a "play" icon. Material in the print book can be viewed on a mobile device by downloading the Springer Nature "More Media" app available in the major app stores. The media enhancements in the online version of the work can be accessed directly by authorized users.

ISBN 978-3-031-08482-9 ISBN 978-3-031-08483-6 (eBook)
https://doi.org/10.1007/978-3-031-08483-6

This Springer imprint is published by the registered company Springer Nature Switzerland AG
The registered company address is: Gewerbestrasse 11, 6330 Cham, Switzerland

The book is dedicated to all patients whose breasts we could save from an amputation, thanks to pedicled perforator flaps!

Foreword

Moustapha Hamdi is the world's expert on the use of Perforator Flaps in the Breast, and he has now literally written the book on it! This is an invaluable addition to the literature and will be essential reading for anyone who operates on the breast.

Not only does this book describe a host of available chest wall flaps that can be used in partial breast reconstruction, but it also describes how these flaps can be used in breast conserving surgery. Oncoplastic surgery is a combined effort between plastic and breast surgeons. Therefore, having two renowned breast surgeons as Miss Vidya and Mr. Agrawal as co-editors is a unique endeavour for all involved specialists in this field.

Dr. Hamdi and his co-editors have brought together experts from around the world to share their experience and their pearls on every aspect of using these various perforator flaps. However, the book is more than just a compendium of flaps. It contains descriptions of how to choose the best flap for a given defect, how to deal with issues of breast volume replacement, how to achieve a reconstruction with invisible or minimal scarring. Considering the potential effects of postoperative radiation is something we all deal with in our reconstructions and this subject is comprehensively covered here. Of course, a thorough explanation of any procedure is incomplete without a detailed description of complications and how to deal with them. Everyone must deal with complications from time to time so that having a resource to consult on this topic is invaluable. While it is extremely useful to learn the details of a new technique or a new flap, this information is incomplete without the perception of what results can be anticipated. Dr. Hamdi has given us this perspective with the final chapter in the book on Quality and Outcomes.

This book will be invaluable to any surgeon who performs breast reconstruction. It should also be required reading for those in training and it will be a worthwhile resource for anyone involved in breast surgery, whether reconstructive or ablative.

Peter C. Neligan
Division of Plastic Surgery
University of Washington
Seattle, WA, USA

Preface

Breast cancer is the commonest solid cancer amongt women. Surgery is the single best treatment for all biological types of early breast cancer regardless of age. Breast oncological surgery now is not just oncological surgery, nor does it simply add quality of life. Instead, it aims to restore near-normal whole female aesthetics and body image. Hence, breast surgery truly reflects the 'art' of surgery in the form of oncoplastic or is increasingly referred to as onco-aesthetic surgery.

The latest in breast oncological surgery is the technique of partial breast reconstruction with muscle-less chest wall perforator flaps. This enables breast preservation with the maintenance of the breast aesthetics despite excision of larger tumours from breasts that otherwise would have been either left deformed or would have needed a mastectomy.

The first application of this technique in breast surgery was about 20 years ago. However, it has gained traction mainly in the last decade, albeit in limited global breast geography. Therefore, most breast and plastic surgeons need a comprehensive compendium of individual techniques within the broader remit of chest wall perforator flaps. Thus, this book attempts to fill in the yawning gap in the breast surgery literature. We hope it will help breast and plastic surgeons provide an equitable range of oncoplastic procedures in their practice.

The book collates experiences from surgeons worldwide who perform this surgery and do not just write or talk hearsay on the topic. Their extensive experience has led them to teach or publish in the technique. Thus, the book reflects true and honest practice and thoughts.

The discussions amongst editors started pre-pandemic more than two years ago, and much like everything during the Covid-19 pandemic, the pace was affected due to the clinical service pressures of surgeons who put in stupendous effort in seeing this book through to the light of the day that publisher and editors are truly grateful for.

Brussels, Belgium
Wolverhampton, UK
Cambridge, UK
November 2022

Moustapha Hamdi
Raghavan Vidya
Amit Agrawal

Acknowledgements

When I finished my fellowship at Canniesburn Hospital Glasgow in Scotland in 1997, I was confident that muscle sparing techniques using perforator flaps should be the way forward in reconstructive surgery.

When I started in Gent, the Mecca of perforator flaps for total breast reconstruction, I felt I had to make a difference in my reconstructive approach to partial breast reconstruction. Most breast cancer patients with small breasts had to undergo mastectomy because of the limited options for breast conserving surgery. At that time, the mini latissimus dorsi flap was popular among British breast surgeons but it was not well accepted among plastic surgeons because of the sacrifice of the latissimus dorsi muscle.

It is thanks to my colleague Prof. Herman Depypere from the Department of Surgical Oncology in Ghent that I started with perforator flaps back in May 2000. Herman referred me the first patient for whom I performed a pedicled thoracodorsal artery perforator (TDAP) flap in immediate partial breast reconstruction. All of us, the patient, my colleague Herman and myself, were pleasantly surprised by the fluent postoperative course for the patient. We were able to remove the drains after 2 days and the patient had a swift rehabilitation without seroma formation at the donor site. The aesthetic result was truly amazing.

Taking this experience forward, both in clinical and academic practice, I was very happy to publicly defend my PhD thesis in July 2007. With no surprise, the title was Pedicled Flaps: A new concept.

During the following 22 years of my practice, I was eager to investigate every vascular pedicle around the breast. This led to the birth of many other pedicled perforator flaps. The indications of these flaps were many and changed with the course of time. I spent hours and hours to teach this technique through cadaver dissections, courses, live surgery demonstrations and national and international meetings with followers and friends worldwide from extending from Japan in the East to Argentina in the West.

Using these perforator flaps revolutionised the surgical approach of breast cancer in small to moderate breasts. Before our techniques, most of these patients were treated by mastectomies. It is therefore a real pleasure to see that pedicled perforator flaps have become a well-established technique in breast surgery.

I would like to thank all the authors who contributed to this book detailing their fabulous surgical techniques. I also would like to express my profound gratitude to my co-editors Vidya and Agrawal who will allow this heritage to be transmitted to the next generation of surgeons. Furthermore, my personal appreciation goes to Leonardo Dias for his unwavering help in preparing this book. Special thanks to Springer Verlag for their support and patience in finishing this new book.

Moustapha Hamdi

Growing up in India, I was fascinated to learn about eminent surgeons such as Sushruta and the origins of plastic surgery (600 bc) in the country. Graduating from the renowned Stanley Medical College, with an institutional history of over 300 years and an exemplary set of dedicated and deeply learned faculty such as Prof. CMK Reddy and Prof. Venkataswami, I developed a lifelong sense of purpose and mission alongside the professional knowledge. I completed a Master's in General Surgery under the guidance of Prof. Nitynanth and Prof. Palanivel who instilled in me a determination to pursue nothing less than a benchmark of excellence in surgery. In the course of training, I found mentors such as Prof. Mike Dixon who instilled confidence in me often saying 'less is more'. I understood the key concepts of integrating oncological safety with plastic techniques during my oncoplastic fellowship guided by Mr. S Harries, Mr. D Clarke, Mr. F Fatah and Mr. G Sterne, each of whom set such exemplary standards which inspire me to this day. Applauds to Prof. Hamdi for introducing the concept of Chest Wall Perforator Flaps to the world which is now getting adopted by surgeons around the UK and Europe. I must also share my sincere gratitude towards my friend Mrs. G Shetty who taught and trained me on the technique. The incorporation of the technique promoted breast conservation, received perfect feedback with high patient satisfaction, and mitigated the need for mastectomy. We have been teaching this technique to colleagues and trainees through cadaveric and live courses. Although the technique is a proven success and continues to further evolve, there is no concise book that explains its concepts. Therefore, I proposed the idea to Prof. Hamdi and Dr. Amit Agrawal to join hands with other eminent global authors to fill the void.

As I glance over the completed manuscript, I feel indebted to thank my family members including my father, late Mr. Raghavan, my mother Annapoorani, my sister Chitra, and brother-in-law Vaidyanthan for always encouraging me to share knowledge and promote innovation. My sincere thanks to my husband Dr. S Venkatachalam and my son Abhinav without whose support and sacrifice (time), this would not be possible.

Finally, my heartfelt and sincere gratitude to my patients and author-colleagues without whose participation and efforts this book would not take its current form.

Raghavan Vidya

Breast cancer surgery is the perfect blend of science and art. Breast surgeons led the way into the science of breast cancer of what it is today. Albert Schinzinger (Surgeon, Germany) in 1889 first proposed oophorectomy for treating advanced breast cancer. George Beatson (Surgeon, Scotland) in 1895 proved the concept by performing oophorectomy on a few patients. These led to the concept of breast cancer treatment with systemic therapy. A few decades later, in the 1970s, the importance of art in breast surgery and what better place to come from...Milan, the fashion capital. Umberto Veronesi (Surgeon, Italy) led to the concept of breast conservation as an oncological equivalent to mastectomy for treating early breast cancer. The early millennium saw the explosion of oncoplastic techniques leading up to the latest innovation that this book caters to.

Who inspired me? Well, these leaders, they all did besides parents. Particularly, Veronesi's name somehow stuck in my head since my third-year medical school. I did have my fanboy moment in 2005 at the European breast cancer meeting in Nice when he gave a plenary lecture. Alas, selfies weren't invented then!

It's been a long-winding journey and many more miles to go. At least, for one agenda, there should be unanimity amongst surgeons that we all have busy surgical practice and most with none or least amount of paid time for academic work. Still, we put in our soul for the best patient outcomes, not just quantitively but also qualitatively. Proactively and enthusiastically, we keep up with the pace of uniquely both the science and art of breast oncology, which we should be proud of. I initiated a cadaveric course in chest wall perforator flaps a few years ago in Cambridge. It's been successful with the grateful and enthusiastic support of co-editors (Prof. Hamdi, Vidya) and many authors, i.e., faculty, who spend unpaid time to share skills and knowledge with colleagues so that we all can provide the best for our patients. The alternative was to continue with age-old practice without the stresses of initiating new with inherent inertia and resistance.

Therefore, as much as our individual enthusiasm for the best possible care for our patients may or may not be recognised. However, we do consistently fail to recognise the toll it takes on our personal physical and mental health, family, and financial health. Innovations come at the cost of diverted time away from family and friends; and sadly, there is no evaluation of surgeon or surgeon's family health or robust support. I remain grateful to Priyanka and daughters, Anya, and Alisha, my parents (Shri LP and Shrimati Chinta), extended family, and friends for their forbearance and somewhat unrequited understanding, and yet unbridled love and unflinching support.

Amit Agrawal

Contents

List of Video

The online version contains supplementary material available at https://doi.org/10.1007/978-3-031-08483-6_9

History of Pedicled Perforator Flaps for Breast Reconstruction

1

Leonardo Pires Novais Dias, Marzia Salgarello, and Moustapha Hamdi

Contents

1.1 Breast Reconstruction Historical Background

Breast cancer first records are outlined in the surgical papyri of Edwin Smith, allegedly dated from 2500 to 3000 BC [1]. Until the last decades of the 1800s, treatment followed unreliable medical opinions without any background over the disease's biological behaviour. William Halsted filled this knowledge hiatus, inspired by Virchow's theory on the origin of breast cancer. He established the thought that breast cancer started as a limited locoregional phenomenon [2]. Therefore, in 1894, Halsted described the radical mastectomy technique, which became the standard treatment for breast cancer (Fig. 1.1) [3]. Originally, Halsted left the mastectomy wound open for second intention healing and strongly criticised any attempt to breast reconstruction, which he considered an oncological risk [3, 4].

L. P. N. Dias
Head of the Breast Surgery Department, Mater Dei Hospital, Salvador, Brazil
e-mail: leonardo.dias@materdei.com.br

M. Salgarello
Head of the Plastic Surgery Department, Agostino Gemelli University Hospital Foundation, Rome, Italy

M. Hamdi (✉)
Head of the Plastic Surgery Department, Brussels University Hospital, Vrije Universiteit Brussel, Brussels, Belgium
e-mail: moustapha.hamdi@uzbrussel.be

M. Hamdi et al. (eds.), *Pedicled Flaps in Partial Breast Reconstruction*,
https://doi.org/10.1007/978-3-031-08483-6_1

a

b

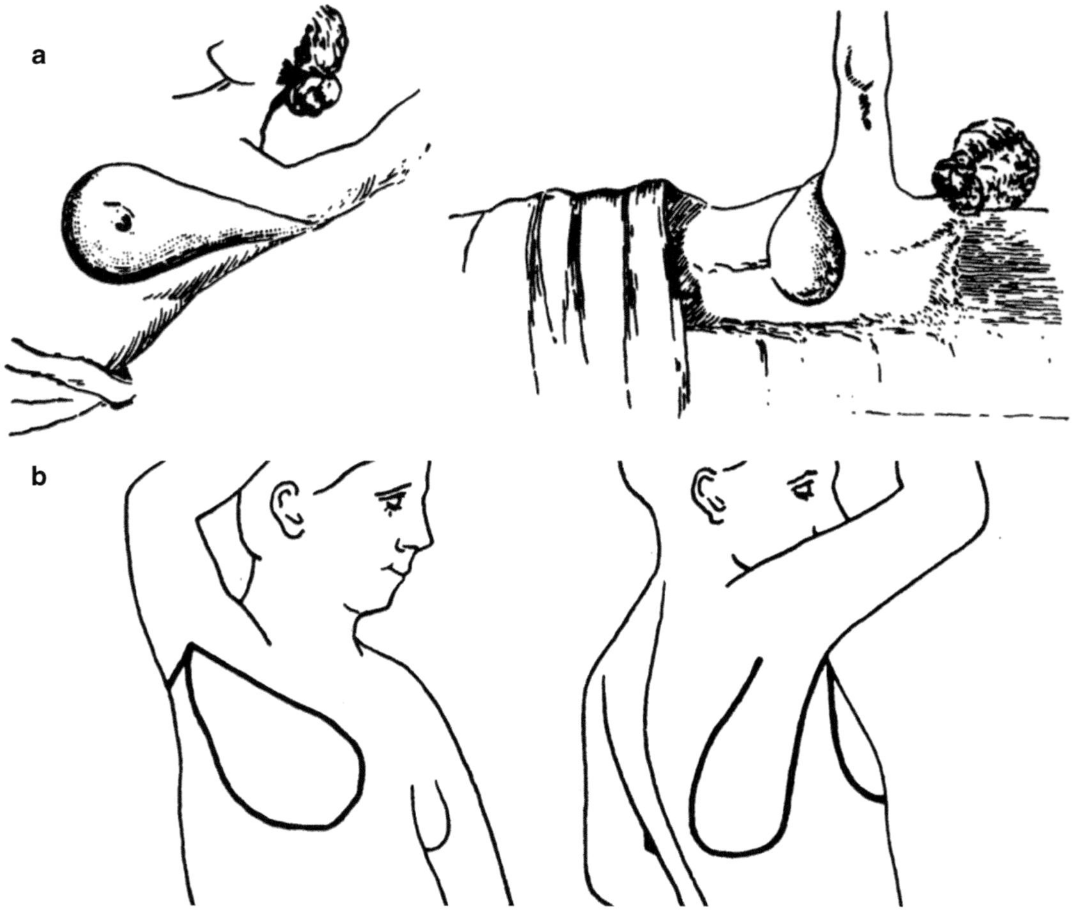

Fig. 1.1 Latissimus Dorsi Flap described by Iginio Tansini (1855–1943). (**a**) Dorsal skin flap design as shown in Tansini's original article (Redrawn from I. Tansini, Nuovo processo per l'amputazione della mammella per cancre. *Reforma Medica*, 12:3,1896). (**b**) Tansini's revised procedure showing the area of the skin to be excised and the design of the latissimus dorsi musculocutaneous flap used for coverage (Redrawn from F. Purpura, Tansini method for cure of cancer of the breast, *Lancet*, 1:634, 1908). *Note*. Adapted from "Iginio Tansini and the Origin of the Latissimus Dorsi Musculocutaneous Flap," by G. P. Maxwell, 1980, Plastic and Reconstructive Surgery, 65 (5), pg. 687, figs. 2 & 3. 686-692. Reprinted with permission

The radical mastectomy technique is a mutilating procedure with several associated dilemmas. For instance, this procedure favoured significant lymphedema, shoulder movement impairment, chronic pain syndrome, and severe local deformity [5, 6]. Therefore, facing these surgical outcomes from the radical mastectomy, the Italian surgeon Iginio Tansini proposed to cover the wound with a pedicled flap harvested from the dorsal area of the trunk. However, as one might expect from Tansini's skin flap design, he consistently experienced distal necrosis [7]. A few years later, after reviewing the vascular area of the trunk, Tansini described in detail the first pedicled musculocutaneous flap for breast reconstruction in 1906 (Fig. 1.1) [8]. Nevertheless, what seemed a natural path stopped on Halsted's concept of oncological safety. Hence, women had to wait almost a century before they were offered favourable circumstances for breast reconstruction [9].

Halsted's negative influence on breast reconstruction began to change with the introduction of modified radical mastectomies techniques between the 1940s and 1970s. A few years later, the advent of quadrantectomy, followed by radiotherapy in 1981, demonstrated the oncological safety of less mutilating procedures. Alongside, screening programmes permitted patients to have early diagnosis and adjuvant systemic treatment allowed downstaging the tumour prior to resection. Finally, the development of skin/nipple-sparing mastectomies and oncoplastic breast-conserving techniques led to a new era for breast reconstruction [10, 11].

Besides the oncological dogma, the first attempts of breast reconstruction showed unsatisfactory results. For instance, contralateral breast sharing, tubed and racquet-shaped flaps had poor design and delivered high donor site morbidity. Gradually, adjustments in understanding the vascular supply to muscles and skin permitted the rediscovery of the latissimus dorsi flap in 1976. One year later, it was successfully used to cover silicone prosthesis on a new attempt for breast reconstruction. In parallel, the abdominal wall flaps were gradually refined, and in 1982 Hartrampf et al. described the first characteristics of what became a standard of care from breast reconstruction, the transverse rectus abdominis myocutaneous flap [12]. The simplicity of the procedure and these encouraging results changed breast reconstruction perspective, helping it gain popularity and acceptance among the population and surgeons [10].

Alongside the improvement in the knowledge over breast cancer behaviour, several vital impediments to breast reconstruction were resolved during the second half of the twentieth century. The feasibility of immediate breast reconstruction stimulated patients to request the procedure and delivered notable psychological benefits [13, 14]. The rediscovery of anatomical superficial vascular territories in the 1980s launched the background for microsurgery, which was followed by the description of a variety of new autologous reconstructive techniques. Eventually, microsurgery faced some obstacles to become eligible since it has a longer duration and is technically more demanding, especially free flaps. On the other hand, the progression of anaesthesia protocols was crucial to increase indications. Consequently, surgeons could safely perform these longer and more challenging interventions [10, 15].

1.2 Perforator Flaps Historical Background

The word “flap” originates from the Dutch word “Flappe”, which means something that hangs loose, connected only on one side. In medical terms, a flap is a unit of tissue that is transferred from a donor site to another recipient area while maintaining its blood supply. There are several types of flaps, with different tissue components, shapes, and forms. They range from simple skin advancements to pedicled or also free tissue transfer.

The history of reconstructive perforator flap surgery began in 1889, when Carl Manchot described the first studies over the superficial vascular system of the body [16]. Manchot explored the description of cutaneous vessels pathways crossing muscles and fissures and their interconnections. In 1936, Salmon extended the knowledge on these superficial vessels with a report based on anatomical investigations centred on static radiographic imaging and cadaver dissection [17]. Besides the innovative description, these studies had limited influence on the scientific community at that time. Only in the 1980s these works were reviewed and had their value recognised [18, 19]. These were translated and served as a backdrop for the further development of the perforator flap technique (Fig. 1.2).

Besides some isolated attempts, the progress of the reconstruction flap surgery underwent a time hiatus until the late 1960s [9]. Then, in 1970, Milton reported the relation between skin flap design and adequate blood supply, which depended on a pedicle containing a large skin vessel [20]. In fact, at that time, the design of skin flaps was randomly selected based on proximity to the defect and geometry, with no specific assessment of perfusion beyond the general knowledge of the subdermal plexus. Thus, a significant source of blood supply was still totally neglected, and flaps were restricted to rigid length/width relationships to ensure viability [21].

In 1972, McGregor and Jackson described the groin flap, recognised as the first axial pattern flap to be reported [22]. Their studies

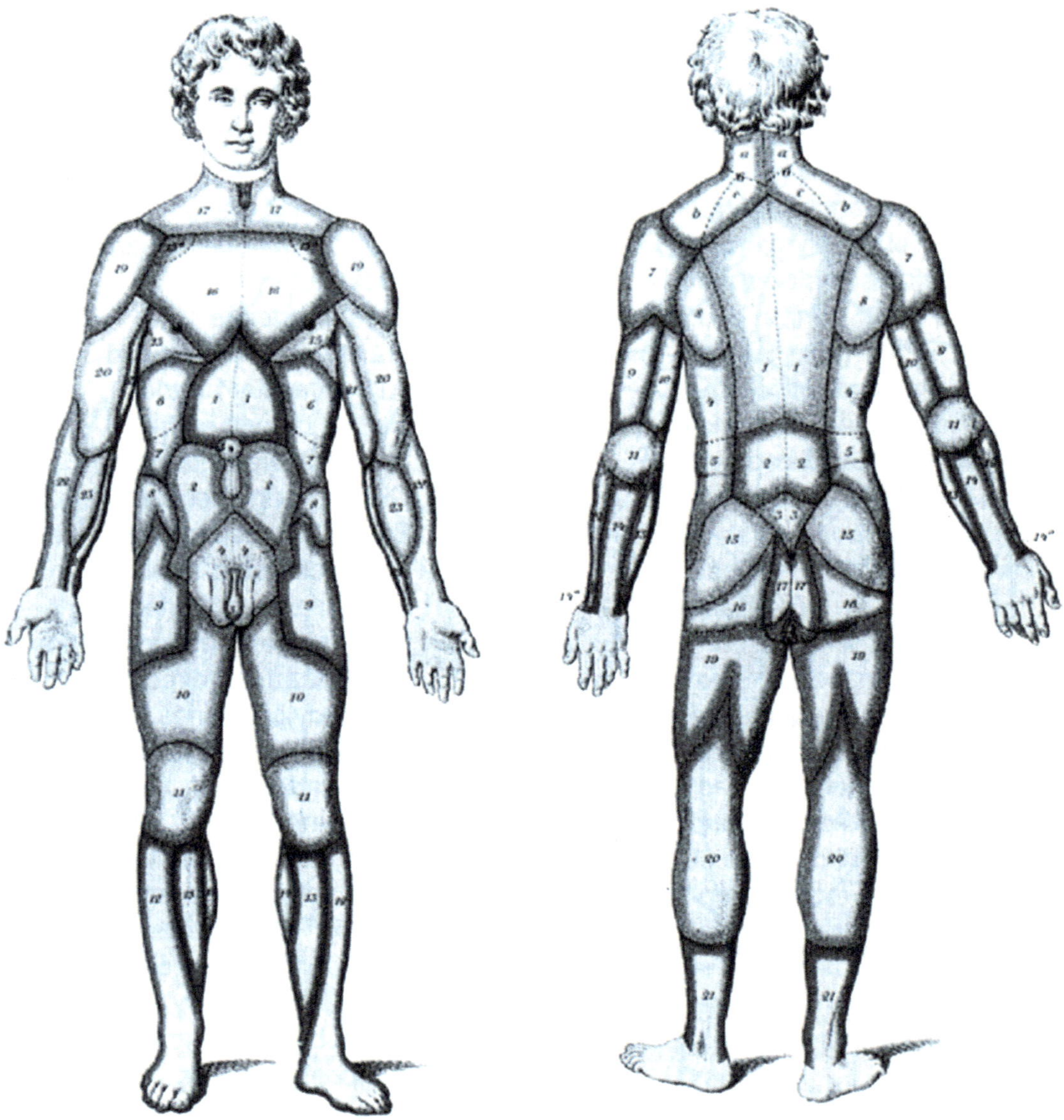

Fig. 1.2 The vascular territories of the body as described by Carl Manchot in 1889. *Note.* Adapted from "The Anatomic Basis of Perforator Flaps," by S. F. Morris et al., 2010, *Clinics in Plastic Surgery*, 37(4), p. 554, fig. 1. Copyright 2010 by Elsevier. Reprinted with permission

demonstrated the predictable orientation of vessels in axial flaps, which supported the report from Milton. Subsequently, the vaster reliability of axial flaps compared with previous techniques stimulated the description of new techniques and increased the number and type of flaps available. A few years later, in 1977, McGregor described the basic principles of the physiology of the flap [23]. In 1981, Pontén stated that blood flow in the cutaneous flap increases by including the deep fascia. With that, the surgeon may have better length/width ratios for the flap design. However, the author limited himself to a restricted anatomical description and did not demonstrate the rationale for the before-mentioned improvement [24].

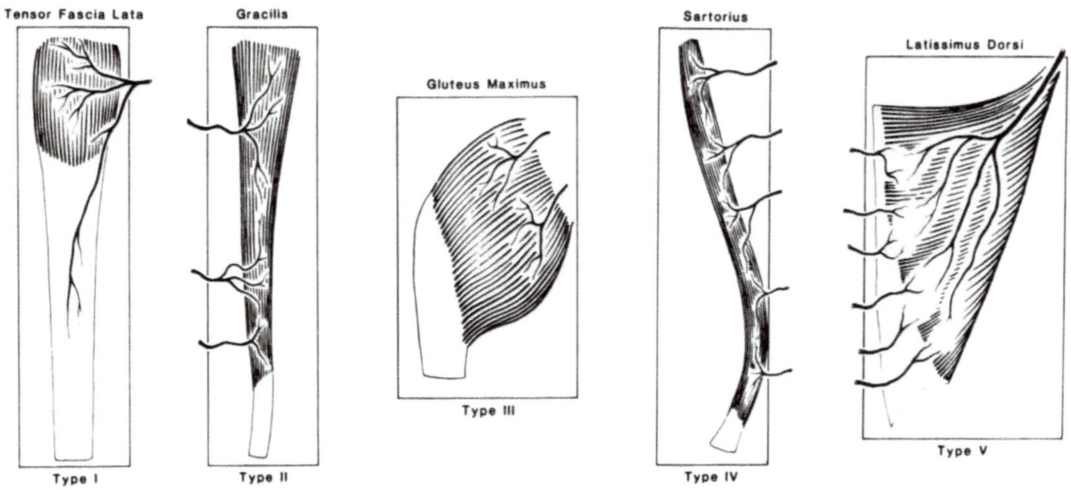

Fig. 1.3 Illustration of Mathes and Nahai Classification for Musculocutaneous Flaps. Type I: one vascular pedicle; Type II: dominant pedicle(s) plus minor pedicles; Type III: two dominant pedicles; Type IV: segmental vascular pedicles; Type V: dominant pedicle plus secondary segmental pedicles. *Note*. Adapted from "Classification of the vascular anatomy of muscles: experimental and clinical correlation," by S. J. Mathes and F. Nahai, 1981, *Plastic and reconstructive surgery, 67(2)*, p. 178, fig. 2. Copyright 1981 by Wolters Kluwer Health. Reprinted with permission

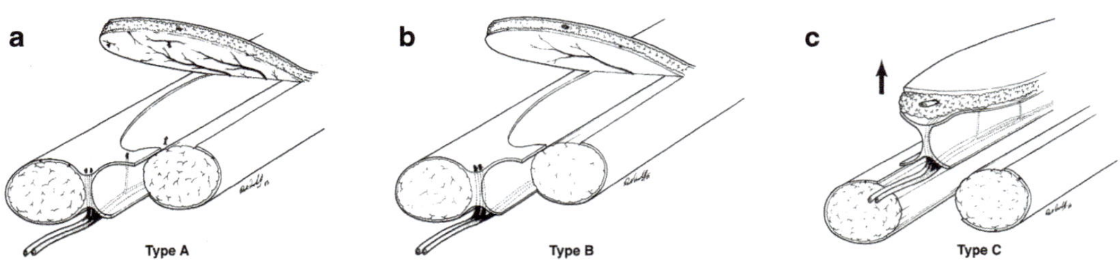

Fig. 1.4 Cormack and Lamberty classification for fasciocutaneous flaps. Type A: A pedicled fascia-cutaneous flap dependent on multiple fascia-cutaneous perforators at the base and orientated with the long axis of the flap in the predominant direction of the arterial plexus at the flap; Type B: A pedicled or a free flap depending on a single sizeable and consistent fascia-cutaneous perforator feeding a plexus at the level of the deep fascia; Type C: The ladder type. The skin's support is dependent upon the fascial plexus supplied by multiple small perforators along its length. Note. Adapted from A classification of fasciocutaneous flaps according to their patterns of vascularisation, by Cormack, G. C., and Lamberty, B. G., 1984, *British journal of plastic surgery*, *37*(1), p. 82, fig. 4; p. 83, fig. 5; p. 84, fig. 7. Copyright 1984 by Elsevier. Reprinted with permission

Higher detailed knowledge of vascular anatomy allowed better flap selection and refinement. Therefore, in 1981, Mathes and Nahai proposed a classification system for muscle flaps based on their vascularity, including predictions of the overlying skin blood supply (Fig. 1.3) [25]. At that time, the blood supply to the skin was considered to be composed of direct cutaneous and musculocutaneous vessels. However, in 1984, Cormack and Lamberty pondered the existence of another category: the fasciocutaneous perforators. These vessels supply the skin by passing along the fascial septa between adjacent muscles. Based on the relevance of fasciocutaneous perfo-

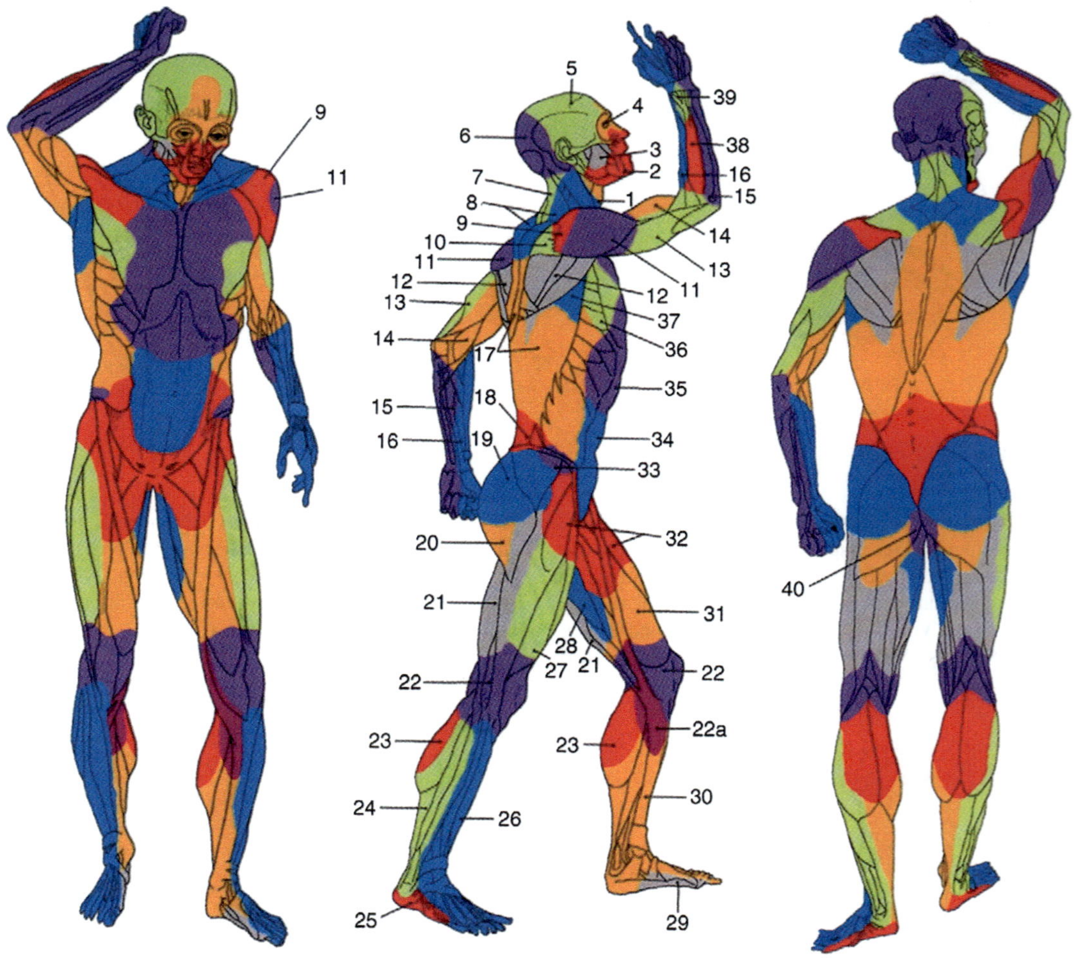

Fig. 1.5 The superficial vascular territory—Angiosomes concept. *Note*. Adapted from "The Anatomic Basis of Perforator Flaps," by S. F. Morris et al., 2010, *Clinics in Plastic Surgery*, *37 4*, p. 556, fig. 3. Copyright 2010 by Elsevier. Reprinted with permission

rators' pattern of vascularisation, Cormack and Lamberty classified these skin flaps into three categories (Fig. 1.4) [26]. In 1986, Nakajima proposed a classification for these skin flaps with six subtypes [27].

To overcome the possible incoherence amidst classification, Taylor and Palmer published in 1987 an innovative work explaining the superficial vascular territories and their arteries origins, termed angiosomes. Their study divided the body into 40 individual skin sections that were nourished by a specifically named source vessel and considered independent from the others (Fig. 1.5). Taylor and Palmer were inspired by the concept that every artery to the skin can be regarded as a direct or indirect branch from the underlying named source vessel. In fact, following this rationale, a direct branch always runs towards the skin, whether they pass between, along with or through the muscle. On the other hand, an indirect branch emerges throughout the deep fascia and supplies muscles and surrounding tissues. This report was a foundation for the subsequent development of perforator flaps [28].

The study of angiosomes revealed a new concept to be explored [28]. As a result, the literature became flooded with papers describing new flaps, variations in the technique, terminology, and classifications. In 1989, Koshima and Soeda coined the term perforator flap mainly to differentiate these from fasciocutaneous flaps. This perception was emphasised by their belief that the suprafascial plexus did not contribute to the vascularisation of the flap [29]. Since the first applications, the concept of perforator flaps has become trendier over the last decades. Its expanding acceptance is primarily related to the significant decrease in donor site morbidity due to the preservation of innervation, vascularisation, and functionality of the donor's muscle. According to Kroll and Rosenfield (1988), the perforator flap combined musculocutaneous flaps' reliability and vascular safety with the lower donor site morbidity of simple cutaneous flaps [30].

In 2003, Hallock defined a perforator as any vessel that enters the skin layer between a limited aperture in the deep fascia, despite its origin. Hallock differentiated direct and indirect perforators due to the specific source of the vessels that nourish the area and the structures they cross before penetrating the deep fascia [31]. Direct perforators pierce the deep fascia without traversing any other structural tissue. Indirect perforators first travel through deeper tissues, mainly muscle and septum.

Table 1.1 Gent consensus

	Definitions
1	A perforator flap is a flap comprising skin and/or subcutaneous fat. The vessels that supply blood to the flap are isolated perforator (s). These perforators may pass either through or in between the deep tissues (mostly muscle)
2	A muscle perforator is a blood vessel that traverses muscle to supply the overlying skin
3	A septal perforator is a blood vessel that traverses only the septum to supply the overlying skin
4	A flap that is vascularised by a muscle perforator is called a muscle perforator flap
5	A flap vascularised by a septal perforator is called a septal perforator flap
6	A perforator flap should be named after the nutrient artery or vessels, not the underlying muscle. If there is a potential to harvest multiple perforator flaps from one vessel, the name of each flap should be based on its anatomical region or muscle

At this point, the original classification of Cormack and Lamberty [26] became out-of-date, and the one from Nakajima et al. [27] was considered too complex for clinical purposes. Therefore, at the beginning of the twenty-first century, a group of surgeons from Gent proposed a new classification. In 2003, the Gent consensus summarised and created a nomenclature with six definitions concerning perforator flaps, which were widely accepted. The main idea was to develop a terminology that would provide sufficient anatomical and surgical detail to promote these new flap techniques' diffusion, reproduction, and popularisation (Table 1.1) [32].

In 2009, Saint-Cyr M. et al. advanced the understanding regarding distinct vascular territories of each perforator vessel and described the perforasome concept. In a series of cadaveric specimens, the study demonstrated the arterial territorial pattern of individual perforators and its multidirectional flow dynamics (Fig. 1.6). The report described the direct and indirect interconnections in the perforator territory. It stated that the bidirectional flux depended on the perfusion pressure (Fig. 1.7) [33]. A year later, the findings of the perforasome study were proved to be applicable in an in vivo analysis [34].

The perforasome concept provided an additional step for the surgical evolution of perforator flaps. Nowadays, suprafascial dissection is preferred to subfascial dissection and cutaneous-subcutaneous flaps over those that include the deep fascia. The amount of soft tissue that can safely be harvested in a pedicled perforator flap is based on the perforasome dynamics. The perforasome territory can be intraoperatively assessed by clinical examination or using indocyanine green angiography (ICG). The ICG gives a real-time evaluation of tissue perfusion and plays a crucial role in evaluating the maximum area of flap perfusion, allowing intraoperative flap adjustments [35].

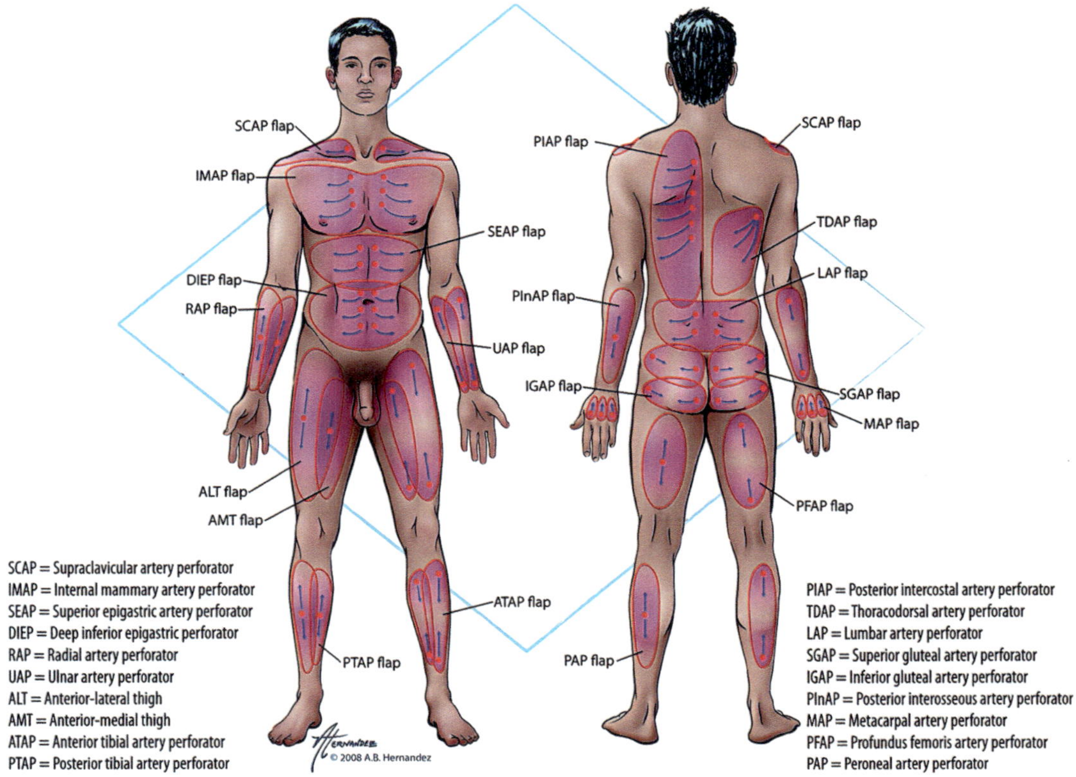

Fig. 1.6 Perforasomes of the body—Direction of the axial linking vessels. *Note.* Adapted from "The perforasome theory: vascular anatomy and clinical implications," by M. Saint-Cyr, et al., 2009, *Plastic and reconstructive surgery*, *124*(5), p. 1543, fig. 21. Copyright 2009 by Wolters Kluwer Health. Reprinted with permission

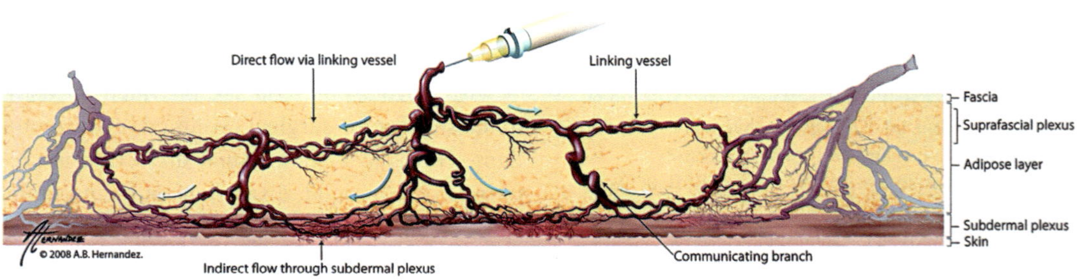

Fig. 1.7 Illustration of the perforasome concept with interperforator direct and indirect flow. Note. Adapted from "The perforasome theory: vascular anatomy and clinical implications," by M. Saint-Cyr, et al., 2009, *Plastic and reconstructive surgery*, *124*(5), p. 1533, fig. 2. Copyright 2009 by Wolters Kluwer Health. Reprinted with permission

1.3 History of Surgical Planning of Perforator Flaps

Evolution also affected the surgical planning of perforator flaps: the perforator location and its characteristics can be studied by multimodal techniques. However, the cheapest and easiest unidirectional Doppler gives an estimation of perforator presence only. In contrast, the other imaging methods, i.e., B-mode and colour-Doppler ultrasound (CDUS) [36] (Fig. 1.8), computed tomographic angiography (CTA) [37]

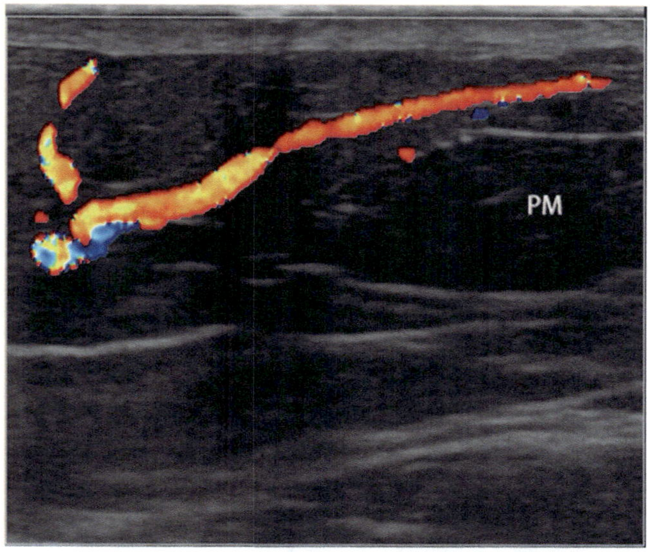

Fig. 1.8 Coloured Doppler Ultrasound findings of the superficial branch of the lateral thoracic artery. PM: pectoralis muscle. *Note*. Adapted from "Preoperative color Doppler ultrasound assessment of the lateral thoracic artery perforator flap and its branching pattern," by K. Tashiro, 2015, *J Plast Reconstr Aesthet Surg*, Jun;68(6):e120–5. Copyright 2015 by Elsevier. Reprinted with permission

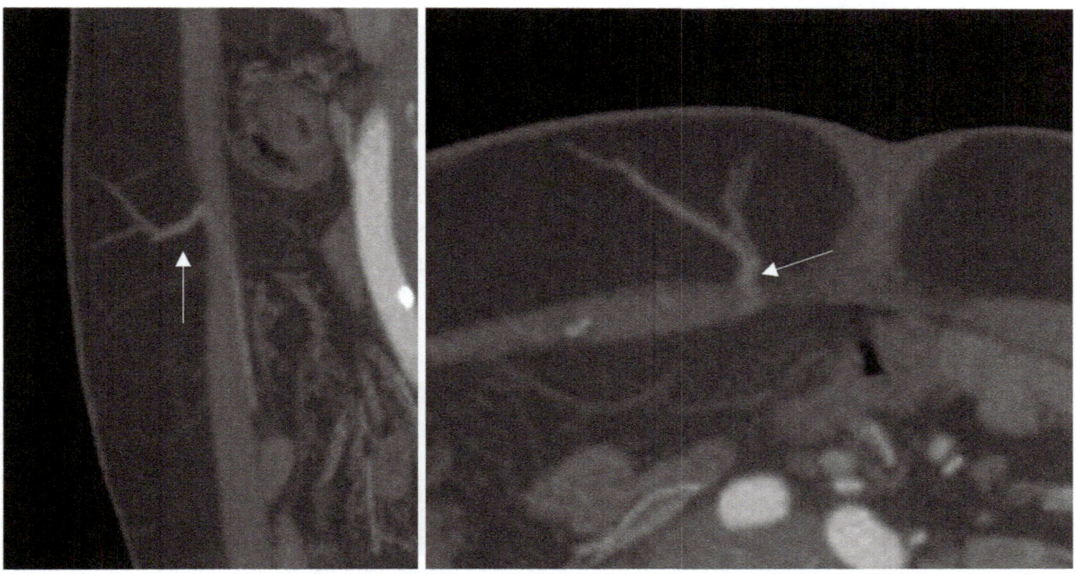

Fig. 1.9 Sagittal and axial 5 mm MIP reconstructions from a CTA. Right paramedian perforator with 2 mm calibre arising medial to the rectus abdominis muscle (white arrows). *Note*. Adapted from "CTA in preoperative planning for DIEP breast reconstruction: what the reconstructive surgeon wants to know. A modified Delphi study.," by K. K. Wong et al., 2019, *Clin Radiol*, Dec;74(12):973.e15–973.e26. Copyright 2019 by Elsevier. Reprinted with permission

(Fig. 1.9), and magnetic resonance angiography [38] (Fig. 1.10), can expand knowledge in terms of the measurement of perforator calibre, analysis of its course below the fascia up to the main vessels and its flow dynamics.

Among the various imaging methods, preoperative ultrasound-based planning allows one to know the vascular anatomy, select the best perforator vessel closest to the defect, and plan the surgery. The CDUS is the operative surgeon's tool for mapping the flap perforators and appropriately planning each flap [39]. The latest promising technology is ultra-high frequency ultrasonography (UHF-US), which allows evalu-

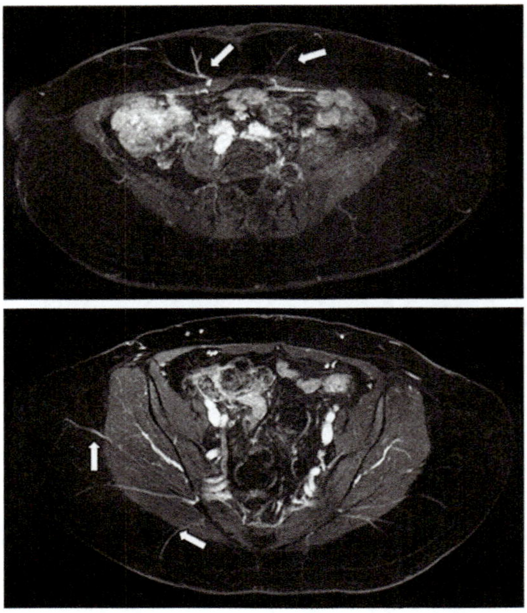

Fig. 1.10 Magnetic Resonance Angiography axial images show several perforators (white arrows) from the abdomen (top) and gluteal areas (bottom). *Note*. Adapted from "Perforator flap magnetic resonance angiography for reconstructive breast surgery: a review of 25 deep inferior epigastric and gluteal perforator artery flap patients," by T. M. Newman et al., 2010, *J Magn Reson Imaging*, May;31(5):1176–84. Copyright 2010 by John Wiley & Sons. Reprinted with permission

ating perforator course within the subcutaneous tissue up and within the dermis (Fig. 1.11). It aids in pre-operative perforator selection, allows the pre-operative planning of thin and super-thin flaps, and precisely shows superficial microvascular anatomy, which permits tailoring the flap thickness to the recipient needs [40–44].

1.4 Perforator Flap Era

Interestingly, some perforator flaps were described before the angiosomes report in 1987 (Table 1.2) [28]. For instance, Taylor and Daniel reported several superficial perforator flaps in an anatomical report in 1975, including the superficial inferior epigastric artery perforator (SIEAP) flap [45]. However, the SIEAP flap was only used for breast reconstruction in 1991 by Grotting [46]. Based on a subcutaneous vascular pedicle, the SIEAP flap allows the same inferior abdominal flap to be transferred as a deep inferior artery perforator (DIEAP) flap without incising the fascia. Although it completely preserves the abdominal muscular wall, the superficial inferior epigastric artery flap is rarely indicated because

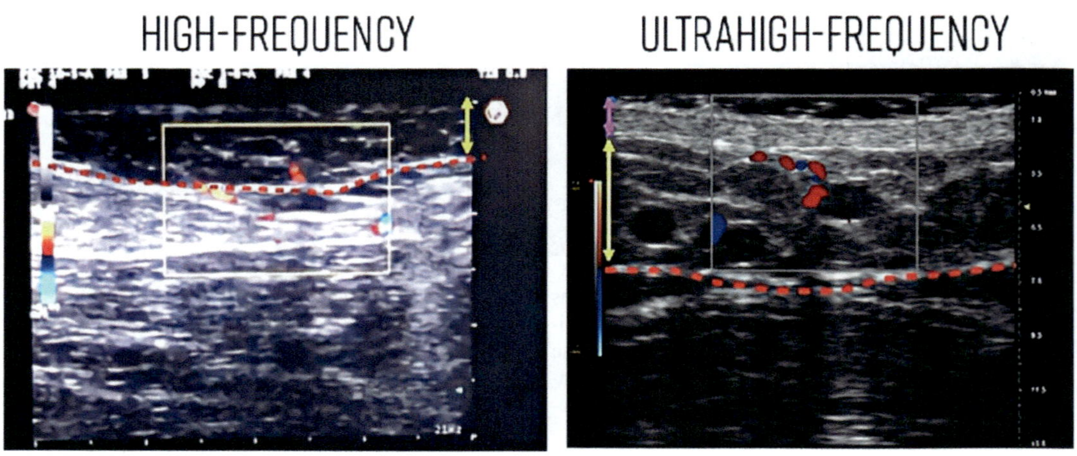

Fig. 1.11 Comparison of High-Frequency and Ultra High-Frequency Ultrasound of perforator of profunda femoral artery. The High-Frequency ultrasound gives a reasonable estimation of perforator exit point and intramuscular course but cannot visualise its subcutaneous course up to the dermis as it is possible to visualise with UHF-US. Red dotted line is muscular fascia, subcutaneous tissue depth is indicated by yellow arrows. The dermis, clearly visualisable with UHF-US, is shown with a pink arrow

Table 1.2 Timeline of the perforator flaps used for breast reconstruction

Year of publication	Authors	Perforator Flap	Breast Reconstruction	Authors
1975	Taylor and Daniel	SIEAP flap	1991	Grotting
1984	Song et al.	ALT flap	2002	Wei et al.
1989	Koshima and Soeda	DIEAP flap	1994	Allen and Treece
1993	Koshima et al.	SGAP flap	1995	Allen and Tucker
1993	Paletta et al.	PAP flap	2012	Allen et al.
1995	Angrigiani et al.	TDAP flap	1995	Angrigiani et al.
2000	Deiler et al.	Tensor fascia latae perforator flap	2011	Kind and Foster
2002	Peek et al.	Gracilis perforator flap	2002	Peek et al.
2002	Higgins et al.	IGAP flap	2004	Guerra et al.
2002	Feinendegen and Klos	SCAP flap	2019	Delchet et al.
2004	Hamdi et al.	LICAP flap	2004	Hamdi et al.
2005	Hallock	SEAP flap	2014	Hamdi et al.
2006	Pittet et al.	SAAP flap	2008	Hamdi et al.
2006	Hamdi et al.	AICAP flap	2011	Munhoz et al.
2011	Kim et al.	LTAP flap	2015	McCulley et al.
2015	Angrigiani et al.	Extended TDAP flap	2015	Angrigiani et al.

Note. SIEAP superficial inferior epigastric artery perforator, *ALT* anterolateral thigh perforator, *DIEAP* deep inferior epigastric artery perforator, *SGAP* superior gluteal artery perforator, *PAP* profunda artery perforator, *TDAP* thoracodorsal artery perforator, *IGAP* inferior gluteal artery perforator, *SCAP* subcostal artery perforator, *LICAP* lateral intercostal artery perforator, *SEAP* superior epigastric artery perforator, *SAAP* serratus anterior artery perforator, *AICAP* anterior intercostal artery perforator, *LTAP* lateral thoracic artery perforator

of its vascular pedicle's anatomical variety and the vessel's small diameter, which may increase the risk of flap failure.

Another perforator flap published before 1987 is the anterolateral thigh artery perforator (ALT) flap. In 1984, Song et al. described the ALT flap. This versatile and reliable flap has achieved popularity in head and neck surgery and reconstructive surgery of the hand and upper and lower extremities. The ALT flap can be used as a flow flap to reconstruct soft tissue and significant vessel defects in the extremities and as an adipofascial flap [47]. In 2002, Wei et al. were the first to use the ALT flap for breast reconstruction [48].

Despite the publications detailed above, for most of the microsurgeons, the perforator flap era began in 1989, when Koshima and Soeda described the deep inferior epigastric artery perforator (DIEAP) flap to reconstruct the floor of mouth and groin defects, noting that a large flap without muscle could survive with a single muscle perforator flap [29]. A few years later, Allen and Treece first described the DIEAP flap for breast reconstruction in 1994 [49].

In 1993, Koshima et al. described the gluteal artery perforator flap based on parasacral perforators [50] and in 1995, Allen and Tucker described the superior gluteal artery perforator (SGAP) flap for breast reconstruction [51]. The SGAP flap is often an option for patients with unsuitable abdominal donor site tissue. The SGAP has a longer vascular pedicle, and its main advantages for breast reconstruction include low donor site morbidity, excess adipose tissue even in thin patients and a hidden scar.

In 1993, Paletta et al. described the profunda artery perforator (PAP) flap that was initially used to repair defects of the lower extremity and pressure wounds [52]. In 2012, Allen et al. illustrated its use in autologous breast reconstruction [53]. The advantages of the flap area are reliable blood supply, an excellent pedicle length, and a favourable donor site location.

The thoracodorsal artery perforator (TDAP) flap was first reported by Angrigiani et al. in 1995. This report described a partial breast reconstruction with a TDAP flap in a 16-year-old female with a burned sequela on the lateral chest wall area. The TDAP flap is a highly versatile flap with a long pedicle and abundant donor site area. It is one of the first options for partial breast reconstruction of the lateral quadrants of the breast [54].

In 2000, Deiler et al. described the tensor fascia latae perforator flap to cover defects on the lower limb [55]. A decade later, in 2011, Kind and Foster reported the tensor fasciae latae perforator flap for breast reconstruction. The main advantage of this flap is the longer pedicle. However, its weakness comprises the high risk of wound dehiscence at the donor site if the skin harvested paddle is excessively large [56].

In 2002, Peek et al. described the gracilis perforator flap as an alternative for autologous breast reconstruction. The purpose of this study was to outline the anatomy of the medial thigh and assess musculocutaneous and septocutaneous perforators and intramuscular conduits. Peek reported six successful breast reconstructions, including two bilateral procedures [57].

In 2002, Higgins et al. described the inferior gluteal artery perforator (IGAP) flap and used it to cover an ischial pressure sore [58]. The dissection of a lateral perforator down to the origin of the inferior gluteal artery permits harvest of a well-vascularised fasciocutaneous flap on a long pedicle. In 2004, Guerra et al. described its use for breast reconstruction. This flap provided adequate tissue to perform the reconstruction but caused an exposure to the sciatic nerve and was found to have significant disadvantages compared to the SGAP flap [59]. In 2006, Allen et al. placed the donor site scar of the IGAP in the lower buttock crease, which increased the donor site cosmetic result [60].

In 2002, Feinendegen and Klos described the subcostal artery perforator (SCAP) flap to cover a significant lumbar defect. The long pedicle allowed for a large arc of rotation and the midline defect in the lower back could be covered with no tension [61]. Delchet et al. in 2019 reported a feasibility study on a cadaver with SCAP for breast reconstruction. The drawback is a long, unpleasant scar on the flank area [62].

Hamdi pioneered several versatile flaps for breast reconstruction. For instance, in 2004, he described the lateral intercostal anterior perforator (LICAP) flap based on the perforating arteries, which originate in the costal segment of the intercostal arteries. The LICAP flap provides an elegant option to fill a defect in the outer breast quadrants (Fig. 1.12) [63].

The abdominal skin flaps represent one of the earliest areas to be explored for flaps. After publishing the DIEAP flap in 1989, Koshima and Soeda [29], describing the SEAP flap was a matter of time. Hallock, as defined by himself, "self-fulfilled the prophecy". In 2005, Hallock described the superior epigastric artery perforator (SEAP) flap and used it to cover a chest wall defect (Fig. 1.13) [64]. However, only in 2014, Hamdi et al. published the application of a SEAP flap for breast reconstruction [65].

In 2006, Pittet described the serratus anterior artery perforator (SAAP) flap [66]. However, Pittet et al. did not visualise direct communication between the muscular branches from the intercostal artery perforator vessels and the thoracodorsal pedicle of the serratus anterior. Therefore, in 2008, Hamdi et al. found the vascular connections between the serratus anterior artery and intercostal perforators in 10/47 cadavers (21%) [67]. Later, these communications were recognised as crucial to characterise the SAAP flap (Fig. 1.14).

In 2006, Hamdi described the anterior intercostal artery perforator (AICAP) flap and used it for sternal wound repair after a Mohs procedure [68]. The AICAP has a long pedicle originating from the muscular or rectal segment of intercostal arteries. In 2011, Munhoz et al. reported using the AICAP flap for breast reconstruction (Fig. 1.15) [69].

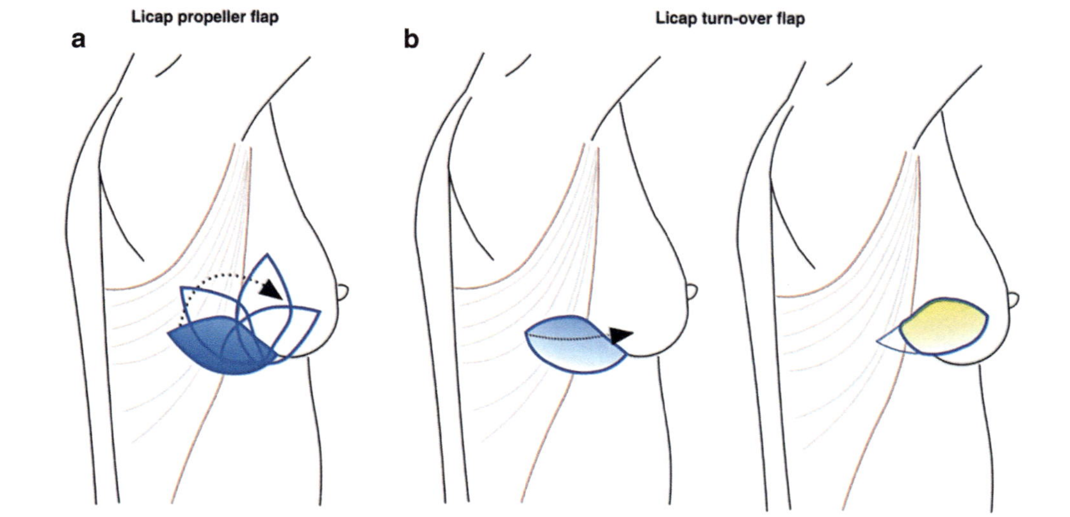

Fig. 1.12 (**a**) LICAP propeller flap design. (**b**) LICAP turn-over flap design. *Note*. Adapted from "Breast Reconstruction Using the Lateral Thoracic, Thoracodorsal, and Intercostal Arteries Perforator Flaps," M. L. Mangialardi et al. 2021, *Plastic and reconstructive surgery, Global open*, *9*(1), p. 6, fig. 6. Copyright 2021 by Wolters Kluwer Health. Reprinted with permission

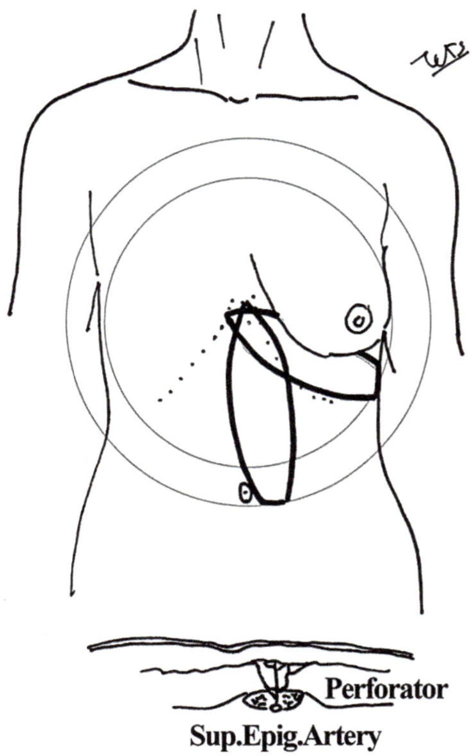

Fig. 1.13 Superior epigastric artery perforator flap. *Note*. Adapted from "Superior epigastric artery perforator flap: preliminary report,"by T. Uemura, 2007, *Plastic and reconstructive surgery*, *120*(1), p. 5e, fig. 9. Copyright 2007 by Wolters Kluwer Health. Reprinted with permission

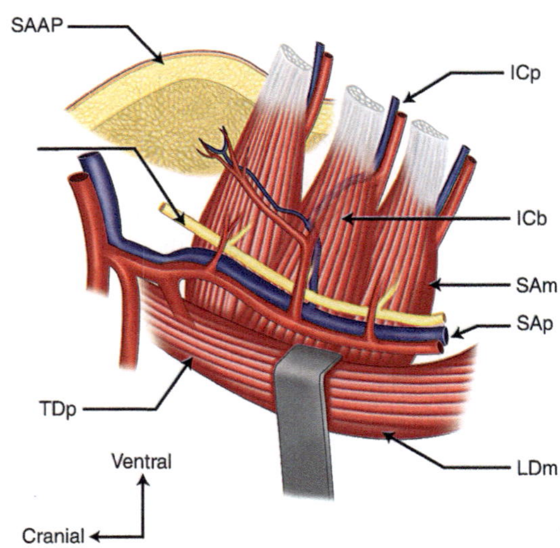

Fig. 1.14 Illustration of the connection between serratus and intercostal perforators. *SAAP* serratus anterior perforator flap, *TDp* thoracodorsal perforator, *LDm* latissimus dorsi muscle, *SAp* serratus anterior perforator, *SAm* serratus anterior muscle, *ICb* intercostal branch, *ICp* intercostal perforator. *Note*. Adapted from TAP, LICAP, SAAP, and AICAP Flaps, by E. Mecham, J. Park and L. Phillips. In V. Klimberg, T. Kovacs, I. Rubio (Eds.), Oncoplastic Breast Surgery Techniques for the General Surgeon, Springer, 2020, p. 513, fig. 29.11. Copyright 2020 by Springer Nature. Reprinted with permission

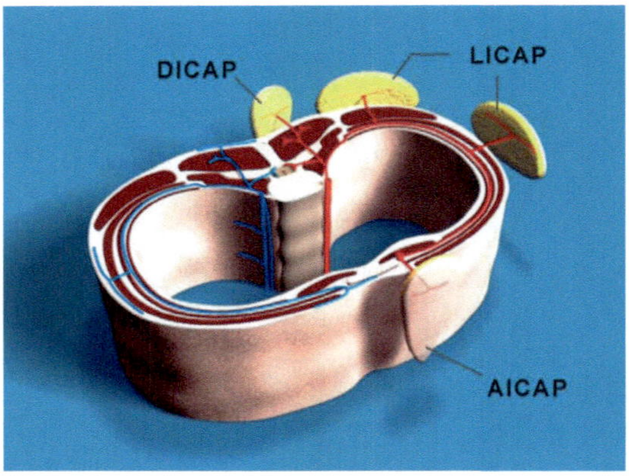

Fig. 1.15 Perforators flaps raised from the intercostal vascular arcade. *DICAP* dorsal intercostal artery perforator flap, *LICAP* lateral intercostal artery perforator flap, *AICAP* anterior intercostal artery perforator flap. *Note.* Adapted from "The versatility of the inter-costal artery perforator (ICAP) flaps," by M. Hamdi et al., 2006, *Journal of plastic, reconstructive and aesthetic surgery: JPRAS*, *59*(6), p. 646, fig. 2. Copyright 2006 by Elsevier. Reprinted with permission

In 2011, Kim et al. described the lateral thoracic artery perforator (LTAP) flap. This flap shares similar versatility to the other two perforator flaps based on the thoracodorsal system [70]. Later on, in 2015, McCulley et al. described the pedicled LTAP flap as a new flap for partial breast reconstruction. The flap is based on single or multiple perforators of the lateral thoracic vessels (Fig. 1.16) [71].

In 2015, Angrigiani described the extended TDAP flap. The TDAP flap blood supply derives from the proximal perforator of the descending branch of the thoracodorsal artery, and according to anatomic studies, there is an exceptionally high prevalence of the proximal branch of the thoracodorsal artery in the human body. Hence, Angrigiani hypothesised that the before-mentioned thoracodorsal proximal perforator branch reliably irrigates fat tissue that encompasses the area of the standard TDAP. Therefore, surgeons can harvest an ample adjacent volume to the former TDAP flap and perform a total breast reconstruction of a patient with small-to-moderate-sized breasts [72].

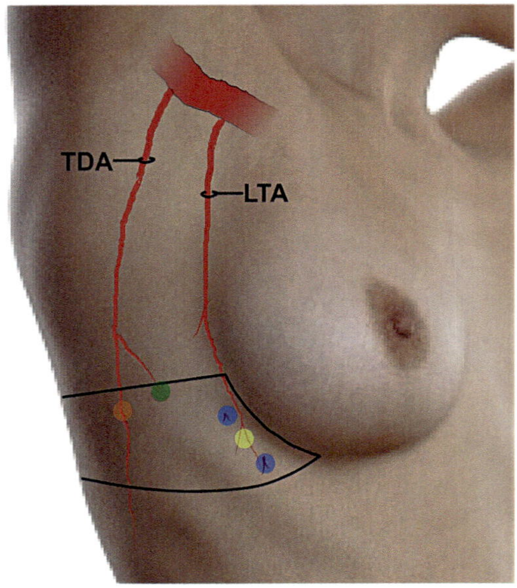

Fig. 1.16 Lateral thoracic artery perforator flap. *Note.* Adapted from "Lateral thoracic artery perforator (LTAP) flap in partial breast reconstruction" by S. J. McCulley et al., 2015, *Journal of plastic, reconstructive and aesthetic surgery: JPRAS*, *68*(5), p. 687, fig. 1. Copyright 2015 by Elsevier. Reprinted with permission

1.5 Pedicled Perforator Flaps: Tissue Transfer Evolution

By definition, pedicled perforator flaps (PPF) are perforator flaps transposed locally using their pedicle as a pivot. Therefore, they can reach the defect by rotating on the perforator axis in propeller mode, by advancing the perforator vessels in VY, in keystone and turnover mode, and transposition using the whole pedicle as a carrier, as frequently happens in the TDAP flap [73].

The pedicle obviates the need for microsurgical anastomosis and offers a potentially more straightforward and faster harvest than free flaps [74]. respecting the ideal like-for-like tissue reconstruction principle represents an excellent local option for reconstruction. Similarly to free perforator flaps, pedicled perforator flaps are also named after their nutrient artery, the source vessel, which is well defined anatomically.

TC Teo defined propeller flap as a local island fasciocutaneous flap based and pivoted on a single dissected perforator. It was designed like a propeller with two blades of unequal length, with the perforator as the pivot, enabling a rotation of each blade up to 180° [75, 76]. Propeller flap was then redefined by the Tokyo Consensus (2011) as an island flap moved to the recipient site employing an axial rotation [77]. The propeller flap is a single perforator flap with significant rotational capability based on the location of the perforator entry within the skin paddle. An elliptical flap that perforator entry point is eccentrical and close to the defect allows a significant rotation and reach [73]. The pedicle has to be traditionally dissected to its source vessel to increase flap mobility and decrease the possibility of twisting and kinking by distributing rotational forces along its vascular axis and then inserted by rotating the flap towards the least vessel twisting and kinking (conventional perforator flap).

Pedicle dissection is unnecessary when the perforator entry is close to the defect and the patient shows laxity. The flap dissection stops close to the perforator emergence point as soon as the peduncle is glimpsed, without skeletonising it. The undissected tissue surrounding the main perforator, with the other tiny vascular connections and nerves, represents a security anchor, as it protects the perforator from tension and twisting (perforator-based flap) without compromising its mobility. It frequently happens with lateral thoracic wall perforator flaps.

Whenever the perforator is very close to the flap edge, it does not require skeletonising to turn the flap into the defect. This manoeuvre protects the pedicle from twisting and increases its reaching. It also keeps the sensate nerve and many tiny vessels within the flap pedicle, sacrificing only those structures limiting the flap movement. Then the flap is rotated into the defect. The donor site closure also pushes the lateral tissue excess at the anterior axillary line (the turning point of the pedicle) inside the breast. Thus, the flap movement is through rotation and advancement in this scenario, named "translation" [39].

In summary, the conventional perforator flap requires perforator skeletonization [78], in contrast the perforator-based island flap (PBIF) avoids pedicle skeletonization to protect the pedicle. Paradoxically, this preserves the pedicle from twisting when turning the pedicled flap and allows a more distant reach.

1.6 Conclusion

In the last three decades, pedicled perforator flaps have emerged. Despite the unfolding of microsurgical techniques, many clinical situations have been elegantly solved by local and regional perforator flaps. Their evolution was based on previous extensive anatomical studies, and different radiological pre-operative mapping established feasibility with better planning. Finally, the freestyle design and transfer have enhanced their popularity.

References

1. Breasted JH. The Edwin Smith surgical papyrus: published in facsimile and hieroglyphic transliteration with translation and commentary in two volumes. Chicago, IL: University of Chicago Press; 1930.
2. Sakorafas GH, Safioleas M. Breast cancer surgery: an historical narrative. Part II. 18th and 19th centuries. Eur J Cancer Care. 2010;19(1):6–29. https://doi.org/10.1111/j.1365-2354.2008.01060.x.
3. Halsted WS. I. The results of operations for the cure of cancer of the breast performed at the Johns Hopkins Hospital from June, 1889, to January, 1894. Ann Surg. 1894;20(5):497–555.
4. Halsted WS. Developments in the skin-grafting operation for cancer of the breast. JAMA. 1913;60(6):416–8. https://doi.org/10.1001/jama.1913.04340060008004.
5. Ki Kissin MW, Querci della Rovere G, Easton D, Westbury G. Risk of lymphoedema following the treatment of breast cancer. Br J Surg. 1986;73(7):580–4. https://doi.org/10.1002/bjs.1800730723.
6. Yeoh EK, Denham JW, Davies SA, Spittle MF. Primary breast cancer. Complications of axillary management. Acta Radiol Oncol. 1986;25(2):105–8. https://doi.org/10.3109/02841868609136386.
7. Tansini I. Nuovo processo per l'amputazione della mammaella per cancre. Reforma Med. 1896;12:3.

8. Tansini I. Sopra il mio nuovo processo di amputazione della mammella. Gazz Med Ital. 1906;12:757.
9. Homsy A, Rüegg E, Montandon D, Vlastos G, Modarressi A, Pittet B. Breast reconstruction: a century of controversies and progress. Ann Plast Surg. 2018;80(4):457–63. https://doi.org/10.1097/SAP.0000000000001312.
10. Champaneria MC, Wong WW, Hill ME, Gupta SC. The evolution of breast reconstruction: a historical perspective. World J Surg. 2012;36(4):730–42. https://doi.org/10.1007/s00268-012-1450-2.
11. Sakorafas GH. Breast cancer surgery--historical evolution, current status and future perspectives. Acta Oncol. 2001;40(1):5–18. https://doi.org/10.1080/028418601750070984.
12. Hartrampf CR, Scheflan M, Black PW. Breast reconstruction with a transverse abdominal island flap. Plast Reconstr Surg. 1982;69(2):216–25. https://doi.org/10.1097/00006534-198202000-00006.
13. Noone RB, Murphy JB, Spear SL, Little JW 3rd. A 6-year experience with immediate reconstruction after mastectomy for cancer. Plast Reconstr Surg. 1985;76(2):258–69. https://doi.org/10.1097/00006534-198508000-00012.
14. Vinton AL, Traverso LW, Zehring RD. Immediate breast reconstruction following mastectomy is as safe as mastectomy alone. Arch Surg (Chicago, Ill: 1960). 1990;125(10):1303–8. https://doi.org/10.1001/archsurg.1990.01410220087012.
15. Mavrogenis AF, Markatos K, Saranteas T, Ignatiadis I, Spyridonos S, Bumbasirevic M, Soucacos PN. The history of microsurgery. Eur J Orthop Surg Traumatol. 2019;29(2):247–54. http://dx.doi.org.bibliosan.clas.cineca.it/10.1007/s00590-019-02378-7.
16. Manchot C. Die Hautarterien des Menschlichen Körpers. Leipzig: F.C.W. Vogel; 1889.
17. Salmon M. Arte'res de la Peau. Paris: Mason et Cie; 1936.
18. Manchot C. The cutaneous arteries of the human body. New York: Springer-Verlag; 1983.
19. Salmon M. In: Taylor GI, Tempest M, editors. Arteries of the skin. London: Churchill Livingstone; 1988.
20. Milton SH. Pedicled skin-flaps: the fallacy of the length: width ratio. Br J Surg. 1970;57(7):502–8. https://doi.org/10.1002/bjs.1800570705.
21. Geddes CR, Morris SF, Neligan PC. Perforator flaps: evolution, classification, and applications. Ann Plast Surg. 2003;50(1):90–9. https://doi.org/10.1097/00000637-200301000-00016.
22. McGregor IA, Jackson IT. The groin flap. Br J Plast Surg. 1972;25(1):3–16. https://doi.org/10.1016/s0007-1226(72)80003-1.
23. McGregor IA. Basic principles in skin flap transfer. Surg Clin North Am. 1977;57(5):961–76. https://doi.org/10.1016/s0039-6109(16)41336-8.
24. Pontén B. The fasciocutaneous flap: its use in soft tissue defects of the lower leg. Br J Plast Surg. 1981;34(2):215–20. https://doi.org/10.1016/s0007-1226(81)80097-5.
25. Mathes SJ, Nahai F. Classification of the vascular anatomy of muscles: experimental and clinical correlation. Plast Reconstr Surg. 1981;67(2):177–87.
26. Cormack GC, Lamberty BG. Fasciocutaneous vessels. Their distribution on the trunk and limbs, and their clinical application in tissue transfer. Anat Clin. 1984;6(2):121–31. https://doi.org/10.1007/BF01773164.
27. Nakajima H, Fujino T, Adachi S. A new concept of vascular supply to the skin and classification of skin flaps according to their vascularisation. Ann Plast Surg. 1986;16(1):1–19. https://doi.org/10.1097/00000637-198601000-00001.
28. Taylor GI, Palmer JH. The vascular territories (angiosomes) of the body: experimental study and clinical applications. Br J Plast Surg. 1987;40(2):113–41. https://doi.org/10.1016/0007-1226(87)90185-8.
29. Koshima I, Soeda S. Inferior epigastric artery skin flaps without rectus abdominis muscle. Br J Plast Surg. 1989;42(6):645–8. https://doi.org/10.1016/0007-1226(89)90075-1.
30. Kroll SS, Rosenfield L. Perforator-based flaps for low posterior midline defects. Plast Reconstr Surg. 1988;81(4):561–6. https://doi.org/10.1097/00006534-198804000-00012.
31. Hallock GG. Direct and indirect perforator flaps: the history and the controversy. Plast Reconstr Surg. 2003;111(2):855–66. https://doi.org/10.1097/01.PRS.0000040462.38363.C7.
32. Blondeel PN, Van Landuyt KH, Monstrey SJ, Hamdi M, Matton GE, Allen RJ, Dupin C, Feller AM, Koshima I, Kostakoglu N, Wei FC. The "Gent" consensus on perforator flap terminology: preliminary definitions. Plast Reconstr Surg. 2003;112(5):1378–87. https://doi.org/10.1097/01.PRS.0000081071.83805.B6.
33. Saint-Cyr M, Wong C, Schaverien M, Mojallal A, Rohrich RJ. The perforasome theory: vascular anatomy and clinical implications. Plast Reconstr Surg. 2009;124(5):1529–44. https://doi.org/10.1097/PRS.0b013e3181b98a6c.
34. Rozen WM, Ashton MW. Re: the perforasome theory: vascular anatomy and clinical implications. Plast Reconstr Surg. 2010;125(6):1845–6. https://doi.org/10.1097/PRS.0b013e3181d51450.
35. Burnier P, Niddam J, Bosc R, Hersant B, Meningaud JP. Indocyanine green applications in plastic surgery: a review of the literature. J Plast Reconstr Aesthet Surg. 2017;70(6):814–27. https://doi.org/10.1016/j.bjps.2017.01.020.
36. Kehrer A, Sachanadani NS, da Silva N, Lonic D, Heidekrueger P, Taeger CD, Klein S, Jung EM, Prantl L, Hong JP. Step-by-step guide to ultrasound-based design of alt flaps by the microsurgeon - basic and advanced applications and device settings. J Plast Reconstr Aesthet Surg. 2020;73(6):1081–90. https://doi.org/10.1016/j.bjps.2019.11.035.
37. Masia J, Clavero JA, Larrañaga JR, Alomar X, Pons G, Serret P. Multidetector-row computed tomography in the planning of abdominal perforator flaps. J Plast

Reconstr Aesthet Surg. 2006;59(6):594–9. https://doi.org/10.1016/j.bjps.2005.10.024.
38. Masia J, Navarro C, Clavero JA, Alomar X. Noncontrast magnetic resonance imaging for preoperative perforator mapping. Clin Plast Surg. 2011;38(2):253–61. https://doi.org/10.1016/j.cps.2011.03.004.
39. Salgarello M, Visconti G. Designing lateral thoracic wall perforator flaps for breast reconstruction using the ultrasound. J Reconstr Microsurg. 2021;38(3):228–32. https://doi.org/10.1055/s-0041-1740127.
40. Narushima M, Yamasoba T, Iida T, Matsumoto Y, Yamamoto T, Yoshimatsu H, Timothy S, Pafitanis G, Yamashita S, Koshima I. Pure skin perforator flaps: the anatomical vascularity of the super-thin flap. Plast Reconstr Surg. 2018;142(3):351e–60e. https://doi.org/10.1097/PRS.0000000000004698.
41. Yoshimatsu H, Hayashi A, Yamamoto T, Visconti G, Karakawa R, Fuse Y, Iida T. Visualisation of the "intradermal plexus" using ultrasonography in the dermis flap: a step beyond perforator flaps. Plast Reconstr Surg Glob Open. 2019;7(11):e2411. https://doi.org/10.1097/GOX.0000000000002411.
42. Visconti G, Bianchi A, Hayashi A, Salgarello M. Pure skin perforator flap direct elevation above the subdermal plane using pre-operative ultra-high frequency ultrasound planning: a proof of concept. J Plast Reconstr Aesthet Surg. 2019;72(10):1700–38. https://doi.org/10.1016/j.bjps.2019.06.016.
43. Visconti G, Hayashi A, Yoshimatsu H, Bianchi A, Salgarello M. Ultra-high frequency ultrasound in planning capillary perforator flaps: preliminary experience☆. J Plast Reconstr Aesthet Surg. 2018;71(8):1146–52. https://doi.org/10.1016/j.bjps.2018.05.045.
44. Hong JP, Choi DH, Suh H, Mukarramah DA, Tashti T, Lee K, Yoon C. A new plane of elevation: the superficial fascial plane for perforator flap elevation. J Reconstr Microsurg. 2014;30(7):491–6. https://doi.org/10.1055/s-0034-1369807.
45. Taylor GI, Daniel RK. The anatomy of several free flap donor sites. Plast Reconstr Surg. 1975;56(3):243–53. https://doi.org/10.1097/00006534-197509000-00001.
46. Grotting JC. The free abdominoplasty flap for immediate breast reconstruction. Ann Plast Surg. 1991;27(4):351–4. https://doi.org/10.1097/00000637-199110000-00011.
47. Song YG, Chen GZ, Song YL. The free thigh flap: a new free flap concept based on the septocutaneous artery. Br J Plast Surg. 1984;37(2):149–59. https://doi.org/10.1016/0007-1226(84)90002-x.
48. Wei FC, Jain V, Celik N, Chen HC, Chuang DC, Lin CH. Have we found an ideal soft-tissue flap? An experience with 672 anterolateral thigh flaps. Plast Reconstr Surg. 2002;109(7):2219–30. https://doi.org/10.1097/00006534-200206000-00007.
49. Allen RJ, Treece P. Deep inferior epigastric perforator flap for breast reconstruction. Ann Plast Surg. 1994;32(1):32–8. https://doi.org/10.1097/00000637-199401000-00007.
50. Koshima I, Moriguchi T, Soeda S, Kawata S, Ohta S, Ikeda A. The gluteal perforator-based flap for repair of sacral pressure sores. Plast Reconstr Surg. 1993;91(4):678–83. https://doi.org/10.1097/00006534-199304000-00017.
51. Allen RJ, Tucker C Jr. Superior gluteal artery perforator free flap for breast reconstruction. Plast Reconstr Surg. 1995;95(7):1207–12. https://doi.org/10.1097/00006534-199506000-00010.
52. Paletta C, Bartell T, Shehadi S. Applications of the posterior thigh flap. Ann Plast Surg. 1993;30(1):41–7. https://doi.org/10.1097/00000637-199301000-00006.
53. Allen RJ, Haddock NT, Ahn CY, Sadeghi A. Breast reconstruction with the profunda artery perforator flap. Plast Reconstr Surg. 2012;129(1):16e–23e. https://doi.org/10.1097/PRS.0b013e3182363d9f.
54. Angrigiani C, Grilli D, Siebert J. Latissimus dorsi musculocutaneous flap without muscle. Plast Reconstr Surg. 1995;96(7):1608–14. https://doi.org/10.1097/00006534-199512000-00014.
55. Deiler S, Pfadenhauer A, Widmann J, Stützle H, Kanz KG, Stock W. Tensor fasciae latae perforator flap for reconstruction of composite Achilles tendon defects with skin and vascularised fascia. Plast Reconstr Surg. 2000;106(2):342–9. https://doi.org/10.1097/00006534-200008000-00016.
56. Kind GM, Foster RD. Breast reconstruction using the lateral femoral circumflex artery perforator flap. J Reconstr Microsurg. 2011;27(7):427–32. https://doi.org/10.1055/s-0031-1281527.
57. Peek A, Müller M, Exner K. Der freie Grazilis-Perforator-Lappen zur autologen Brustrekonstruktion [The free gracilis perforator flap for autologous breast reconstruction]. Handchir Mikrochir Plast Chir. 2002;34(4):245–50. https://doi.org/10.1055/s-2002-36292.
58. Higgins JP, Orlando GS, Blondeel PN. Ischial pressure sore reconstruction using an inferior gluteal artery perforator (IGAP) flap. Br J Plast Surg. 2002;55(1):83–5. https://doi.org/10.1054/bjps.2001.3713.
59. Guerra AB, Metzinger SE, Bidros RS, Gill PS, Dupin CL, Allen RJ. Breast reconstruction with gluteal artery perforator (GAP) flaps: a critical analysis of 142 cases. Ann Plast Surg. 2004;52(2):118–25. https://doi.org/10.1097/01.sap.0000095437.43805.d1.
60. Allen RJ, Levine JL, Granzow JW. The in-the-crease inferior gluteal artery perforator flap for breast reconstruction. Plast Reconstr Surg. 2006;118(2):333–9. https://doi.org/10.1097/01.prs.0000227665.56703.a8.
61. Feinendegen DL, Klos D. A subcostal artery perforator flap for a lumbar defect. Plast Reconstr Surg. 2002;109(7):2446–9. https://doi.org/10.1097/00006534-200206000-00042.
62. Delchet O, Majoulet L, Avisse C, Stroumza N. Experimental study of pedicled subcostal artery perforator (SCAP) flap: a new application in breast

reconstruction. J Plast Reconstr Aesthet Surg. 2019;72(8):1299–303. https://doi.org/10.1016/j.bjps.2019.03.030.
63. Hamdi M, Van Landuyt K, Monstrey S, Blondeel P. Pedicled perforator flaps in breast reconstruction: a new concept. Br J Plast Surg. 2004;57(6):531–9. https://doi.org/10.1016/j.bjps.2004.04.015.
64. Hallock GG. The superior epigastric (RECTUS ABDOMINIS) muscle perforator flap. Ann Plast Surg. 2005;55(4):430–2. https://doi.org/10.1097/01.sap.0000174621.49158.b4.
65. Hamdi M, Craggs B, Stoel AM, Hendrickx B, Zeltzer A. Superior epigastric artery perforator flap: anatomy, clinical applications, and review of literature. J Reconstr Microsurg. 2014;30(7):475–82. https://doi.org/10.1055/s-0034-1376399.
66. Pittet B, Mahajan AL, Alizadeh N, Schlaudraff KU, Fasel J, Montandon D. The free serratus anterior flap and its cutaneous component for reconstruction of the face: a series of 27 cases. Plast Reconstr Surg. 2006;117(4):1277–88. https://doi.org/10.1097/01.prs.0000208297.02556.a5.
67. Hamdi M, Spano A, Landuyt KV, D'Herde K, Blondeel P, Monstrey S. The lateral intercostal artery perforators: anatomical study and clinical application in breast surgery. Plast Reconstr Surg. 2008;121(2):389–96. https://doi.org/10.1097/01.prs.0000298317.65296.cf.
68. Hamdi M, Van Landuyt K, de Frene B, Roche N, Blondeel P, Monstrey S. The versatility of the intercostal artery perforator (ICAP) flaps. J Plast Reconstr Aesthet Surg. 2006;59(6):644–52. https://doi.org/10.1016/j.bjps.2006.01.006.
69. Munhoz AM, Montag E, Arruda E, Brasil JA, Aldrighi JM, Gemperli R, Filassi JR, Ferreira MC. Immediate conservative breast surgery reconstruction with perforator flaps: new challenges in the era of partial mastectomy reconstruction? Breast. 2011;20(3):233–40. https://doi.org/10.1016/j.breast.2011.01.001.
70. Kim JT, Ng SW, Naidu S, Kim JD, Kim YH. Lateral thoracic perforator flap: additional perforator flap option from the lateral thoracic region. J Plast Reconstr Aesthet Surg. 2011;64(12):1596–602. https://doi.org/10.1016/j.bjps.2011.06.048.
71. McCulley SJ, Schaverien MV, Tan VK, Macmillan RD. Lateral thoracic artery perforator (LTAP) flap in partial breast reconstruction. J Plast Reconstr Aesthet Surg. 2015;68(5):686–91. https://doi.org/10.1016/j.bjps.2015.01.008.
72. Angrigiani C, Rancati A, Escudero E, Artero G. Extended thoracodorsal artery perforator flap for breast reconstruction. Gland Surg. 2015;4(6):519–27. https://doi.org/10.3978/j.issn.2227-684X.2015.04.20.
73. Abraham JT, Saint-Cyr M. Keystone and pedicle perforator flaps in reconstructive surgery: new modifications and applications. Clin Plast Surg. 2017;44(2):385–402. https://doi.org/10.1016/j.cps.2016.12.005.
74. Lecours C, Saint-Cyr M, Wong C, Bernier C, Mailhot E, Tardif M, Chollet A. Freestyle pedicle perforator flaps: clinical results and vascular anatomy. Plast Reconstr Surg. 2010;126(5):1589–603. https://doi.org/10.1097/PRS.0b013e3181f02ee3.
75. Teo TC. Reconstrucción de la extremidad inferior con colgajos de perforantes locales. Cirugía Plástica Ibero-Latinoamericana. 2006;32(4):287–92. Recuperado en 28 de septiembre de 2021, de http://scielo.isciii.es/scielo.php?script=sci_arttext&pid=S0376-78922006000400008&lng=es&tlng=es.
76. Teo TC. The propeller flap concept. Clin Plast Surg. 2010;37(4):615–vi. https://doi.org/10.1016/j.cps.2010.06.003.
77. Pignatti M, Ogawa R, Hallock GG, Mateev M, Georgescu AV, Balakrishnan G, Ono S, Cubison T, D'Arpa S, Koshima I, Hyakusoku H. The "Tokyo" consensus on propeller flaps. Plast Reconstr Surg. 2011;127(2):716–22. https://doi.org/10.1097/PRS.0b013e3181fed6b2.
78. Kim JT. Evolution and revolution of perforator flaps. 1st ed. Byeong-Hoon Jang; 2017.
79. Halsted WS. I. The results of radical operations for the cure of carcinoma of the breast. Ann Surg. 1907;46(1):1–19. https://doi.org/10.1097/00000658-190707000-00001.

Pre-operative Mapping and Imaging of Perforator Flaps

2

Carola Brussaard

Contents

2.1 Introduction

Imaging techniques are widely used to provide a pre-operative overview of the surgical possibilities before reconstructive microsurgery. The pre-operative overview allows the surgeon to choose and discuss the options of the donor site autograft with the patient. This approach reduces the time in the operating room since, besides the location, the suspected quality of the vascular bundle is evaluated in advance. Ultrasound (US) with color and power doppler mode, computed tomography (CT scan), and magnetic resonance imaging (MRI) are available for this purpose. The sophisticated US with high-frequency probes (9–15 MHz) has a voxel size of 0.18 mm, the best spatial resolution compared to CT scan and MRI. However, the main disadvantages of the US are the lack of a complete overview of all the available perforators, the limited in-depth visibility (max. 2 cm), and the operator dependency. Angio-CT and Angio-MR overcome these disadvantages. After post-processing, a sufficient field of view (FOV) and a complete in-depth visualization (3D) are depicted. The result of the examination is only limited operator or

C. Brussaard (✉)
Department of Radiology, Universitair Ziekenhuis Brussel, Brussels, Belgium
e-mail: carola.brussaard@uzbrussel.be

M. Hamdi et al. (eds.), *Pedicled Flaps in Partial Breast Reconstruction*,
https://doi.org/10.1007/978-3-031-08483-6_2

patient dependent. Angio-CT and Angio-MR both use intravenous contrast administration. In Angio-MR, a series in the arterial phase and a second one in the equilibrium phase depicts first the artery and then the combined vascular bundle consisting of an artery and an accompanying vein. However, the 3D reconstructions of MRI are inferior to those of CT due to the better spatial resolution of CT compared to MRI. The nearly isotropic voxel size of CT is 0.6 mm and MRI 1.2 mm. As CT is more available than MRI, a CT scan is, despite the use of radiation, in most hospitals, the working horse for pre-operative imaging of perforator flaps [1].

The fatty tissue for breast reconstruction is typically harvested from the abdominal wall, the medial side of the upper leg, or the backside. The place of harvesting is decided by sufficient, shape-able fat in combination with a valuable vascular branch. For all regions, the procedure for the Angio-CT scan is comparable.

2.2 Procedure for Angio-CT Examination for Mapping of Perforators

The patient is asked to remove underwear and put on a surgical shirt. Therefore, the position of the perforators will not change by impressions of elastic bands in cloths on the skin and subcutis. The patient is positioned supine on the scanning table. The arms might be aside from the corps to scan in the same position as in the operating room. We prefer to scan with the arms softly bend above their head as the position of the perforators does not change significantly by this maneuver. This position avoids streaking artifacts caused by the arms and prevents a rise in radiation up to 40% [2]. The patient will be warned of the effects of the iodinated contrast as the injection causes a warm sensation, which disappears in less than a minute. The explanation prevents an unintended movement due to an unanticipated effect. The scan time lasts one breath-hold.

The scan operator chooses a scan range in agreement with the requesting physician. When the request is to have both a pre-operative screening for malignancies and an image of both donor and receptor vessels, scanning is performed from the base of the neck to 6 cm inferior of the pubis branches. When donor vessels of the thighs are considered, the scan range is extended to the knees. With the possibilities of dose reduction on modern CT equipment, the effective dose radiation for CT scan of thorax-abdomen is already reduced by 50% in the last decade to an average of 7.7 mSv [3], comparable with a natural background radiation of 2.6 years [4]. A volume of 120 mL iodine intravenous contrast (350/400 mg/mL) followed by 40 mL 0.9% NaCl is delivered at a flow rate of 5 mL/s. The optimal moment to perform the scan is in the late arterial phase. We monitor the enhancement of the descending thoracic aorta after the injection until a threshold of 220 Hounsfield units (HUs) is reached. Then the scan table displaces to the starting point. In our institution, the scan direction is from top to bottom. The exact delay between the start of the contrast injection and the start of the scan to achieve this late arterial phase differs from one CT type of equipment to the other one as, for instance, the time needed for the table to reach the starting point differs.

The source images are post-processed to a stack of images with almost isotropic voxels. In the CT scan, the voxel size is approximately $0.7 \times 0.7 \times 0.6$ mm, where 0.6 mm represents the minimum slice thickness. Each voxel is represented by a density expressed in HU depending on the proportion of the different substances in the voxel. In this way, a thin disk of 0.6 mm thickness with a raster of different HU is created. For example, a disk of 6 mm thickness represents a volume of 10 voxels on top of each other. In maximum intensity projection (MIP), the highest density measured in a voxel in that column will be displayed. As a result, the vessel is visible over a longer length with increasing slice thickness. The volume rendering technique (VRT) completes the post-processing by images of the body surface and its reference point for mapping [5]. The post-processing for various free flaps using MIP is described in the subchapters.

2.3 Perforators in the Abdominal Wall

2.3.1 Deep Inferior Epigastric Artery Perforator (DIEAP) Flap

The most common type of autologous breast reconstruction is realized with the DIEAP flap. The DIEAP flap uses perforators that originate from the distal part of the external iliac artery. The branch has three anatomical variants [6]: a single branch, a bifurcation, and a division in three or more branches. A coronal MIP series of the abdominal wall with a slice thickness of 50 mm, highlights the present anatomical variant. The source images (slice thickness 0.6 mm) are loaded in a workstation and processed in a 3D viewer using the MIP. The site of the break-through of the arterial perforators through the fascia of the abdominal rectus muscle is searched on MIP reconstructions with a slice thickness of 15 mm. Next, the radiologist describes the arterial perforators in relation to an anatomical landmark, the umbilicus (Fig. 2.1). The radiology report mentions the most relevant perforators based on their suspected sufficient caliber for microsurgery (1–3 mm), taking into account the desire for the presence of mobilizable fat. The ultimate judgment of the most valuable perforator is, of course, made by the plastic surgeon, as he is not only interested in the largest caliber of a vessel but also in the possible central position of the vessel in to harvest fatty tissue and the presence of a relevant venous drainage system. Typically, at least three vessels inferior of the umbilicus and one above on each side is noted in with *x*- and *y*-coordinates in millimeters with their specification (visible accompanying venous structures, division of the perforators in the subcutaneous fat, lateral course of the perforator superficial or deep from the fascia) [7, 8].

2.3.2 Superficial Inferior Epigastric Artery Perforator (SIEAP) Flap

Superficial inferior epigastric artery originates from the common femoral artery about 1 cm inferior to the inguinal ligament and has a course more lateral in the subcutis of the abdominal wall than the DIEAP and superficial of the abdominal rectus muscle. The vessel might be suitable when the caliber is over 1 mm. The size of the vessel might be prognostic for the size of the nurtured area. The vessel usually has a long pedicle. The artery is congenital absent in one-third of the patients or might be destructed, e.g., after a caesarian section. The post-processing on the radiological workstation runs identical to the described method for DIEAP, with *x*- and *y*-coordinates relative to the umbilicus [8].

2.3.3 Superior Epigastric Artery Perforator (SEAP) Flap

The superior epigastric artery (SEA) originates from the internal mammary artery. The main terminal branch is named SEA and follows a course through the abdominal muscles. Therefore, it supplies blood to the upper abdominal rectus muscle and the subcutis of the abdominal wall. The perforators, blood suppliers for the skin, are visible from 1 to 20 cm inferior to the xiphoid on both sides of the midline, where they leave the fascia of the abdominal muscle. The perforator is described with the umbilicus as their reference point (Fig. 2.2). Usually, the area is in the scan range for DIEAP/SIEAP flap orientation. The vessel can be highlighted by MIP reconstruction. Coronal MIP reconstructions with a moderate thickness (5–10 mm) are recommended, as high dens bony structures from the ribs might otherwise mask the tiny vessels [9].

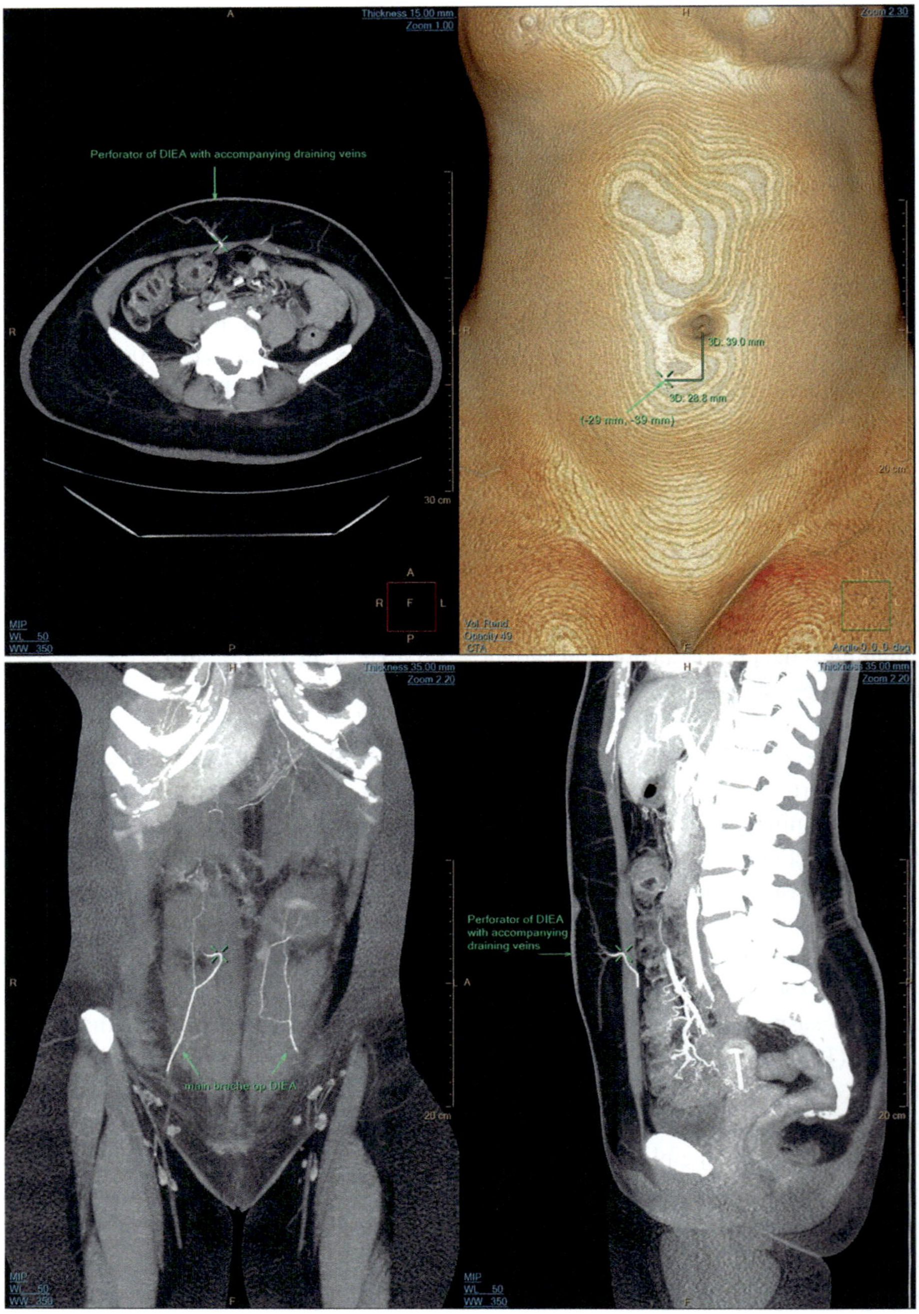

Fig. 2.1 Image composition after post-processing for preoperative localization of perforators of the deep inferior epigastric artery (DIEA). The images in the three orthogonal planes are crosslinked. A good overview is maintained in MIP reconstructions with a slice thickness of 15 mm while searching for suitable perforators. Fine-tuning of the localization is achieved by revisiting the MIP reconstructions with a slice thickness of 3 mm, after which a limited correction on the axial and sagittal images leads to more accurate localization. Finally, an image composition meaningful for clinical use is created with MIP reconstructions in three orthogonal planes with a supplementary VRT image. In this case study, the MIP slice thickness for the axial image is 15 mm. The MIP slice thickness for the coronal and sagittal image is obligatory the same in the image composition as illustrated (workstation: PhilipsPortal IntelliSpace). The coronal MIP reconstructions with a slice thickness of 30–50 mm provide a global view of the branching of the DIEA. The final measurements of the position of the perforator are made in millimeters on the VRT image using the *x*- and *y*-coordinate system with the umbilicus as the reference point

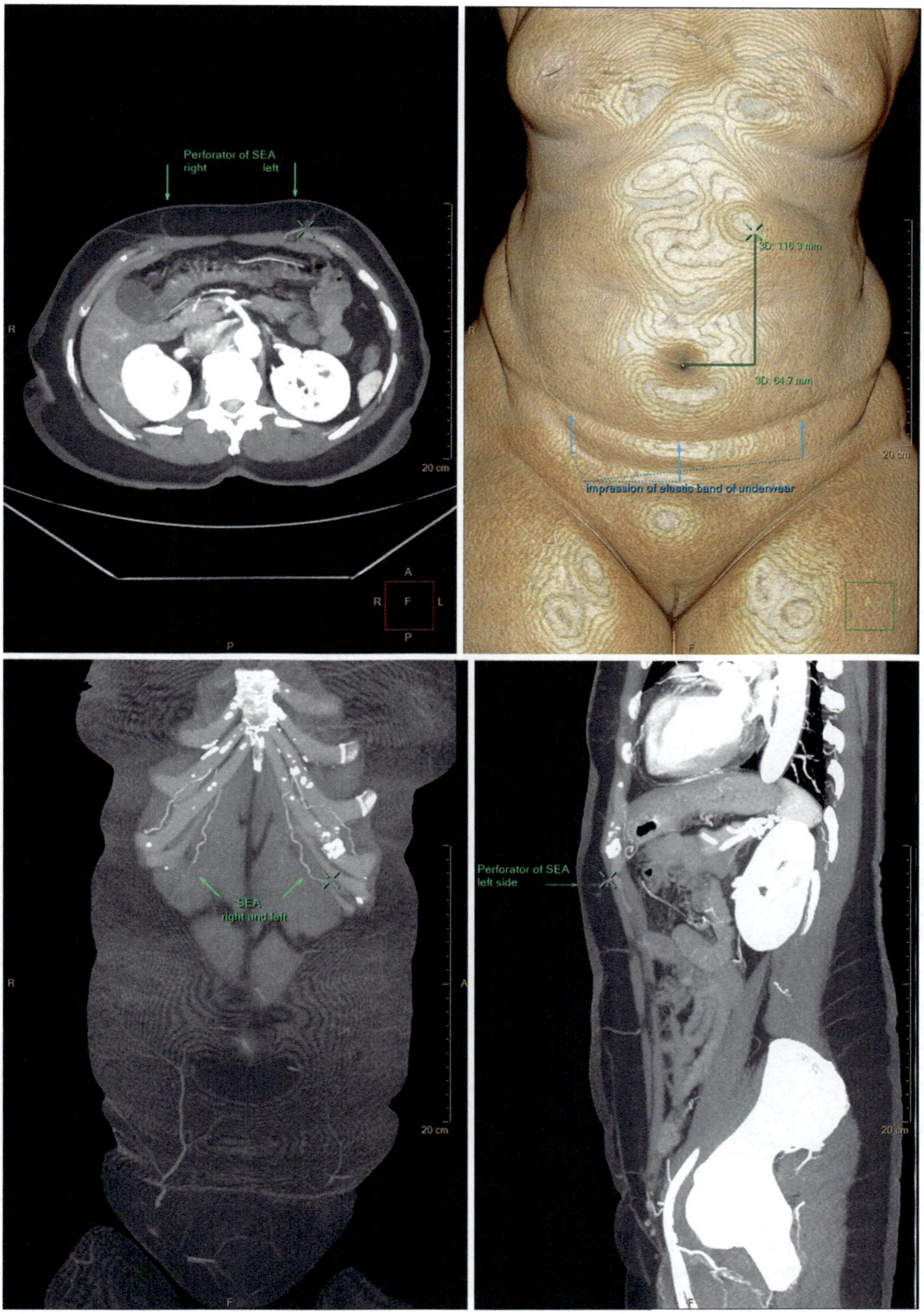

Fig. 2.2 Image composition after post-processing for pre-operative localization of perforators of the SEA. The same procedure is followed as described for DIEA perforator localization with the umbilicus as a reference point as indicated on the VRT image. Note the impression of the elastic band of underwear, which might influence the position of perforators of DIEA/SIEA perforators, but not of the SEA ones

2.4 Perforators of the Tight

2.4.1 Profunda Artery Perforator (PAP) Flap

After the DIEAP, the perforators of the Artery Profunda are next in line desired for breast reconstructions. The perforators at the medial site are most attractive as they are accessible with the patient in supine position with the leg in frog position during surgery. The scan can be performed in a prone position where the inferior gluteal crest can serve as a landmark. In our institution, a CT scan is performed in the same way as described for the perforators of the abdominal wall in a supine position. The post-processing is different as the anatomical landmark of the umbilicus can no longer be used. The source images are uploaded to a workstation in a 3D viewer. The MIP post-processing is used with a 5 mm slice thickness. First, we draw a horizontal line perpendicular to the symphysis pubis. Next, a line perpendicular to that horizontal line will connect with the middle of the superior patella border. In a carefully positioned patient (supine, the toes of both feet against each other), that line courses usually straight downward (Fig. 2.3a). We scroll down in an axial plane.

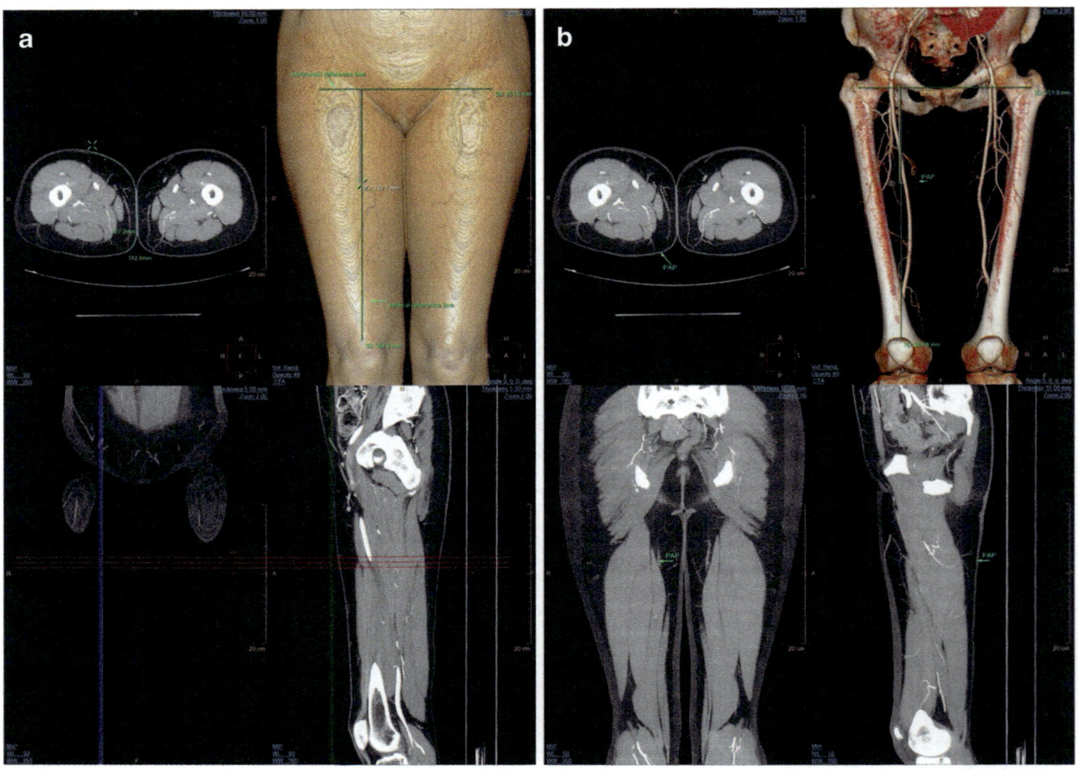

Fig. 2.3 Image composition after post-processing for pre-operative localization of perforators of the Profunda Artery. The horizontal reference line is the line parallel to the symphysis pubis. The vertical reference line departs perpendicularly from this horizontal line to the middle part of the upper patellar border. Both lines are drawn on the VRT image. Then, crosslink the images with MIP reconstructions with a slice thickness of 5 mm in the three orthogonal planes at the interception of the two reference lines on the skin as visible on the VRT image. Scroll caudally in the axial image series until a perforator of the profound femoral artery is seen. On the VRT image, the cross subsequently relocates caudally over the vertical reference line. On the VRT image, the distance is measured along the vertical reference line from the point where the perforator is detected to the horizontal reference line (coordinate 1). The distance from the cross on the skin to the perforator is measured on the axial image in the medial direction (coordinate 2) (**a**). Finally, the vessel's depth is measured perpendicular from the skin to the muscle fascia in millimeters (coordinate 3) (**b**)

When we see a perforator, we note the distance from that point to the horizontal line. Next, we measure the distance over the skin of the leg in the medial direction until we are closest to the perforator and specify the vessel's depth. Now, relocate the linked position on the orthogonal MIP images to the exact position of the perforator. A nice overview shows the perforator in the three orthogonal planes in MIP mode and on the adapted, more transparent VRT image (Fig. 2.3b). Finally, we mention their intramuscular or interseptal course. Cadaver studies have demonstrated that the perforators of the profound femoral artery on the medial side are positioned on a line at the posteromedial side of the tight [10, 11].

2.5 Perforators of the Back

2.5.1 Lumbar Artery Perforator (LAP) Flap

Perforators of the back are less used. Harvesting autologous tissue from the back might be an alternative when intervention on the abdominal wall or the tight will not be successful (e.g., burns).

The perforators of the lumbar arteries are visible on every Angio-CT scan performed for preparation of the abdominal wall perforators. Therefore, the scan does not have to be repeated when the treatment plan favors harvesting autologous tissue from the back. As the marks on the patient's skin are now made on the back, reproducible anatomical landmarks on the backside are necessary. We propose as x-axis a horizontal line that connects the uppermost part of the iliac crest right and left. The y-axis is the line connecting the spinal processes and might be somewhat curved in case of scoliosis (Fig. 2.4). With MIP reconstructions of 15 mm, the dominant perforator is detected on the left and right sides. Most commonly, the L3 and L4 perforators are dominant. The ipsilateral perforator is planned as the patient is placed in lateral decubitus for breast reconstruction. By planning the ipsilateral perforator, two teams can work simultaneously on both the donor and receptor sides [12].

2.5.2 Gluteal Artery Perforators

Perforators of gluteal arteries exist both from the superior and inferior arteries. However, the harvested autologous fatty tissue is less pliable and more firm than fatty tissue with blood supply by perforators of lumbar arteries. This donor site is less used for breast reconstruction [8, 12].

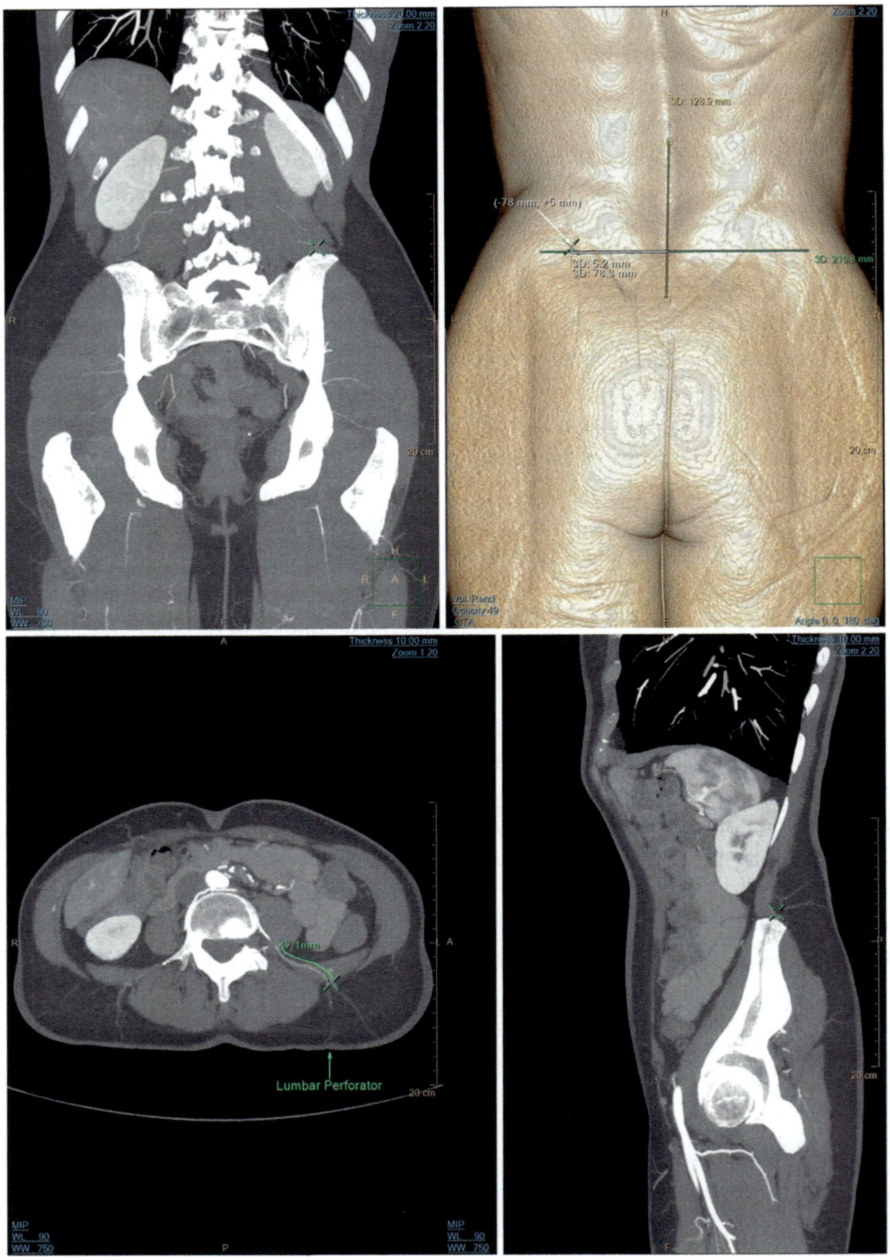

Fig. 2.4 Image composition after post-processing for pre-operative localization of perforators of the Lumbar Arteries. The reference lines are drawn on the VRT image. The horizontal reference line connects the uppermost part of the iliac crest right and left. The vertical reference line follows the curve of the spinal processes of the lumbar vertebrae. The reference point is the intersection of the two lines. In the 3D viewer, the usual 2 × 2 format is used. We recommend viewing the coronal MIP reconstruction and the VRT image side by side in the upper half of the screen and the axial and sagittal MIP reconstruction in the lower half. First, search in the coronal plane with MIP reconstruction with a slice thickness of 15–25 mm for the dominant perforator. Then, crosslink the three orthogonal planes and determine with MIP reconstructions with a slice thickness of 3 mm the precise localization of the lumbar perforator. The final measurements are again made on the VRT image. In step 1, the distance from the reference point along the horizontal axis is determined, and in step 2, the distance in the craniocaudal direction. The pedicle length is estimated on the axial image by changing the slice thickness of the images in MIP reconstruction to 5–10 mm (47 mm). To notice: the scan is performed in a supine position. The image volume of the VRT is rotated along the long axis over 180 degrees to obtain a VRT view of the back of the patient. This rotation implicates a right-left change in the coronal images in the MIP reconstruction vs. the VRT images

Tips and Tricks

How to Judge the Diameter of the Donor and Receptor Vessel?

In the report, usually, a subjective score about the diameter is mentioned. In our institution, a score from + to +++ is noted. We give a score (+) to a perforator with a small diameter (< 1 mm) and a density clearly lower than the feeding vessel and a score (+++) to a perforator with an expected diameter over 1 mm and a density comparable with the feeding vessel. However, little data are available concerning the reliability of the measurement of the diameter of a perforator on CT compared to the diameter of the vessel as found by the surgeon [13]. This uncertainty is inherent to the technical aspect of CT. The pixel size in the FOV of the scan is divided by the matrix size (512 × 512), meaning in the case of a FOV of 35 cm, a pixel value of 0.7×0.7 mm^2. The thickness of the source images is usually 0.6 mm. The substances in the voxel (volume of $0.7 \times 0.7 \times 0.6$ mm^3) determine the density of the voxel in HU. When an enhanced perforator of 0.7 mm hits only one voxel, the voxel density is the same as the density of the vessel (e.g., 200 HU). The vessel is displayed with a diameter of 0.7 mm. When the same vessel fills two adjacent voxels, the two voxels are partially filled with an enhanced vessel and partially by fat, which has a far lower density of −30 HU). The mean density of the two adjacent voxels is far less (e.g., 85 HU), but the vessel is displayed with a diameter of two voxels (1.4 mm). Therefore, besides the diameter of the vessel, the radiologist is also interested in the density of the displayed vessel compared to surrounding vessels. The larger the vessel is and the denser the vessel is compared to surrounding vessels, the more likely it is that the vessel fills a larger proportion of those adjacent voxels and will have a diameter of up to 1.4 mm. In MRI, the images of the vessels seem to be even nicer. Nevertheless, the voxel size of an MRI is at least 1.2 × 1.5 mm in the axial plane, so the vessels all look bigger than on CT, but the estimation of the actual diameter is more difficult. To remember: the measurement of the diameter of a vessel will always be a multiple of the pixel size. Given the limited size of the vessels sought, density is also an important factor in deciding on the diameter of the perforator.

Which Other Factors Influence the Density of the Vessels?

Each pre-operative imaging needs a quality check about the actual vascular phase in which the scan is made. The perforators are the terminal branches of arteries and are prone to a reduced opacification due to underfilling with contrast. A late arterial phase is recommended to opacify those terminal branches. Bolus tracking is a method that allows measurements of the enhancement of a vessel (e.g., descending thoracic aorta) in real time, showing a steep rise in density. After a certain threshold is reached (220 HU), the arterial phase is reached. Machine dependent, the scan will start 12–15 s later to scan in a late arterial phase. A late arterial phase is recognized on the still inhomogeneous enhancement of the spleen and on the portal vein, which is only slightly opacified, mimicking a filling defect. In cardiac failure, the rise in HU with relapsing time after injection will not be that steep. The threshold for the progress of the scan procedure is reached later or even not at all. Then, the scan will start too late. As a result, the arteries will not enhance as much as desired. This non-optimal timing is recognizable on the spleen, which is then homogenous, and a fully opacified portal vein. To remember: check the presence of the late arterial scan phase. If not present, be aware that perforators with lower HU are possibly part of good vascular branches.

References

1. A. Cina, L. Barone-Adesi, P. Rinaldi, et al. All the radiologist should know about multidetector CT, magnetic resonance imaging, and color-Doppler US planning of free flaps for reconstructive surgery. ECR 2012/C-1693. https://doi.org/10.1594/ecr2012/C-1693.
2. Liu H, Gao Y, Ding A, Caracappa PF, Xu XG. The profound effects of patient arm positioning on organ doses from CT procedures calculated using Monte Carlo simulations and deformable phantoms. Radiat Prot Dosim. 2015;164(3):368–75. https://doi.org/10.1093/rpd/ncu284.
3. Patient safety - radiation dose In X-ray and CT exams. https://www.radiologyinfo.org/en/info/safety-xray. Consulted: 24 Aug 2021.
4. Smith-Bindman R, Lipson J, Marcus R, et al. Radiation dose associated with common computed tomography examinations and the associated lifetime attributable risk of cancer. Arch Intern Med. 2009;169(22):2078–86. https://doi.org/10.1001/archinternmed.2009.427.
5. Fishman EK, Ney DR, Heath DG, et al. l. Volume rendering versus maximum intensity projection in CT angiography: what works best, when, and why. Radiographics. 2006;26(3):905–22. https://doi.org/10.1148/rg.263055186.
6. Lam DL, Mitsumori LM, Neligan PC, et al. Pre-operative CT angiography and three-dimensional image post processing for deep inferior epigastric perforator flap breast reconstructive surgery. Br J Radiol. 2012;85(1020):e1293–7. https://doi.org/10.1259/bjr/30590223.
7. Rozen WM, Garcia-Tutor E, Alonso-Burgos A, et al. Planning and optimising DIEP flaps with virtual surgery: the Navarra experience. J Plast Reconstr Aesthet Surg. 2010;63(2):289–97. https://doi.org/10.1016/j.bjps.2008.10.007.
8. Karunanithy N, Rose V, Lim AKP, et al. CT angiography of inferior epigastric and gluteal perforating arteries before free flap breast reconstruction. Radiographics. 2011;31:1307–19. https://doi.org/10.1148/rg.315105089.
9. Hamdi M, Van Landuyt K, Ulens S, et al. Clinical applications of the superior epigastric artery perforator (SEAP) flap: anatomical studies and pre-operative perforator mapping with multidetector CT. J Plast Reconstr Aesthet Surg. 2009;62(9):1127–34. https://doi.org/10.1016/j.bjps.2007.12.078.
10. Ahmadzadeh R, Bergeron L, Tang M, et al. The posterior thigh perforator flap or profunda femoris artery perforator flap. Plast Reconstr Surg. 2007;119(1):194–200. https://doi.org/10.1097/01.prs.0000244848.10434.5f.
11. Haddock NT, Greaney P, Otterburn D, et al. Predicting perforator location on pre-operative imaging for the profunda artery perforator flap. Microsurgery. 2012;32(7):507–11. https://doi.org/10.1002/micr.21980.
12. Hamdi M, Craggs B, Brussaard C, et al. Lumbar artery perforator flap: an anatomical study using multidetector computed tomographic scan and surgical pearls for breast reconstruction. Plast Reconstr Surg. 2016;138(2):343–52. https://doi.org/10.1097/PRS.0000000000002347.
13. Boer VB, van Wingerden JJ, Wever CF, et al. Concordance between pre-operative computed tomography angiographic mapping and intraoperative perforator selection for deep inferior epigastric artery perforator flap breast reconstructions. Gland Surg. 2017;6(6):620–9. https://doi.org/10.21037/gs.2017.09.13.

Choosing the Right Patient and Right Approach in Partial Breast Reconstruction with Pedicled Chest Wall Perforator Flaps

3

Dinesh Thekkinkattil and Tuabin Rasheed

Contents

Patient Selection Chest wall perforator flaps are suitable for small- to medium-sized breasts. The decision to choose these flaps depends on several patient and tumour related factors. Patient preference is very important, and these flaps are useful to avoid any contralateral symmetrisation procedures in majority of patients. These flaps can also be useful in a subset of patients with larger breasts who prefers to keep the current size and volume of their breasts and want to avoid contralateral procedures. Alternative options of therapeutic mammoplasty and therapeutic mastopexy in moderate to large sized breasts often requires contralateral procedures to correct volume disparity, shape, and nipple position. Chest wall perforator flaps are robust and well perfused, and smoking is not considered as a contraindication. The main contra indications are lack of adequate tissue at donor site and lack of any suitably placed perforators at the donor site because of previous surgery.

D. Thekkinkattil (✉)
Lincoln County Hospital, United Lincolnshire Hospitals NHS Trust, Lincoln, UK
e-mail: dinesh.thekkinkattil@ulh.nhs.uk

T. Rasheed
Nottingham University Hospital NHS Trust, Nottingham, UK
e-mail: Tuabin.Rasheed@nuh.nhs.uk

M. Hamdi et al. (eds.), *Pedicled Flaps in Partial Breast Reconstruction*,
https://doi.org/10.1007/978-3-031-08483-6_3

3.1 Preoperative Perforator Mapping

During planning these flaps, it is essential to locate the perforators preoperatively and helps to design the suitable skin paddle and reduce operating time and complication rate. Potential perforators are identified using a unidirectional handheld doppler (8 Hz) and the paddle is designed to incorporate these perforators. Perforators are mapped with patient lying down simulating intraoperative position [1, 2]. Usually, preoperative image guided localisation of perforators is not required.

Flap Design Lateral chest wall-based flaps (LICAP, LTAP, and TDAP) are designed on the lateral chest wall by pinching the redundant roll of fat with variable extension to the back. The flap width and length depend on the volume needed to fill the breast defect permitting tension free closure of donor site defect [3]. The flaps are generally oriented parallel to skin tension lines with the tip curving up posteriorly along the underlying ribs following the angiosome distribution. Some surgeons prefer to use a modified incision with 'two lazy S' incisions starting from inframammary crease [4] (Figs. 3.1 and 3.2). Lateral flaps are based mainly on the perforators found between anterior border of LD muscle and lateral border of breast from third to seventh intercostal spaces. The flaps can be mobilised to the defects either as a transposition propeller flap or a flip over or turn over flaps. Propeller flap is needed if a skin paddle is needed in reconstruction. Utmost care is needed, while turning the flap to defect and not to cause any torsion of the perforators. It is not always necessary to skeletonise the perforators, if flaps have enough mobility and can be transposed to the defect without any tension.

Patient Position and Intraoperative Approach Most of these lateral chest wall perforator flap (LTAP and LICAP) surgeries can be carried out by keeping the patient in supine position with ipsilateral arm abducted at 90° and with a sand bag or inflatable device beneath the ipsilateral paraspinal area to give a tilt of patient achieving good exposure of donor site area permitting comfortable flap harvesting [5]. If further exposure needed because of the flap length or design such as TDAP, patient should be kept in lateral decubitus position leaving the upper limb in neutral abduction (90° of shoulder abduction and 90° of elbow flexion). Resection of breast tumour is usually carried out through an incision in the lateral breast crease. After tumour resection, the flap is raised from lateral to medial direction and the dissection is carried out in the supra fascial or sub-facial plane identifying all perforators and special attention is needed while

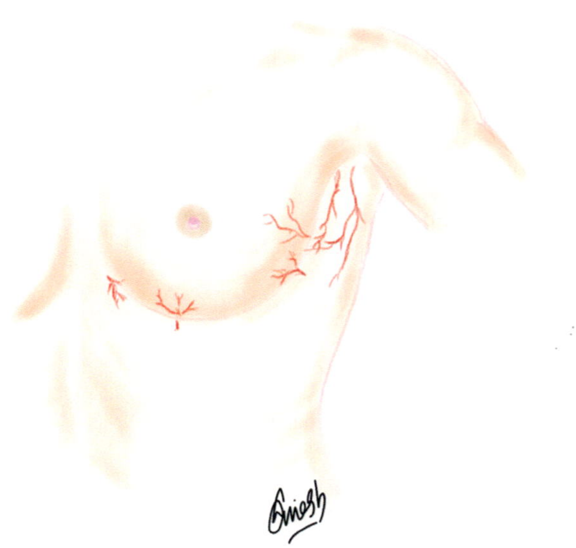

Fig. 3.1 Perforators in anterior and lateral chest wall for pedicled flap procedures

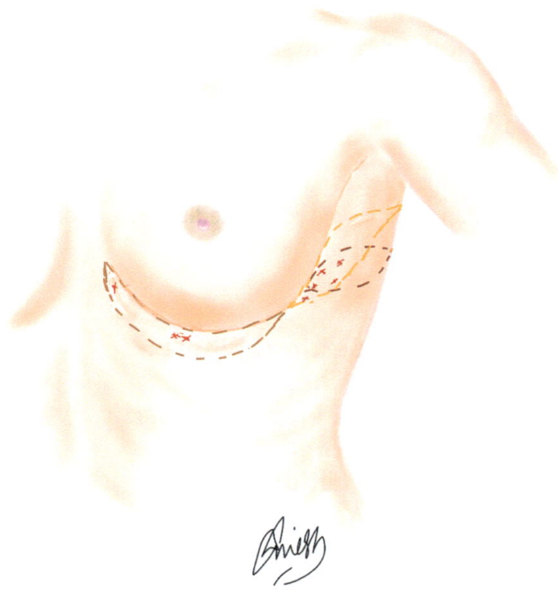

Fig. 3.2 Flap designs for lateral intercostal, lateral thoracic, anterior intercostal, and medial intercostal artery perforator flaps

dissecting the flap in the superior border to avoid any damage to LTAP pedicle. Intraoperative doppler can be used to check the position of perforators during surgery. It is advisable to use bipolar forceps to avoid any collateral damage to the perforators when dissection is carried out medially in proximity to the perforators. The usual practice is not to sacrifice any preoperatively doppler marked perforators and to preserve LTAP pedicle in the initial stages of operation. Once the flap is fully mobilised, some of the perforators may need to be sacrificed to allow transposition of the flap into the defect either as a propeller or as a turnover flap without any tension. Flaps are de-epithelised and anchoring sutures can be used to inset the flap in the defect. Some surgeons prefer not to anchor the flap to the breast tissue and the flap is held is position just by closure of the lateral breast crease wound. If a skin island is needed to reconstruct any defect after tumour resection, flap needs to be propelled to the defect, rather than turned over. Axilla can usually be accessed through the superior incision for the flap. Use of drain for the donor site is not mandatory and depends upon the extent of skin flap mobilisation and flap volume. Closure of the donor site is in layers.

TDAP is usually harvested in the lateral decubitus position as described above. The skin is usually incised in the anteroinferior border of flap allowing identification of anterior border of LD muscle. Skin and subcutaneous tissue are incised to the level of the muscle fascia, bevelling outwards to include more fat. Supra fascial dissection is carried out cranially above the LD fascia until preoperatively identified perforators are encountered. Once a suitable perforator is identified, LD muscle is split around the perforator in the direction of muscle fibres. Perforator is freed from the surrounding muscle fibres, ligating any branches to the muscle with clips or bipolar diathermy under loupe magnification. The main thoracodorsal pedicle is dissected free until required pedicle length is obtained. When the dissection of perforator is complete, flap is detached from serratus fascia and from the LD muscle and any intercostal artery perforators anteriorly. Flap is passed through the split LD muscle and then either transposed to the breast defect through a subcutaneous tunnel. Utmost care is taken during this step to avoid any damage to the perforator. Where a longer pedicle is required, the horizontal branches are divided, and the thoracodorsal vessels are dissected out preserving the nerves.

Donor site is closed in layers with or without a drain. Patient is turned to supine position for flap inset. Flap is partially or completely de-epithelised depending on the need for skin paddle.

AICAP flaps are carried out in supine position and the flap is either based on medial perforators or anterior perforators.

3.2 Clinical Settings Where Pedicled Chest Wall Perforator Flaps Are Used in Partial Breast Reconstruction

Chest wall perforator flaps can be carried out in three different settings for partial breast reconstruction. Firstly, a one stage Immediate reconstruction when the flap surgery is combined with wide local excision. Secondly, it can be done as a two staged procedure where initial surgery involves cancer resection and appropriate axillary procedure, and flap reconstruction is done 2–3 weeks later once histology confirms clear resection margins and finally these flaps can also be used to correct deformities and volume deficit from breast conservation surgery and adjuvant treatment in the delayed setting.

In one stage approach, flap reconstruction is done at the time of wide local excision of breast cancer and most of the studies confirm this approach as the preferred option in their clinical practice. A two-stage approach is described and adopted in patients where the chest wall perforators flap reconstruction is considered in a subset of patients where preoperative estimation of disease extent is challenging such as lobular cancers, extensive DCIS and in Post Neoadjuvant Chemotherapy patients [1]. In this approach, during initial surgery, wide local excision with appropriate axillary procedure is carried out and the wide local excision cavity is maintained by filling it with normal saline or water. Once the histology confirms, adequate resection margins, perforator flap procedure is carried out as a second stage procedure. These patients are at high risk for needing a potential mastectomy if resection margins are not clear on attempted breast conservation procedure. Hence deferring the flap procedure till histological confirmation, allows all possible reconstructive options if patient needs a completion mastectomy. Disadvantage of this approach is the challenges with logistics of arranging two operations with limitation of the permissible period between the two procedures due to implications of saline absorption and possibility of more scars if wide local excision incision cannot be incorporated as part of planned procedure.

3.3 Lateral Thoracic Artery Perforator Flap (LTAP)

The lateral thoracic artery originates from the second part of the axillary artery and variably from the subscalpular artery and runs along the lateral border of pectoralis major muscle within 2 cm of lateral breast crease (Figs. 3.1 and 3.2). One of the advantages of flap based on LTAP vessel is the ability to dissect the pedicle partially or entirely to allow greater flap mobility.

3.4 Lateral Intercostal Artery Perforator Flap (LICAP)

Lateral intercostal artery perforators are more inferior and lateral to LTAP perforators. LICAP perforators are located fourth to eighth intercostal spaces at a mean distance of 3.5 cm anterior to anterior border of LD muscle [6] (Figs. 3.1 and 3.2). These perforators are variable in their size and position. It is advisable to take extra care and not to damage the LTAP pedicle while dissecting the superior aspect of the flap and this in most situations give the flexibility of combining the LTAP and LICAP perforators to perfuse the flap [7].

3.5 Anterior Intercostal Artery Perforator Flap (AICAP), Medial Intercostal Artery Perforator Flap (MICAP)

Anterior intercostal artery perforator flaps are defined as the flap perfused from perforators arising from intercostal artery between anterior axillary line and xiphoid process (Figs. 3.1 and 3.2). Lower pole defects in a small to moderate sized breast is challenging if the patient is not suitable for mammoplasty or mastopexy. Defects in this area is notorious for creating worst deformities such as bird's beak appearance. Hence volume replacement with tissue from the inframammary fold is very useful for this subset of patients. Flap is based on the perforators in the inframammary fold area and can be based either perforators in the medial intercostal space (MICAP) or anterior intercostal space in the breast meridian area (AICAP). Carrasco-Lopez et al. suggested that the perforators consistently located in medial, middle, and lateral thirds of anterior thorax [8]. Usually, a crescent of tissue in the inframammary fold is raised based on the perforator and moved to the lower pole defects in the breast. Denning et al. suggested a modification of crescentic flap with inferior extension to add volume to the flap [9]. Advantage of anterior and medial intercostal artery perforator flaps are the ease of dissection, reduced time for surgery and minimal donor site morbidity. However, the inframammary fold usually gets lowered to include the perforator. These flaps are also useful in patients with cancer in the lower pole of breast and had previous breast reduction surgery who are not a suitable candidate for further therapeutic reduction mammoplasty or therapeutic mastopexy (Figs. 3.3 and 3.4).

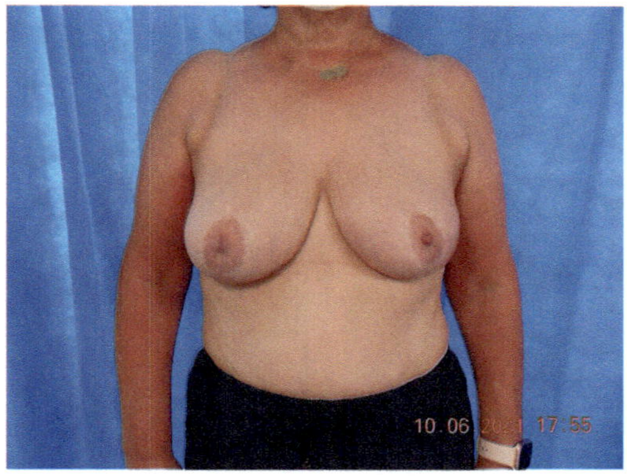

Fig. 3.3 Anterior intercostal artery perforator flap reconstruction in a patient who had previous bilateral breast reduction (preoperative)

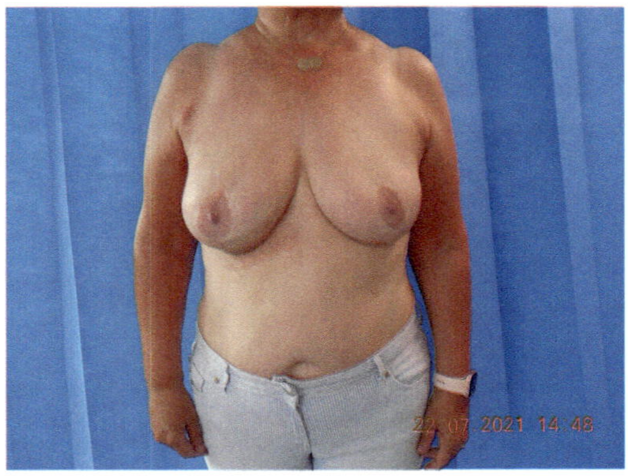

Fig. 3.4 Anterior intercostal artery perforator flap eeconstruction in a patient who had previous bilateral breast reduction (postoperative)

3.6 Thoracodorsal Artery Perforator Flap (TDAP)

TDAP flap is a fasciocutaneous flap based on musculocutaneous or septocutaneous perforators that arise from thoracodorsal artery (Figs. 3.5 and 3.6). Main pedicle of LD is the thoracodorsal artery which divides into descending and transverse branches. Descending branch is the preferred choice for TDAP flap as the perforators take on a more direct perpendicular intramuscular course and makes dissection easier [10]. The musculocutaneous perforators are located within

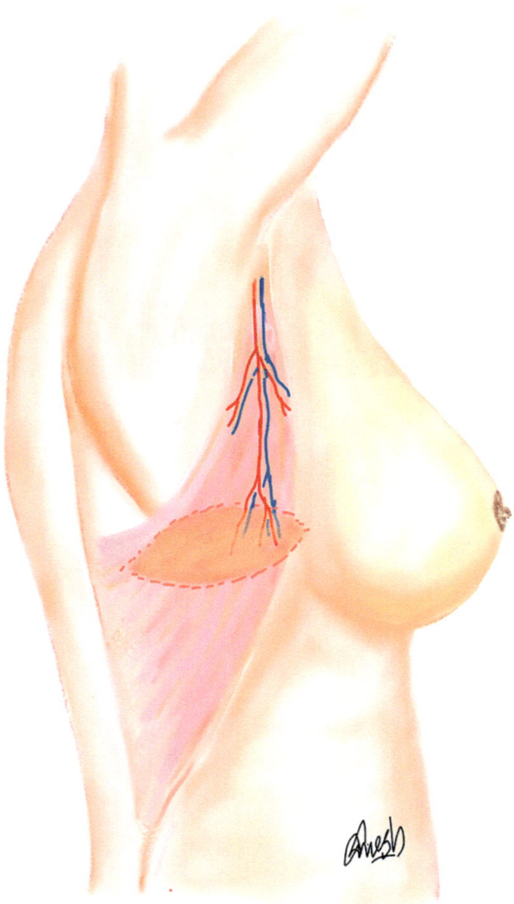

Fig. 3.5 Thoracodorsal artery perforator flap

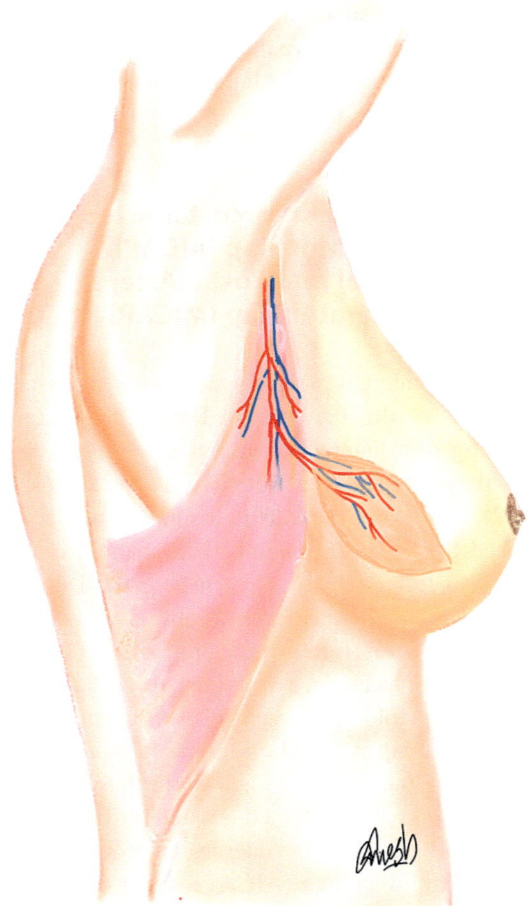

Fig. 3.6 Thoracodorsal artery perforator flap transposed to breast defect

an area of 5 cm posterior to anterior border to LD muscle at a level of 8 to 13 cm caudal to axillary crease. In 55% of patients, septocutaneous perforator arises from the thoracodorsal artery and runs anterior to the border of LD muscle avoiding intramuscular dissection. To include this perforator skin paddle needs to extend beyond anterior border of LD muscle [11]. At least 1 perforator can be found in 80% of cases in a quadrant created by intersection of 4 lines: 2 horizontal lines 9 cm and 11 cm below the posterior axillary fold and 2 vertical lines 1 cm and 4 cm medial to anterior border of LD muscle.

Levine suggested an algorithm of lateral to medial dissection considering thoracodorsal perforator as first option, and then to move medially to consider LTAP and LICAP perforator flaps. However, as LTAP and LICAP flaps are not sacrificing thoracodorsal pedicle, they are considered expendable and McCulley et al. suggested that both LTAP and LICAP flaps are the best option for partial breast reconstruction in the lateral quadrants [7, 12]. Both LICAP and LTAP flaps permit a further reconstruction with an LD flap with moderate skin paddle if required for oncological reasons in the future.

These chest wall perforator fasciocutaneous flaps are associated with minimal donor site morbidity, and its increasing popularity among oncoplastic breast surgeons is helping to broaden the scope of breast conservation surgery [13–15].

References

1. Roy PG. One-stage vs. two-stage approach for partial breast reconstructionwith lateral chest wall perforatorflaps. Cancer Treat Res Commun. 2016;9:56–61.
2. Hamdi M, Van Landuyt K, de Frene B, Roche N, Blondeel P, Monstrey S. The versatility of the inter-costal artery perforator (ICAP) flaps. J Plast Reconstr Aesthet Surg. 2006;59(6):644–52.
3. Mangialardi ML, Baldelli I, Salgarello M, Raposio E. Breast reconstruction using the lateral thoracic, thoracodorsal, and intercostal arteries perforator flaps. Plast Reconstr Surg Glob Open. 2021;9(1):e3334.
4. Neamonitou F, Thekkinkattil D, Sukumar A, Prusty L, Vidya R. A multicentric prospective cohort study of modified lateral intercostal artery perforator flap in partial breast reconstruction. Ann Plast Surg. 2022;88(1):14–9.
5. Hong S, Wang S, Liu J, Qiang Z, Zheng X, Chen G. Usefulness of lateral thoracic adipofascial flaps after breast-conserving surgery in small-to moderate-sized breasts. Clin Breast Cancer. 2019;19(5):370–6.
6. Hamdi M, Spano A, Landuyt KV, D'Herde K, Blondeel P, Monstrey S. The lateral intercostal artery perforators: anatomical study and clinical application in breast surgery. Plast Reconstr Surg. 2008;121(2):389–96.
7. McCulley SJ, Schaverien MV, Tan VK, Macmillan RD. Lateral thoracic artery perforator (LTAP) flap in partial breast reconstruction. J Plast Reconstr Aesthet Surg. 2015;68(5):686–91.
8. Carrasco-Lopez C, Julian Ibanez JF, Vila J, Rodriguez-Baeza A, Carrera-Burgaya A, Reina-de-la-Torre F, et al. The anterior intercostal artery flap: anatomical and radiologic study. Plast Reconstr Surg. 2017;139(3):613e–9e.
9. Denning M, Hayes P, Tsang F, Leff D, Thiruchelvam P, Hadjiminas D. The modified crescenteric anterior intercostal perforator flap. Plast Reconstr Surg Glob Open. 2020;8(5):e2785.
10. Hamdi M, Van Landuyt K, Hijjawi JB, Roche N, Blondeel P, Monstrey S. Surgical technique in pedicled thoracodorsal artery perforator flaps: a clinical experience with 99 patients. Plast Reconstr Surg. 2008;121(5):1632–41.
11. Hamdi M, Rasheed MZ. Advances in autologous breast reconstruction with pedicled perforator flaps. Clin Plast Surg. 2012;39(4):477–90.
12. Levine JL, Soueid NE, Allen RJ. Algorithm for autologous breast reconstruction for partial mastectomy defects. Plast Reconstr Surg. 2005;116(3):762–7.
13. Hamdi M, Van Landuyt K, Van Hedent E, Duyck P. Advances in autogenous breast reconstruction: the role of preoperative perforator mapping. Ann Plast Surg. 2007;58(1):18–26.
14. Lee KT, Mun GH. A systematic review of functional donor-site morbidity after latissimus dorsi muscle transfer. Plast Reconstr Surg. 2014;134(2):303–14.
15. Koh CE, Morrison WA. Functional impairment after latissimus dorsi flap. ANZ J Surg. 2009;79(1–2):42–7.

The Thoracodorsal Artery Perforator (TDAP) Flap

4

Moustapha Hamdi
and Leonardo Pires Novais Dias

Contents

4.1 Anatomy

The perforators that vascularize the TDAP flap often originate from the vertical branch of the thoracodorsal vessels. Usually, 2–3 musculocutaneous perforators from the vertical branch nourish to the skin patch that lays over. These perforators are frequently 2–4 cm apart. The proximal musculocutaneous perforator arises in the subcutaneous plane 8–10 cm below the axillary fold and 2–3 cm from the lateral border of the LD muscle. Regularly, one of these perforators has a direct branch from the thoracodorsal vessel that follows the lateral edge of the LD muscle and goes straight to the skin paddle. Therefore, the harvesting of these septocutaneous branches is frequently easier. However, there are some patients without a reliable perforator. In these cases, the surgical strategy may be changed intra-operatively into a muscle-sparing LD flap. In research from Hamdi et al. [1], the TDAP flap was classified into three categories according to the necessity to harvest a muscle segment with the flap (Fig. 4.1):

M. Hamdi (✉)
Head of the Plastic Surgery Department, Brussels University Hospital, Vrije Universiteit Brussel, Brussels, Belgium
e-mail: moustapha.hamdi@uzbrussel.be

L. P. N. Dias
Head of the Breast Surgery Department, Mater Dei Hospital, Salvador, Brazil
e-mail: leonardo.dias@materdei.com.br

M. Hamdi et al. (eds.), *Pedicled Flaps in Partial Breast Reconstruction*,
https://doi.org/10.1007/978-3-031-08483-6_4

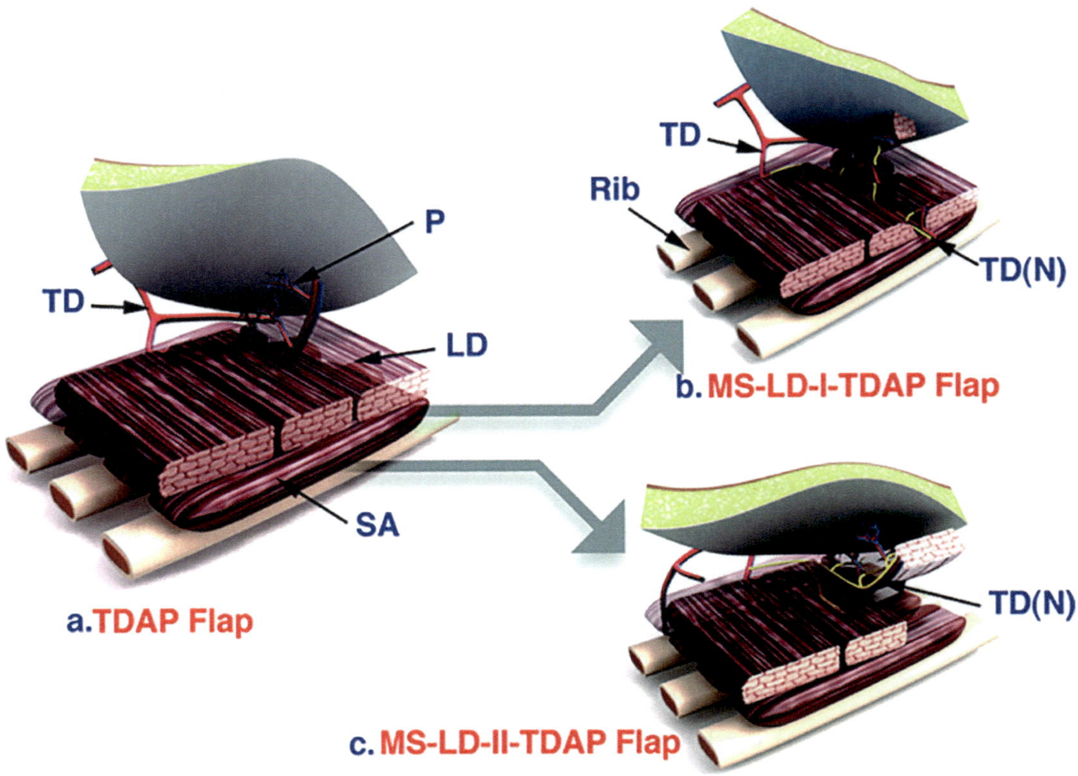

Fig. 4.1 Illustration of the thoracodorsal artery perforator (TDAP) anatomy and subtypes. *TD* thoracodorsal vessels, *P* perforator, *LD* latissimus dorsi, *SA* serratus anterior muscle, *TD(N)* thoracodorsal nerve, *MS-LD-TDAP* muscle-sparing latissimus dorsi thoracodorsal perforator. *Note.* Adapted from "Use of the thoracodorsal artery perforator (TDAP) flap with implant in breast reconstruction," by M. Hamdi et al., 2008, *Annals of plastic surgery*, *61*(2), 143–146. Copyright 2008 by Wolters Kluwer Health. Reprint with permission

- Standard TDAP flap: the flap has no muscle component.
- MS-LD-TDAP I: the flap includes a section of LD muscle (4 cm × 2 cm).
- MS-LD-TDAP II: the flap includes a section of LD muscle up to 5 cm, outlined along the lateral border of the LD muscle.

4.2 Applications

The TDAP flap is the most significant perforator flap in the lateral chest wall area and is considered a natural evolution of the LD flap [2–9]. It is one of the leading surgical options in immediate or delayed partial breast reconstruction when a volume replacement technique is required. It is mainly used when there is a resection of over 20% of the breast parenchyma, and a volume displacement oncoplastic breast reconstruction technique will end in volumetric deformities or asymmetries. The TDAP flap is ideally indicated for partial breast reconstruction of defects on the lateral quadrants of the breast. However, the flap can reach almost all breast quadrants but not the lower median region. The concept is to restore the area by harvesting a flap with a volume similar to the removed tissue, achieving symmetry in a single operative procedure [10]. The primary advantages are the avoidance of microsurgery, the shortness and reliability of the intervention, low morbidity of the donor area, and efficacy of the technique. Absolute contraindication for the TDAP flap includes damage to the thoracodorsal vessels by previous axillary or thoracic surgery. Relative contraindication relies on previous scars and irradiation of the area [11, 12]. The surgeon must review case by case to set a reliable surgical plan.

4.3 Steps

4.3.1 Planning

The flap design starts with the patient in a standing position with the hands on its waist. Then, the surgeon asks the patient to contract the back muscles actively. With that, the anterior lateral border of the LD muscle is identified and marked with a line. Next, a point "A" is marked on the anterolateral muscle line 8 cm down from the axillary fold. The proximal perforator artery often runs parallel and approximately 2 cm lateral to the muscle margin.

Further, the patient lay down on lateral decubitus, leaving the side to be operated towards up. Then the patient places the free arm with a shoulder abduction of 90 degrees and an elbow flexion of 90 degrees. This pose is similar to the final surgical position and is crucial to increase the accuracy between the marked area of the perforators on the skin and their exact location. Then, the surgeon uses a unidirectional 8 MHz hand-held Doppler ultrasonography to locate the thoracodorsal perforators.

After the perforators are correctly pointed and marked along the patient's chest wall, the TDAP flap is outlined, including the traced perforators. Thereat, the drawing must follow the directions of the skin lines and, if possible, set under the area where the bra can cover the scar. In fact, the average flap length is 20 cm and extends horizontally towards to medial portion of the back. The skin island length is always extended over the lateral border of the latissimus dorsi muscle to include the septocutaneous perforators, if present. The flap width average is 8 cm and is designed according to the possibility of immediate closure of the donor site. Finally, the redundant lateral tissue is pinched with the thumb and index finger to mark the desired width.

4.3.2 Harvesting

The TDAP flap is frequently harvested from the posterior access, and the dissection proceeds diagonally through the supra fascial plane down to the LD muscle. First, the diagonal plane is dissected away from the flap to recruit part of the fat compartments around it. Then, the surgeon lifts the flap from the back area towards the axillary region. The dissection shall continue under loupe magnification until the perforator vessel is found.

When the chosen perforator is identified, the surgeon must assess if the vessel has a visible pulsation and an adequate caliber of at least 0.5 mm. The dissection shall proceed along the perforator course up to the main thoracodorsal pedicle if the perforator is reliable. In case the perforator has an intramuscular course, the dissection advances towards the LD muscle fibers. If two perforators are found along the same row, they can be included within the flap, sacrificing no muscle fibers. All the perforator side branches within the muscle fibers are ligated or coagulated, and nerves that may come across should be preserved.

In case of inadequate perforator dimension, the flap is converted to a muscle-sparing LD. Therefore, the flap is raised, maintaining a small cuff of muscle around the perforator's space. In every case, the thoracodorsal nerve must be isolated and preserved. Hamdi et al. described this arrangement to the technique as type I and type II TDAP flaps. It is also valuable when a wider flap is planned since preserving some LD muscle fibers around the perforators would lessen the jeopardy of some tension at the perforator insertion into the flap [1].

4.3.3 Transference

The surgeon has four alternatives, and the final judgment is based on the position and extent of the breast defect. Deformities located towards the medial area or that require a large skin patch usually are treated by the conventional technique. With that, the flap will be released entirely from the donor site, and harvesting shall continue towards the axilla up to its subscapular origin, leaving the flap connected only to its vascular pedicle. This dissection is more sophisticated and will provide a longer pedicle to the flap that will reach the inner quadrants of the breast. In the

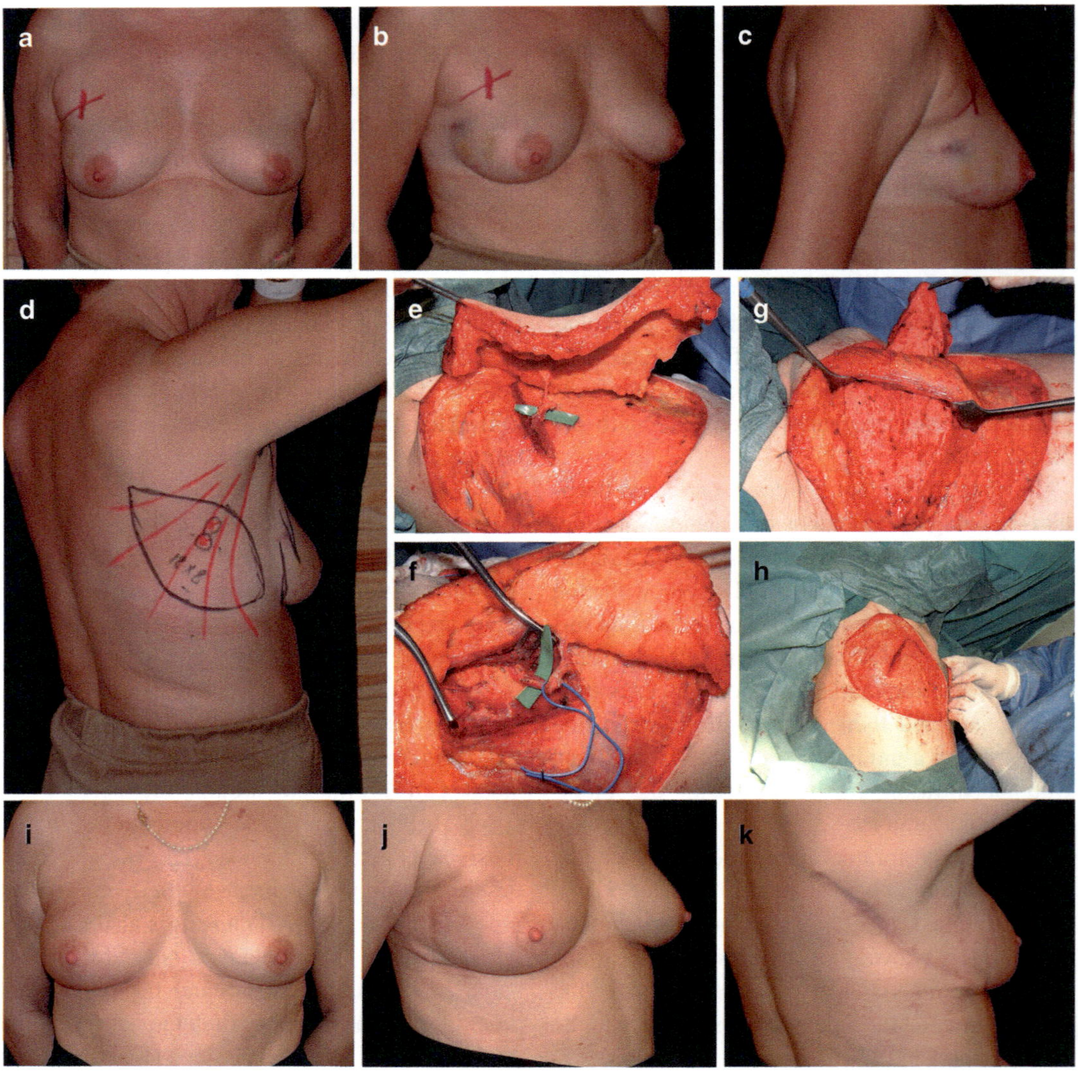

Fig. 4.2 (**a**) Pre-operative anterior view. Red marking outlines the tumor location on the right breast. (**b**) Pre-operative oblique right side view. (**c**) Pre-operative right lateral view. (**d**) Pre-operative marking of an oblique upward TDAP flap measuring 18 × 8 cm² with the identified hot spots of two thoracodorsal perforators, which were detected with a hand-held Doppler probe. (**e**) Dissection of the thoracodorsal musculocutaneous perforator from the LD muscle. (**f**) Thoracodorsal perforator isolated and dissected over and under the LD muscle. Next to the perforator pedicle, there is the preserved thoracodorsal nerve. (**g**) The de-epithelized TDAP flap is then passed through the LD muscle to be set on the breast defect. (**h**) Final wound on the donor site area. (**i**) Anterior view. Overview of the eventual result after partial breast reconstruction on the right side with TDAP flap showing pleasing contour and symmetry. (**j**) Oblique view after partial breast reconstruction with de-epithelized TDAP flap based on one perforator. (**k**) Donor site scar after TDAP flap harvesting

case of a musculocutaneous perforator, the flap is then tunneled through a "window" cut on the LD fibers with a parallel orientation to decrease the damage on the muscle. Next, the flap transfer is performed through a subcutaneous tunnel dissected by the surgeon under the skin island between the lateral breast footprint and the TDAP flap. The surgeon must meticulously follow the flap through the tunnel to avoid any injury to the pedicle (Fig. 4.2).

The second option is described as a propeller flap transfer. It is used when the lack is on the lateral quadrants of the breast. The dissection of the perforator may stop merely after the skin flap is freed from the LD muscle. The flap then should be rotated up to 180° and inserted in the defect area. A notable portion of the flap remains behind the anterior axillary line with this technique and does not entirely reach the breast footprint area. This plan is straightforward and is the preferred one by surgeons. On the other hand, the outlined skin patch creates a more extensive scar range, which produces a worse aesthetic outcome when compared to the conventional flap.

The third is the muscle-sparing technique. When small pulsative perforators are found, a muscle-sparing technique (MS-LD-TDAP I) is used to harvest the flap with a 2-cm width LD-muscle piece. Here, the perforators will be "deroofed" within the split LD muscle. The posterior side of the perforator is kept attached to the muscular part, which will be included in the flap. This strategy requires including the muscle under direct visualization of the perforators to prevent damage during harvesting the muscular segment. Thus, only a tiny nerve branch to the muscle is sacrificed. This technique can also be used when the flap is planned to reach more medial defects in the breast. A safer flap in-sitting can be obtained without direct traction on the perforator by keeping the perforator attached to the muscle segment. Suppose the perforators are very tiny and non-pulsating. In that case, the flap should be converted to (MS-LD-TDAP II) flap to incorporate a maximum number of perforators within the flap. The principal nerve of the rest of the LD muscle is always preserved. In these specific cases, the (MS-LD-TDAP I or II) flap enables the surgeon to safer harvest the flap [1].

The fourth option is the flip over technique and is only indicated for volume replacement when no skin transposition is required. Ideal for small to moderate defects right on the edge of the lateral breast footprint. With this technique, the perforators are identified but not entirely isolated from the muscle. The flap is then de-epithelialized and turned to be inserted into the breast defect. The suture of the donor site will maintain the flap in place with no need for further adjustments.

The flap is already at its last position and shall be carefully protected while the drains are placed on the donor site. Then, the donor site defect is closed using three anatomical lines of the suture. Next, the patient is rotated back to the supine position, and the surgeon can define the final contour of the flap while inserting the tissue in the breast defect. Finally, the flap can be partially or entirely de-epithelized if necessary (Fig. 4.3).

Tips

- One frequent issue with the TDAP flap planning is when the surgeon inaccurately pinpoints the thoracodorsal major vessels instead of the perforators while utilizing a unidirectional Doppler during the pre-operative markings. This misplacement happens when the perforators are searched with the patient in orthostasis. Therefore, the patient must be placed similar to the surgical position, laying on lateral decubitus with 90° of shoulder abduction and 90° of elbow flexion. As a result, the thoracodorsal perforators present a more perpendicular orientation when entering the skin, making their Doppler signal more discrete. This maneuver allows one to distinguish the perforator signal from the longitudinally oriented thoracodorsal pedicle. Accurate perforator tones can be distinguished from the thoracodorsal artery by moving the Doppler proximally and distally. If the signal disappears, it belongs to a perforator, while those from the thoracodorsal vessels will be present throughout the length of the LD muscle.
- The surgeon must consider some aspects of partial breast reconstruction related to the timing of the procedure. For immediate breast reconstruction, the drawing of the skin patch must follow the width of the potential defect created on the breast after the extraction of the lesion. However, the final flap design is

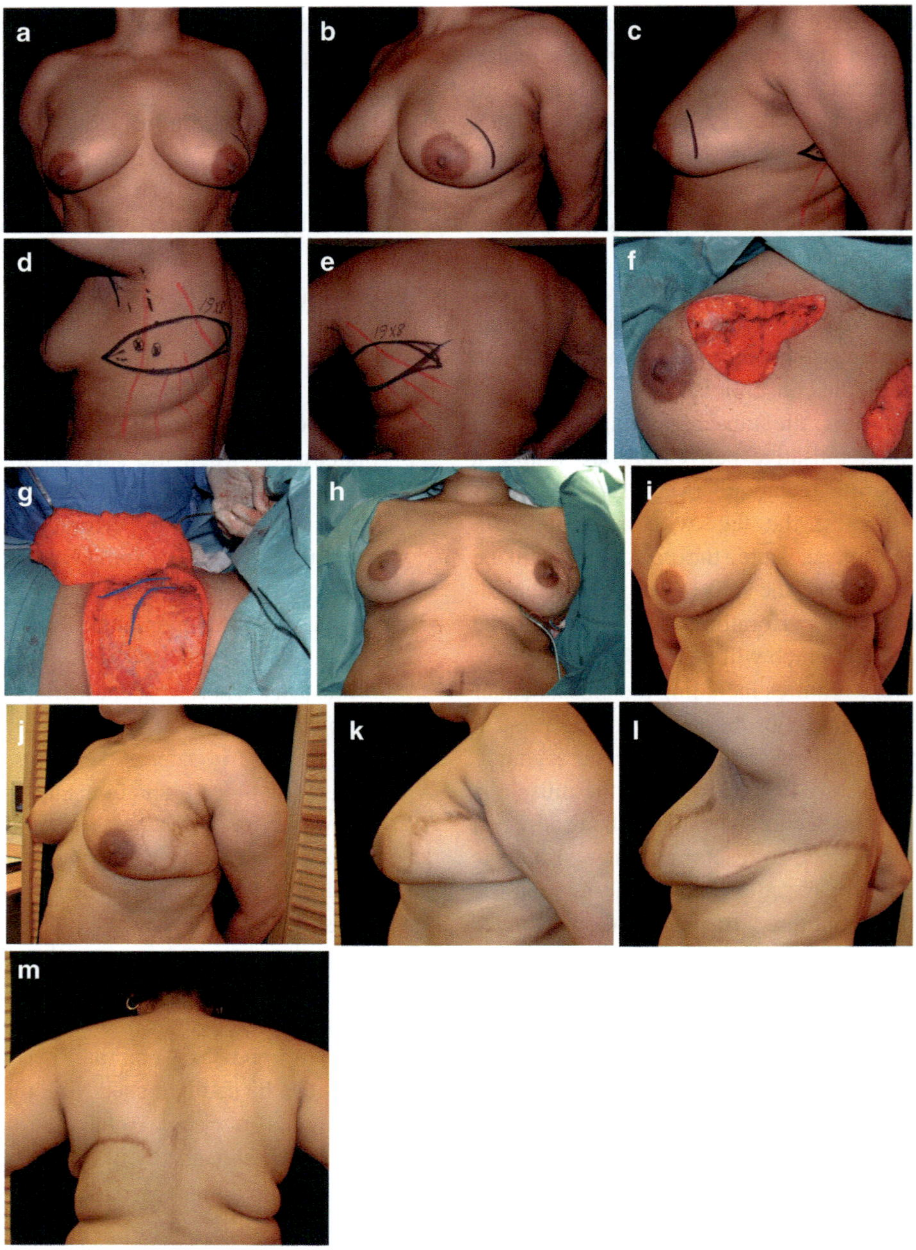

Fig. 4.3 (**a**) Anterior view. (**b**) Oblique view with the marking of the proposed incision for the oncological resection. There is an evident retraction of lower pole skin due to the scarring effect of the tumor over the cooper ligaments of the breast. (**c**) Left lateral view. (**d**) TDAP flap drawing on the left side of the trunk. Planned flap with a horizontal design measuring 19 × 8 cm and two thoracodorsal perforators identified using a hand-held Doppler device. The LD muscle area is outlined with red markings. (**e**) Posterior view of the trunk with the medial drawing of the TDAP flap reaching the area over the erector spinae muscle. (**f**) Defect area on the upper lateral quadrant of the left breast with extensive skin resection. (**g**) TDAP flap entirely harvested based on one thoracodorsal perforator. (**h**) Final intra-op result with the TDAP placed on the defect at the left breast. (**i**) Anterior view after quadrantectomy and lymph node biopsy followed by immediate TDAP flap reconstruction. The color of the skin on the left breast reveals the actinic effect of radiotherapy on the skin. The final result demonstrated symmetry a good contour. (**j**) Left oblique view after immediate partial breast reconstruction using a TDAP flap technique. (**k**) Lateral view. (**l**) Lateral view shows an acceptable result with a moderate dog ear defect, which can be improved with fat a local resection of the surplus tissue. (**m**) Posterior view of the donor site scar after the TDAP flap harvesting

best estimated only when the lesion is resected, weighed, and measured. In secondary or delayed reconstruction, the surgeon must consider the actinic effects on the skin of the breast since the patient has already completed the adjuvant treatment, and every patient presents unique characteristics after being exposed to radiotherapy. Therefore, one of the long-term side effects of radiotherapy is the induced scarring of the soft tissue, which reduces the stretching capacity of the skin. Hence, the final skin patch drawing is delimited intraoperatively after the surgeon releases the retractive scar and exposes the volume deficit.
- The neoadjuvant oncological treatment is another interesting point to consider in patients who will go for immediate partial breast reconstruction with the TDAP flap. The current neoadjuvant protocols have been demonstrated to be effective in surgery de-escalation from mastectomy to breast-conserving surgery in 60% of patients [13]. Patients that were candidates for mastectomies may now be ideal candidates for TDAP flaps. Some patients may also present a complete response to the neoadjuvant treatment, and a type I partial breast reconstruction should be enough to reset the breast mound after the oncological resection [14]. Reconstructive surgeons must work alongside oncological surgeons and preoperatively review all cases submitted to neoadjuvant treatment to set the final surgical plan.

Pitfalls

- Occasionally, the LD muscle contraction is not identified during the test, especially at secondary breast reconstruction. This lack is highly indicative that the previous oncological procedure may have damaged the neurovascular muscle pedicle. The absence of LD muscle contraction represents a lesion on the nerve, and these injuries are often associated with damage to the corresponding vascular vessels. Therefore, the surgeon must rely on the direct assessment of the perforators identified alongside the chest wall. The TDAP flap must be avoided in selected cases, and the surgeon must set a different surgical plan.
- Frequently, the thoracodorsal vessels present a direct septocutaneous perforator to the overlying skin, reaching up 55% of prevalence in some studies [15, 16]. This perforator is in front of the anterior border of the LD muscle and can make the dissection much easier and quicker. However, the pedicle is shorter, and the flap may not reach distant defects. Another critical aspect of the thoracodorsal perforator is that the reconstructive surgeon must know the risk of the perforator being injured during the axillary lymph node dissection. Therefore, it is imperative to verify that it is still pulsating and not coagulated or ligated proximally.

After-Care

- Dressings are placed at the end of the procedure, and no pressure over the flap is deposited. The patient is addressed to the regular ward, with no need for intensive care unit assistance. The TDAP vessels are checked with a unidirectional 8 MHz hand-held Doppler ultrasonography immediately after the procedure and twice a day until the patient is discharged from the hospital unit.
- If the flap has a blood supply impairment during the first 24 h, the first-choice treatment is the surgical review of the flap. The insufficient arterial blood supply or venous drainage occurs primarily because of unpredicted pressure over the pedicled vessels established with the final closure of the skin layers. Customarily, intra-operative adjustments to the flap or pedicle positions should re-establish the regular blood supply.

4.4 Conclusions

Some patients will present inadequate final breast volume or envelope surface after the TDAP flap reconstruction, leading to asymmetry. Therefore, every case must be individually analyzed, and a second procedure can be offered. For example, some patients will need a contralateral breast reduction and others volume or envelope augmentation.

In this scenario, fat grafting is a valuable tool during immediate breast reconstruction and can also be used to augment the TDAP flap. The critical detail is that the flap is still under its resetting after the vascular perfusion was changed, and the fat graft is an avascular tissue that needs a reliable inserting bed to survive. Therefore, only a limited volume can be successfully grafted into the flap. Lipofilling can be done before the flap is harvested, during the initial surgery. For example, 80–100 cc can be safely transferred to an average 250 cc flap. If required, the surgeon may perform subsequent lipofilling sessions, which are safer for the flap.

4.5 Clinical Application

Case 1

A middle-aged female with a breast cancer diagnosis on the upper lateral quadrant of the right breast was submitted to lumpectomy with sentinel lymph node biopsy and immediate reconstruction with a TDAP flap. The lateral view outlines the TDAP marking with the perforator location, performed using a hand-held Doppler device.

Case 2

A middle-age female with a breast cancer diagnosis on the upper lateral quadrant of the left breast. Planning of quadrantectomy and sentinel lymph node biopsy followed by TDAP flap reconstruction.

References

1. Hamdi M, Salgarello M, Barone-Adesi L, Van Landuyt K. Use of the thoracodorsal artery perforator (TDAP) flap with implant in breast reconstruction. Ann Plast Surg. 2008;61(2):143–6. https://doi.org/10.1097/SAP.0b013e318158fd7b.
2. Tansini I. Nuovo processo per l'amputazione della mammaella per cancre. Reforma Med. 1896;12:3.
3. Tansini I. Sopra il mio nuovo processo di amputazione della mammella. Gazz Med Ital. 1906;12:757.
4. Champaneria MC, Wong WW, Hill ME, Gupta SC. The evolution of breast reconstruction: a historical perspective. World J Surg. 2012;36(4):730–42. https://doi.org/10.1007/s00268-012-1450-2.
5. Russell RC, Pribaz J, Zook EG, Leighton WD, Eriksson E, Smith CJ. Functional evaluation of latissimus dorsi donor site. Plast Reconstr Surg. 1986;78(3):336–44. https://doi.org/10.1097/00006534-198609000-00009.
6. Reddick LP. Seroma after latissimus dorsi myocutaneous flap for breast reconstruction. Plast

Reconstr Surg. 1990;85(5):826. https://doi.org/10.1097/00006534-199005000-00042.
7. Taylor GI, Palmer JH. The vascular territories (angiosomes) of the body: experimental study and clinical applications. Br J Plast Surg. 1987;40(2):113–41. https://doi.org/10.1016/0007-1226(87)90185-8.
8. Hallock GG. Evaluation of fasciocutaneous perforators using color duplex imaging. Plast Reconstr Surg. 1994;94(5):644–51. https://doi.org/10.1097/00006534-199410000-00012.
9. Angrigiani C, Grilli D, Siebert J. Latissimus dorsi musculocutaneous flap without muscle. Plast Reconstr Surg. 1995;96(7):1608–14. https://doi.org/10.1097/00006534-199512000-00014.
10. Hamdi M, Van Landuyt K, Monstrey S, Blondeel P. Pedicled perforator flaps in breast reconstruction: a new concept. Br J Plast Surg. 2004;57(6):531–9. https://doi.org/10.1016/j.bjps.2004.04.015.
11. Mangialardi ML, Baldelli I, Salgarello M, Raposio E. Thoracodorsal artery perforator flap in partial breast reconstruction: a systematic review. Plast Reconstr Surg Glob Open. 2020;8(10):e3104. https://doi.org/10.1097/GOX.0000000000003104.
12. Thomsen JB, Rindom MB, Rancati A, Angrigiani C. Thoracodorsal artery flaps for breast reconstruction-the variants and its approach. Arch Plast Surg. 2021;48(1):15–25. https://doi.org/10.5999/aps.2020.01410.
13. Early Breast Cancer Trialists' Collaborative Group (EBCTCG). Long-term outcomes for neoadjuvant versus adjuvant chemotherapy in early breast cancer: meta-analysis of individual patient data from ten randomised trials. Lancet Oncol. 2018;19(1):27–39. https://doi.org/10.1016/S1470-2045(17)30777-5.
14. Clough KB, Kaufman GJ, Nos C, Buccimazza I, Sarfati IM. Improving breast cancer surgery: a classification and quadrant per quadrant atlas for oncoplastic surgery. Ann Surg Oncol. 2010 May;17(5):1375–91. https://doi.org/10.1245/s10434-009-0792-y.
15. Heitmann C, Guerra A, Metzinger SW, Levin LS, Allen RJ. The thoracodorsal artery perforator flap: anatomic basis and clinical application. Ann Plast Surg. 2003;51(1):23–9. https://doi.org/10.1097/01.SAP.0000054189.14799.F3.
16. Miyamoto S, Arikawa M, Kagaya Y, Fukunaga Y. Septocutaneous thoracodorsal artery perforator flaps: a retrospective cohort study. JPRAS. 2019;72(1):78–84. https://doi.org/10.1016/j.bjps.2018.08.026.

Lateral Intercostal Artery Perforator (LICAP) Flap

5

Geeta Shetty and Moustapha Hamdi

Contents

5.1 Anatomy

The LICAP flap is positioned at the lateral area of the chest wall. It is based on a pedicle containing perforators arising laterally to the inframammary fold. These perforators are frequently identified at the fifth to seventh intercostal spaces distant around 3 cm from the anterior margin of the latissimus dorsi (LD) muscle. The LICAP flap perforators originate from the subcostal portion of the intercostal vessels. The vascular intercostal vessels come from a neurovascular arcade composed of a posterior and an anterior neurovascular bundle. The posterior intercostal bundle derives from the aorta. The anterior intercostal bundle emerges from the internal mammary vessels on the —first to sixth intercostal spaces and the musculophrenic artery on the seventh to ninth. A vein of similar diameter accompanies every artery at the intercostal neurovascular bundle lying above it whilst the nerve lies below. The bundle lies deep in the external and internal intercostal muscles and superficial to the inner intercostal muscle and parietal pleura.

G. Shetty
Sandwell and West Birmingham NHS Trust, Birmingham, UK

Edge Hill University, Ormskirk, UK

Manipal Academy of Higher Education (MAHE) and Kasturba Medical College, Mangalore, India
e-mail: g.shetty@nhs.net

M. Hamdi (✉)
Head of the Plastic Surgery Department, Brussels University Hospital, Vrije Universiteit Brussel, Brussels, Belgium
e-mail: moustapha.hamdi@uzbrussel.be

M. Hamdi et al. (eds.), *Pedicled Flaps in Partial Breast Reconstruction*,
https://doi.org/10.1007/978-3-031-08483-6_5

Table 5.1 The intercostal artery perforator (ICAP) flaps classification according to Hamdi et al. [1]

Dorsal intercostal artery perforator flap	*DICAP*	Perforators arise from the *vertebral* segment
Lateral intercostal artery perforator flap	*LICAP*	Perforators arise from the *costal* segment
Anterior intercostal artery perforator flap	*AICAP*	Perforators arise from the *muscular* segment

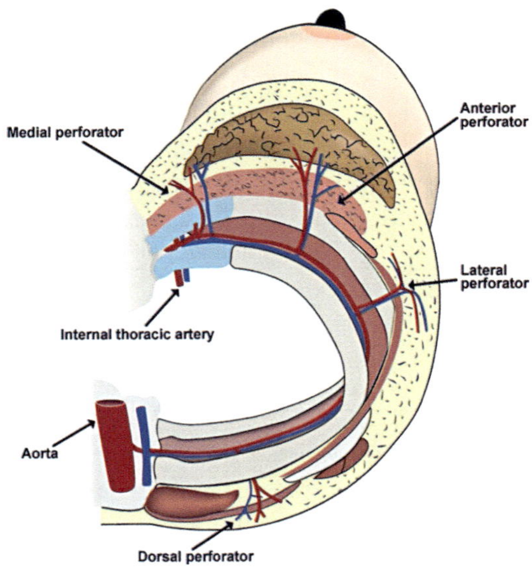

Fig. 5.1 Axial illustration of the anatomy of the neurovascular arcade on the chest area and its main vascular intercostal perforators

The course of the intercostal vessels throughout the arcade was first divided into vertebral, subcostal, intermuscular and rectus. Later on, for clinical purposes, the vascular arcade was divided into three sectors based on the rising area of the perforators: dorsal, lateral and anterior (Table 5.1). The dorsal intercostal perforator flap is based on perforators arising from the posterior area of the trunk, which is overlying the vertebral bones. The LICAP flap is at the lateral costal area. Its nourishing rise from 5 to 7 lateral intercostal perforators at 1–3 cm intervals in a horizontal axis. In addition, 2–5 perforators might be found within 6–8 cm over the mid-axillary line, in a vertical axis. At last, the anterior intercostal artery perforator flap is based on perforators arising from the muscular and rectus segment (Fig. 5.1).

5.2 Applications

The LICAP flap is well suited for tumours on the lateral half of the breast. This procedure allows excising a large volume of breast tissue up to 40% without compromising the cosmetic outcomes [2, 3]. Patients with excess lateral chest wall fasciocutaneous tissue can use this resource with or without skin island to replace the breast defect whilst maintaining its size and shape, often avoiding the contralateral symmetrisation. The redundant tissue on the lateral area of the chest wall offers the ability to replace like to like tissue into the breast without sacrificing the muscle. Additionally, its proximity to the breast borders makes it an excellent choice and does not compromise future options of total breast reconstruction [4].

The LICAP flap is ideal for small to moderate-size breasts with none to minor ptosis and could be extended to upper central tumours with a high tumour to breast ratio [5–7]. This procedure can be performed in either immediate or delayed settings [8, 9]. In the immediate setting, a wide local oncological excision is performed at first, which will assess the estimated defect. With that, the reconstructive surgeon can reshape the flap according to the lack and harvest a proper amount of tissue to perform the partial breast reconstruction. The access for extraction of the tumour could be part of the same incision as for the flap or separate depending on the tumour site to allow adequate access for the oncological procedure. The main advantage of immediate setting is avoiding a second surgery for flap reconstruction and admission to a hospital unless they need further margin excision [10–12].

The LICAP flap is also highly reliable for secondary partial breast reconstruction even after the patient completed breast radiation and axillary lymph node dissection. In a delayed setting, the lumpectomy is performed first, and later they have flap reconstruction as a second operation. A delayed partial breast reconstruction means that the patient already underwent local radiotherapy treatment. Consequently, the reconstructive surgeon might face a lateral chest wall tissue with some actinic effect, such as reduced laxity of the

LICAP flap pedicle, which limits the extension of the flap when rotated towards the breast defect. The LICAP flap might also be indicated as a salvage procedure after a failed reconstruction with another flap and are not a candidate for reconstruction with autologous abdominal flaps. The LICAP flap is also an option for patients with medical co-morbidities that make long free tissue transfer cases risky [13–15].

5.3 Steps

5.3.1 Planning

The LICAP flap marking is preferably performed the day before surgery with the patient standing or sitting. Then, the surgeon marks the prominent landmarks, which are the tumour area, the inframammary fold with its lateral continuation, the lateral breast footprint, the mid-axillary line and the anterior border of the LD. Afterwards, the patient lies down on the contralateral side of the surgery, with the arm raised and supported to simulate the position in the theatre. Then, the lateral chest wall perforators are evaluated using a handheld acoustic Doppler. Next, at the inframammary fold (IMF) level, a 6–8 cm flap pedicle is drawn towards the anterior border LD muscle incorporating one or several identified perforators (Fig. 5.2).

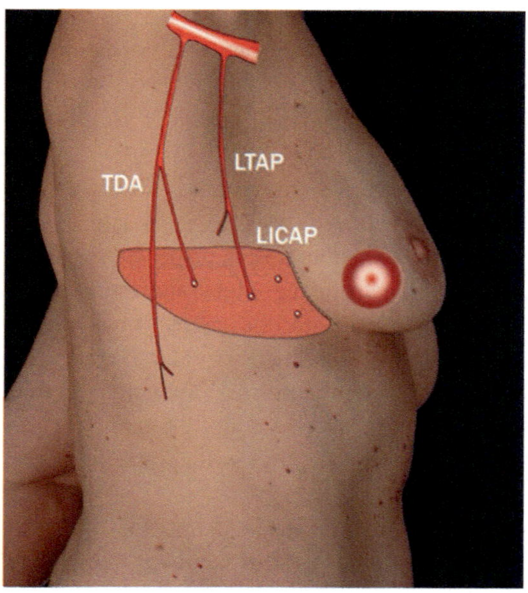

Fig. 5.2 Illustration of the anatomy of a flap on the lateral chest wall and the possible perforators that will nourish the flap. The tumour area on the breast is represented by a red and white circle. *LICAP* lateral intercostal artery perforator, *LTAP* lateral thoracic artery perforator, *TDA* thoracodorsal artery

The LICAP perforators are regularly found between the fifth and seventh intercostal spaces approximately 2.5 and 3.5 cm from the anterior border of LD. The lateral breast crease is used as the initial anterior and superior reference of the flap marking. Then, the skin paddle is drawn based on an assessment of the redundant skin of the lateral chest fold using a manual pinch test. This manoeuvre shows the limits of the flap marking to have a primary closure of the donor site without tension before the flap is harvested. The proximal design of the LICAP flap usually follows the bra line in an elliptical shape, including the perforators. The distal part of the flap is drawn based on the size of flap required, general skin laxity and orientation and such that the scar remains well-hidden within the bra line. There does not appear to be a restriction on the size of the flap compared to the available axillary tissue. Flap height is usually restricted to 10 cm; although more may be achieved, flap length may be up to 30 cm. For one stage procedure, when feasible, a wide local excision is performed through the lateral mammary fold (Fig. 5.3).

5.3.2 Dissection

Patients are positioned in a supine position with the arm extended. A lateral tilt is given for LICAP flap reconstructions, using a saline bag or sandbag placed beneath the scapula and another one beneath the pelvis to avoid traction or twisting. No intra-operative change of position is required. This position is ideal if patients need an axillary procedure in the same setting because axillary orientation is less distorted, unlike in other positions. For the more extended flap, additional access posteriorly can be obtained by positioning the patient laterally with an arm extended at 90° and brought across the chest wall. A single dose

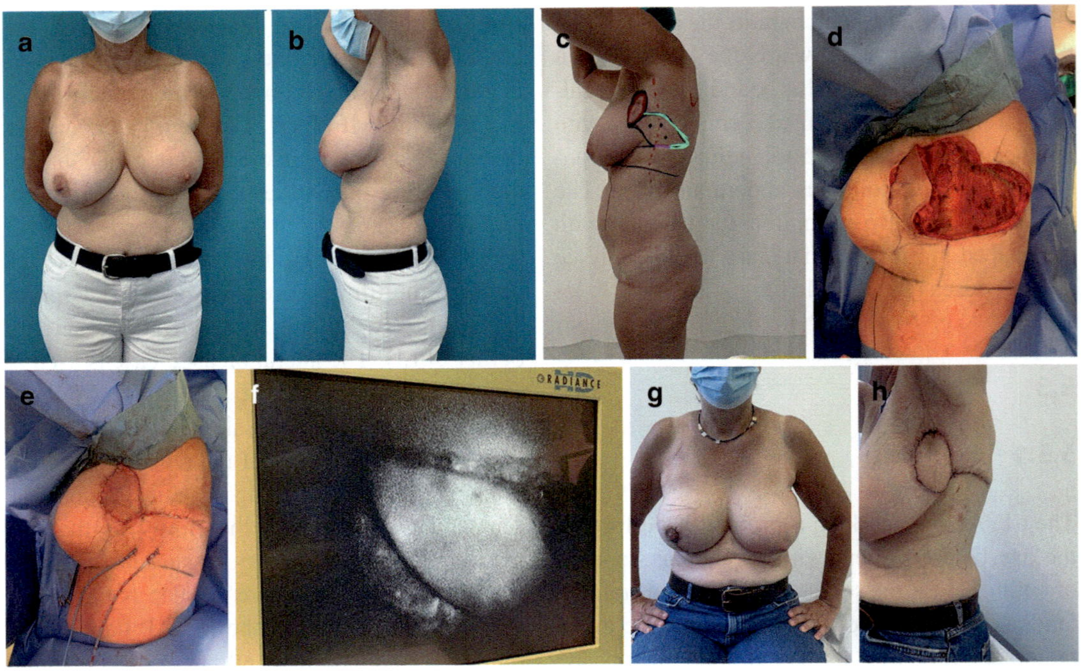

Fig. 5.3 (**a**) Anterior view. (**b**) Left lateral view with arms raised. The previous scar is visible on the Spence tail area surrounded by the marking of the planned tumour resection. (**c**) Left-side view with arms raised. Preoperative markings with the LICAP flap were designed, including the perforators, identified using a handheld Doppler device. The posterior axillary line is outlined with a red dashed marking. (**d**) The LICAP flap often does not require complete dissection of the perforator to reach its final position into the breast footprint. In this case, the flap is rotated 90° and positioned. The skin patch of the flap was preserved to fulfil the lack after oncological dissection. (**e**) The final result immediately after the surgery. (**f**) Indocyanine green angiography was performed to control the blood supply to the flap. (**g**) Postoperative anterior view. Due to the previous asymmetry related to the first treatment protocol which the patient was submitted, a breast reduction was performed on the contralateral breast. (**h**) Left lateral view shows the LICAP flap in place without clinical complications

of antibiotic is preferred preoperatively. In an immediate setting, a single incision is often used for the wide local excision and reconstruction in most cases, irrespective of the type of perforator flap.

In the supine or partial lateral decubitus position, the dissection begins from the most distal flap tip. First, the superior skin edge is incised, and dissection is then carried down to the chest wall. Next, the lateral border of the LD is identified, and dissection continues above the muscle fascia from lateral to medial. Next, the inferior skin edge is incised. The flap is then carefully elevated off the chest wall in the supra fascial plane towards the anterior axillary line. Careful attention is made 6–8 cm from the anterior axillary line at the fifth and sixth intercostal areas. At this stage, the pedicle and the territory of the long thoracic nerve can be easily visualised and protected because it is approached from above. The flap is then inspected for bright red bleeding from the edges and then rotated and transposed into the breast pocket. The intra-operative handheld vascular Doppler can be used to guide the perforators and dissection. Magnification lenses are not essential for this procedure; however, they will aid the dissection of perforators.

The flap can be inserted into the defect by rotation or flopping the tissue over the pedicle. Rotation is the chosen technique when there is a lack of volume and skin on the lateral quadrants. The advancement can go up to 180° from the pivot point at the lateral inframammary crease. After rotation, the skin paddle is inserted in the breast mound or de-epithelialised and buried within the skin envelope to provide vascularised volume. The flap tip can be mobilised to reach the midline of the chest depending on the flap length and how lateral the pivot point is placed. The skin paddle can quickly improve a restricted skin envelope in the lower and lateral areas. Only the volume replacement is necessary, and the defect lies on the inferior lateral quadrant of the breast. The flap can be de-epithelised and inserted in the affected by flopping over its pedicle area.

Finally, tacking sutures are placed to secure the flap to the anterior chest wall with interrupted, absorbable sutures. The skin of the flap can be preserved or completely de-epithelialised based on the defect and reconstruction plan. Afterwards, a capillary drain is placed. Skin incisions are then closed with interrupted dermal sutures and a running subcuticular stitch. The reasonably brief operative time for LICAP flap harvest is an average of 1 h per breast (Fig. 5.4).

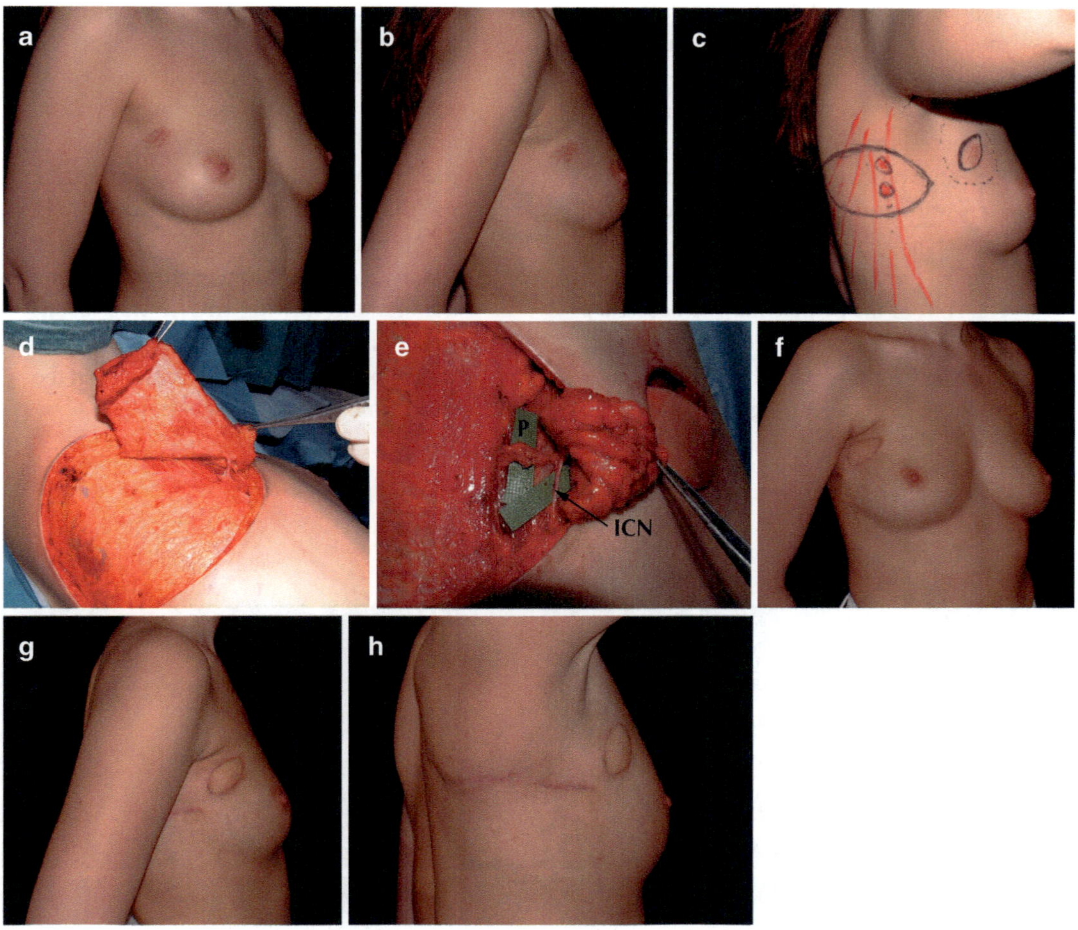

Fig. 5.4 (**a**) Preoperatory oblique right-side view. The previous lumpectomy incision is outlined on the upper lateral quadrant of the breast. (**b**) Lateral right-side view. The previous scar of the lumpectomy is visible on the upper lateral quadrant of the right breast. (**c**) Lateral right-side view. The flap is designed in a horizontal orientation, and two perforators were included in the flap area. The area to the resected on the breast is outlined, including the skin surrounding the scar. The LD muscle is marked in red. (**d**) The SAAP flap was harvested with one lateral intercostal perforator nourishing the flap. (**e**) This intraoperative overview shows the SAAP flap completed harvested based on a musculocutaneous perforator. Due to the close distance between the flap and the breast defect, the flap was rotated 180° and placed into the defect. During the harvesting, one intercostal perforator (P) was dissected and isolated. Also, an intercostal nerve (ICN) was identified and preserved. (**f**) Oblique right-side view. The final result of the SAAP flap used for immediate partial breast reconstruction. (**g**) Lateral right-side view. (**h**) Lateral right-side view with arm raised—donor site with a horizontal scar

Tips

- An interesting consideration is the importance of achieving negative surgical margins during resection. Nevertheless, two crucial situations must be underscored. Frequently, intra-operative assessments using frozen section analysis may minimise the likelihood of delayed re-excision of margins. However, dedicated attention must be given to patients with large tumours submitted to neoadjuvant chemotherapy that became eligible for breast-conserving surgery but did not present a complete pathological response [16–18]. On the other hand, if the entire processing of the tumour specimen warrants re-excision, the perforator flaps can be retracted to re-expose the original tumour defect. Sometimes, a lateral shift of the pedicle may be necessary if a very lateral oncological resection reaches the limits of the lateral breast footprint. Lateral shifting of the pedicle is possible because perforators from the intercostal vessels arise at intervals in the lateral chest fold. Eventually, any immediate partial reconstruction should be delayed if the surgeon is uncertain about the margins or tumour extension despite the preoperative radiological assessment. Therefore, delayed reconstruction can still be performed within a few days after the definitive margins become known (Fig. 5.5).
- Another important tip is related to the closure. The skin and subcutaneous tissue from the lower and upper incision are mobilised to facilitate the closure of the wound. Nevertheless, extensive mobilisation of the lower incision may compromise a future LD skin patch. Finally, often a drain is required at the donor site following LICAP flap reconstructions, especially if the patient has undergone axillary node clearance at the same time.

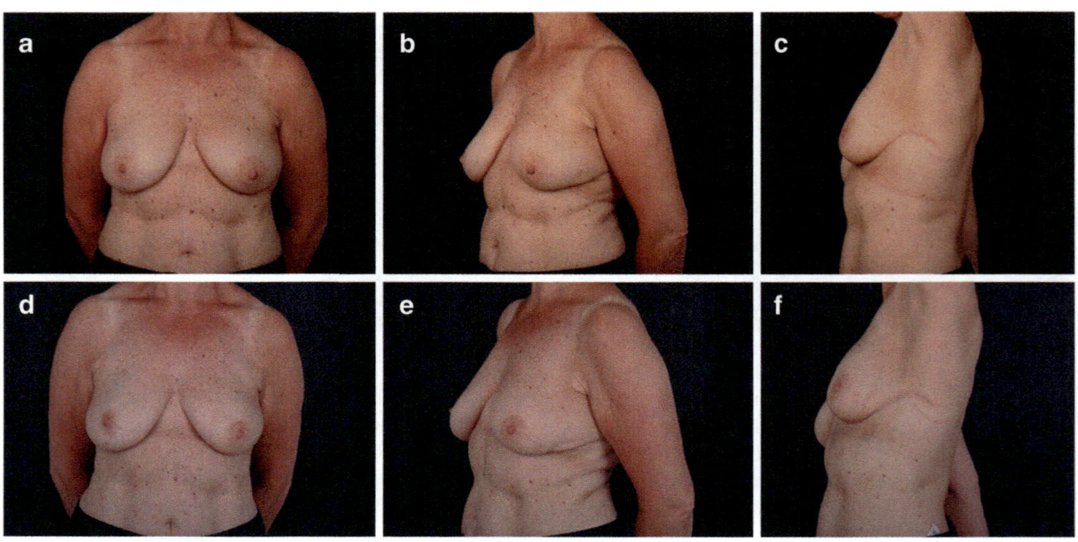

Fig. 5.5 (**a**) Anterior view after 5 months. (**b**) Oblique left-side view after 5 months. (**c**) Lateral left-side view with the arm raised after 5 months. (**d**) Anterior view after 12 months. (**e**) Oblique left-side view after 12 months. (**f**) Lateral left-side view with the arm raised after 12 months

Pitfalls

- A generous pedicle can be maintained to maximise flap viability, especially in early cases, but this will cause a bulky pivot point in the lateral chest, which can be quickly revised as a minor outpatient procedure later. Unfortunately, this situation is frequent for extensive breast resections requiring significant tissue volume for replacement. With that, a large pedicle may not be fully integrated into the breast footprint, delivering a limited cosmetic result.
- Specific issues may limit the mobilisation of adjacent tissue, including prior radiation therapy, morbid obesity, poor skin characteristics and chronic steroid therapy. Therefore, the sign must follow accurate preoperative evaluation with pre-clinical and clinical assessment.

After-Care

- Dressings are placed at the end of the procedure, and no pressure over the flap is set. The patient is addressed to the regular ward, with no need for intensive care unit assistance. The LICAP vessels are checked with a unidirectional handheld Doppler (8 Hz) ultrasonography immediately after the procedure is finished and twice a day until the patient is discharged from the hospital unit.
- If the flap has a blood supply impairment during the first 24 h in the ward, the first-choice treatment is the surgical review of the flap. The insufficient arterial blood supply or venous drainage occurs primarily because of unpredicted pressure over the pedicled vessels established with the final closure of the skin layers. Usually, intra-operative adjustments to the flap or pedicle positions should re-establish the regular blood supply.
- Patients are instructed to refrain from strenuous activity for 4–6 weeks to allow optimal wound healing and reduce the risk of a seroma or contour abnormality at the donor site. Typically, LICAP flap drains are removed after 1 week. Patients are instructed to follow up with the surgeon a few days after discharge from the hospital. They are advised to wear a well-supported bra after day one, which will help to inset the flap. Arm movement is limited to 90° for the first 2–3 weeks, then escalated depending on patient recovery.

5.4 Conclusion

Using pedicled perforator flaps in breast reconstruction was introduced in the literature by Hamdi et al. in 2004 [19]. In his series, he investigated several chest wall perforator flaps. He noted the utility of the LICAP flap specifically for patients with small to moderate-sized breasts with large tumours at the lateral quadrants. However, the ideal concept of this technique is to achieve symmetry with no contralateral procedure, and sometimes, the LICAP flap may not deliver the desired volume replacement. In such cases, he noted that the perforator flaps serve as a vascularised tissue matrix for subsequent fat grafting.

5.5 Clinical Application

Case 2 (M. Hamdi)

A 32-year-old patient with the previous diagnosis of breast cancer on the upper lateral quadrant of the right breast. The first procedure was a lumpectomy with sentinel lymph node biopsy with the immediate closure of the wound. Though the final pathological analysis determined that margins were compromised, and a further re-excision was indicated. The patient presented cup A breast without ptosis, and any further excision without reconstruction would result in a significant breast deformity. Therefore, a LICAP for partial breast reconstruction was planned.

Case 1 (M. Hamdi)

A 59-year-old patient diagnosed with breast cancer recurrence on the spence axillary tail of the left side. The patient was previously submitted to lumpectomy and sentinel lymph node biopsy followed by radiotherapy and chemotherapy. The patient was submitted to neoadjuvant chemotherapy followed by surgical excision of the lesion and partial breast reconstruction with a LICAP flap. The patient presented a volume asymmetry at the pre-op assessment due to the previous oncological treatment with surgery and radiotherapy on the left breast.

Case 3 (G. Shetty)

A 57-year-old patient with partial breast reconstruction with lateral intercostal artery perforator flap, 5 months postop and 12 months postradiotherapy for 35 mm tumour.

References

1. Hamdi M, Van Landuyt K, de Frene B, Roche N, Blondeel P, Monstrey S. The versatility of the intercostal artery perforator (ICAP) flaps. J Plast Reconstr Aesthet Surg. 2006;59(6):644–52. https://doi.org/10.1016/j.bjps.2006.01.006.
2. Fujimoto H, Shiina N, Nagashima T, Sangai T, Sakakibara J, Takada M, Teranaka R, Takishima H, Kawasaki Y, Ohtsuka M. Oncoplastic breast-conserving surgery using chest wall perforator flaps: three-dimensional quantitative analysis of the percentage of breast volume excised and changes over time in flap volume. J Surg Oncol. 2019; https://doi.org/10.1002/jso.25809.
3. Hu J, Cuffolo G, Parulekar V, Chan V, Tenovici A, Roy PG. The results of surveillance imaging after breast conservation surgery and partial breast reconstruction with chest wall perforator flaps; a qualitative analysis compared with standard breast-conserving surgery for breast cancer. Clin Breast Cancer. 2019;19(3):e422–7. https://doi.org/10.1016/j.clbc.2019.01.010.
4. Agrawal SK, Shakya SR, Nigam S, Sharma A, Datta SS, Ahmed R. Chest wall perforator flaps in partial breast reconstruction after breast conservation surgery: an additional oncoplastic surgical option. Ecancermedicalscience. 2020;14:1073. https://doi.org/10.3332/ecancer.2020.1073.
5. Lee JW, Kim MC, Park HY, Yang JD. Oncoplastic volume replacement techniques according to the excised volume and tumor location in small- to moderate-sized breasts. Gland Surg. 2014;3(1):14–21. https://doi.org/10.3978/j.issn.2227-684X.2014.02.02.
6. Yang JD, Ryu DW, Lee JW, Choi KY, Chung HY, Cho BC, Park HY, Byun JS. Usefulness of a lateral thoracodorsal flap after breast conserving surgery in laterally located breast cancer. Arch Plast Surg. 2013;40(4):367–73. https://doi.org/10.5999/aps.2013.40.4.367.
7. Hakakian CS, Lockhart RA, Kulber DA, Aronowitz JA. Lateral intercostal artery perforator flap in breast reconstruction: a simplified pedicle permits an expanded role. Ann Plast Surg. 2016;76(Suppl 3):S184–90. https://doi.org/10.1097/SAP.0000000000000752.
8. Soumian S, Parmeshwar R, Chandarana M, Marla S, Narayanan S, Shetty G. Chest wall perforator flaps for partial breast reconstruction: surgical outcomes from a multicenter study. Arch Plast Surg. 2020;47(2):153–9. https://doi.org/10.5999/aps.2019.01186.
9. Roy PG, Tenovici AA. Staged approach to partial breast reconstruction to avoid mastectomy in women with breast cancer. Gland Surg. 2017;6(4):336–42. https://doi.org/10.21037/gs.2017.03.08.
10. Rainsbury RM. Surgery insight: oncoplastic breast-conserving reconstruction--indications, benefits, choices and outcomes. Nat Clin Pract Oncol. 2007;4(11):657–64. https://doi.org/10.1038/ncponc0957.

11. Clough KB, Kaufman GJ, Nos C, Buccimazza I, Sarfati IM. Improving breast cancer surgery: a classification and quadrant per quadrant atlas for oncoplastic surgery. Ann Surg Oncol. 2010;17(5):1375–91. https://doi.org/10.1245/s10434-009-0792-y.
12. Munhoz AM, Montag E, Gemperli R. Oncoplastic breast surgery: indications, techniques and perspectives. Gland Surg. 2013;2(3):143–57. https://doi.org/10.3978/j.issn.2227-684X.2013.08.02.
13. Youssif S, Hassan Y, Tohamy A, Eid S, Ashour T, Malahias M, Khalil H. Pedicled local flaps: a reliable reconstructive tool for partial breast defects. Gland Surg. 2019;8(5):527–36. https://doi.org/10.21037/gs.2019.09.06.
14. Hamdi M, Spano A, Landuyt KV, D'Herde K, Blondeel P, Monstrey S. The lateral intercostal artery perforators: anatomical study and clinical application in breast surgery. Plast Reconstr Surg. 2008;121(2):389–96. https://doi.org/10.1097/01.prs.0000298317.65296.cf.
15. Meybodi F, Cocco AM, Messer D, Brown A, Kanesalingam K, Elder E, Hsu J, French J. The modified lateral intercostal artery perforator flap. Plast Reconstr Surg Glob Open. 2019;7(2):e2066. https://doi.org/10.1097/GOX.0000000000002066.
16. Sun Y, Liao M, He L, Zhu C. Comparison of breast-conserving surgery with mastectomy in locally advanced breast cancer after good response to neoadjuvant chemotherapy: a PRISMA-compliant systematic review and meta-analysis. Medicine. 2017;96(43):e8367. https://doi.org/10.1097/MD.0000000000008367.
17. Litière S, Werutsky G, Fentiman IS, Rutgers E, Christiaens MR, Van Limbergen E, Baaijens MH, Bogaerts J, Bartelink H. Breast conserving therapy versus mastectomy for stage I-II breast cancer: 20 year follow-up of the EORTC 10801 phase 3 randomised trial. Lancet Oncol. 2012;13(4):412–9. https://doi.org/10.1016/S1470-2045(12)70042-6.
18. Kosasih S, Tayeh S, Mokbel K, Kasem A. Is oncoplastic breast conserving surgery oncologically safe? A meta-analysis of 18,103 patients. Am J Surg. 2020;220(2):385–92. https://doi.org/10.1016/j.amjsurg.2019.12.019.
19. Hamdi M, Van Landuyt K, Monstrey S, Blondeel P. Pedicled perforator flaps in breast reconstruction: a new concept. Br J Plast Surg. 2004;57(6):531–9. https://doi.org/10.1016/j.bjps.2004.04.015.

Serratus Anterior Artery Perforator (SAAP) Flap

6

Moustapha Hamdi
and Leonardo Pires Novais Dias

Contents

6.1 Anatomy

The serratus anterior muscle (SAM) is a type III muscle constituted of seven to ten digitations. The SAM originates from the outer surface of the upper tenth ribs and inserts in the medial margin of the scapula. The vascular supply of the SAM area has three origins: the lateral thoracic artery, the serratus anterior branch of the thoracodorsal artery and the intercostal perforators. The uppermost part of the SAM is mainly supplied by the lateral thoracic artery, which arises directly from the axillary artery. The medial and lower parts are nourished essentially by the serratus branch of the thoracodorsal artery and the intercostal perforators [1].

The serratus anterior vascular pedicle runs superficially to the SAM in its proximal part and is covered by the latissimus dorsi (LD) muscle in this segment (Fig. 6.1). The distal portion of the serratus anterior vessels extends over the SAM and is located directly beneath the skin and subcutaneous tissue. The SAAP flap corresponds to the skin patch overlying the SAM, supplied by interconnections between the serratus anterior vessels and the intercostal perforator branches (Fig. 6.2). Interestingly, this interconnection is

M. Hamdi (✉)
Head of the Plastic Surgery Department, Brussels University Hospital, Vrije Universiteit Brussel, Brussels, Belgium
e-mail: moustapha.hamdi@uzbrussel.be

L. P. N. Dias
Head of the Breast Surgery Department, Mater Dei Hospital, Salvador, Brazil
e-mail: leonardo.dias@materdei.com.br

M. Hamdi et al. (eds.), *Pedicled Flaps in Partial Breast Reconstruction*,
https://doi.org/10.1007/978-3-031-08483-6_6

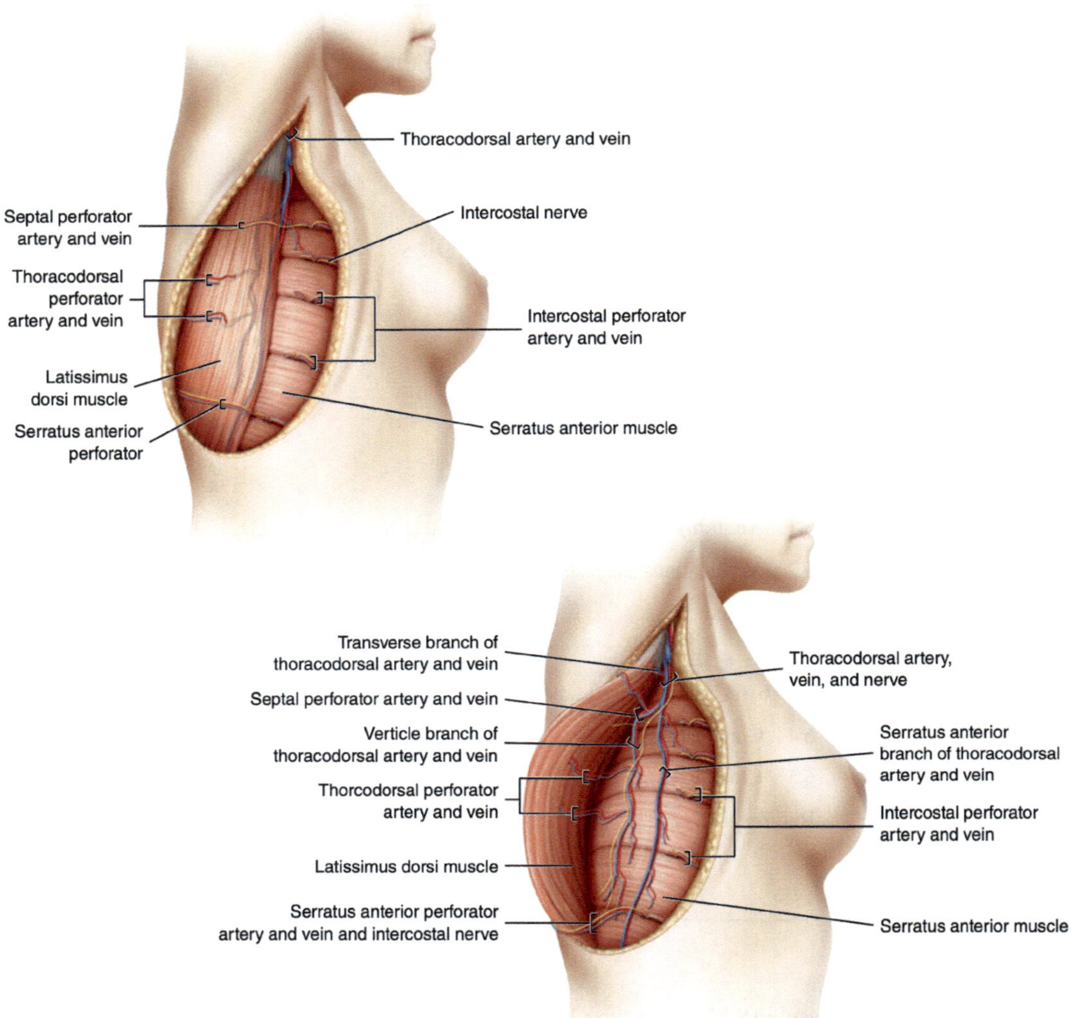

Fig. 6.1 Illustration of the vascular pedicles located on the lateral thoracic wall. *Note.* Adapted from Pedicled Perforator Flap Reconstruction, by M. Hamdi. In A. Losken & M. Hamdi (Eds.), *Partial Breast Reconstruction – Techniques in Oncoplastic Surgery*, 2017 (2nd ed.), p. 390. Thieme. Copyright 2017 by Thieme Publishers. Reprinted with permission

found only in approximately 20% of the patients, essentially in the middle and lower sections of the SAM (Fig. 6.2) [2, 3].

Generally, the skin paddle is designed on the lower part of the SAM, near the inframammary fold (IMF) region. The anatomical landmark to identify the emergence of the SAAP origin is 3–4 cm anterior to the border of the LD muscle in the sixth and seventh intercostal spaces. Hence, the usual boundaries of the skin paddle are the IMF, the anterior border of the LD muscle, the midclavicular line and the ninth rib. If required, the flap can be extended a few centimetres laterally over the LD muscle region. According to studies, the diameter of the vessels varies from 0.5 to 1.0 mm. The perforator length average is 3 cm. When the total length of the pedicle is evaluated, which includes the serratus anterior arterial branch, the pedicle presents from 7 to 11 cm [2].

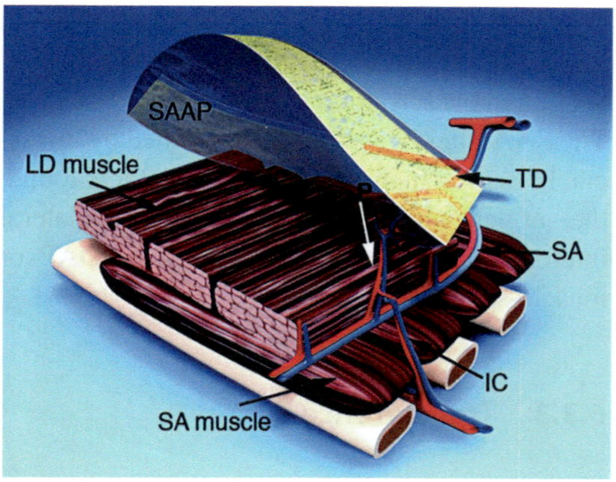

Fig. 6.2 Illustration of the serratus anterior artery perforator flap. *Note.* Adapted from "The Lateral Intercostal Artery Perforators: Anatomical Study and Clinical Application in Breast Surgery, "by M. Hamdi et al., 2008, *Plastic and Reconstructive Surgery, 121* (2), p. 391, fig. 4. Copyright 2008 by Wolters Kluwer Health. Reprinted with permission

6.2 Applications

The SAAP flap is a solid perforator flap that offers a practical approach to reconstruct defects from laterally located breast cancer. It is mainly used when wide resections of the breast parenchyma are performed, which would deliver unfavourable cosmetic results [4]. The typical indication for partial breast reconstruction with the SAAP flap are women with small to moderate-sized breasts that demand volume replacement breast reconstruction on the lateral quadrants with or without skin [5]. This flap has a shorter pedicle and a limited rotation curve when confronted with the thoracodorsal artery perforator (TDAP) flap. Though, it has the convenience of less intramuscular dissection and can be harvested with the patient in a supine position with a lateral bump rather than on a lateral decubitus posture [6].

Pedicled chest wall perforator flaps can be employed in immediate and delayed partial breast reconstructions [7, 8]. The exemplary procedure is to perform immediate reconstruction after the resection of the tumour. Therefore, the surgeon can estimate the lack of parenchyma and restore the deficit by harvesting a properly measured flap in solely one procedure [9]. Besides that, a delayed reconstruction after a partial breast resection implies that the patient underwent radiotherapy, and the actinic impact on the skin can increase the risk of complications [10].

The SAAP flap is a handy, reliable technique that avoids microsurgery procedures and confers limited morbidity to the donor site area. The absolute contraindications for the SAAP flap are when the perforator was previously damaged, or simply the connection between serratus anterior and intercostal perforators are not present. Relative contraindication relies on previous scars, irradiation of the area and extensive breast tissue resection, that even with the SAAP flap, would result in poor cosmetic or excessive asymmetry. In such restricted cases, other autologous techniques are indicated. Surgeons and patients must review safety and expectations to set a reliable plan.

6.3 Steps

6.3.1 Planning

The SAAP flap plan commences by demarcating the resection zone and the regional anatomical landmarks to assist the harvesting. Then, with the patient in the upright position and hands-on its waist, the surgeon identifies the tumour area, the IMF, the lateral footprint limit of the breast and the anterior border of LD. However, in some patients, the LD flap is not evident or palpable. Hence, the surgeon should request the patient to actively contract the LD muscle by forcing her hands towards her hipbones. The subsequent step is to distinguish the perforator vessels on the lateral thoracic wall preoperatively. Therefore, the patients should be placed in a similar position requested for surgery and so the perforators can be identified using an 8 MHz handheld Doppler ultrasonography. Finally, preoperative imaging with a computed tomography angiography is counselled to aid in distinguishing the position, number, and size of perforators due to the reduced prevalence of the interconnection linking the serratus anterior vessels and intercostal perforators.

The anterior border of the flap is placed next to the lateral breast crease, and the other limits are defined by the shape and volume of the defect on the breast. The flap is often drawn in a transversal elliptical shape to set the scar beneath the bra line. However, the SAAP flap can also be outlined vertically, following the lateral breast contour. A pinch test assesses the shortest measure of the flap to allow a safer donor site primary closure. The longest measure is sketched according to the volume requested to restore the breast defect. The SAAP flap area can safely go up to 20×15 cm^2 in corpulent women, depending on the quantity of excess tissue on the lateral thoracic wall area.

6.3.2 Harvesting

The patient can be operated in a supine position with a bump or in a lateral decubitus position. The arm is abducted to 90°, and the elbow is also flexed to 90°. The primary incision is conducted at the posterior marking of the flap, and the subcutaneous tissue is dissected diagonally away from the flap till the border of the LD muscle. The edge of the LD muscle is then blandly raised to reveal the underlying fascia and SAM. Next, harvesting continues under loupes magnification on the gliding fascia over the SAM at the base of the surgical field towards the space where the perforator was beforehand detected with the handheld Doppler. The surgeon ought to be vigilant to distinguish and preserve the lateral thoracic nerve.

When the perforator is selected, the surgeon must evaluate if the vessel is reliable with a satisfactory calibre of a minimum of 0.5 mm and if it has a noticeable pulsation. At this point, the perforator can be isolated, and the flap's position, size, and shape are reviewed for adjustments. If two perforators are found next to each other, both can be isolated and incorporated within the flap. Then, the harvesting goes through the muscle's fascia, following the perforator towards its connection to the serratus anterior vascular branches. The SAAP lies over the SAM, shielded by its fascia. In case of an incompetent perforator is found, the surgical planning can be altered to a lateral intercostal artery perforator (LICAP), TDAP, or muscle-sparing LD flaps.

6.3.3 Transference

After the flap is harvested, the surgeon shall move the flap to the defect area. The manner is directly related to the breast defect's volume, shape, and location. The most used technique is the propeller, which is indicated for flaps with transversal or diagonal orientation. The flap can be safely rotated up to 180° and placed at its ultimate position. With this technique, the surgeon can preserve the intercostal connection to the SAAP, which confers a better blood supply to the flap. The downside of the propeller technique in this area is that the anterior border of the flap is at the lateral limit of the breast defect, and when the skin patch from the SAAP is stored in position, part of the flap still lies out of the breast footprint.

The second alternative is the conventional harvesting of the serratus anterior arterial branch and the complete release of the flap. This technique is mainly indicated to flaps with a vertical orientation. The flap can be moved directly to its final position on the breast since the anterior border of the flap is the lateral breast footprint. With the conventional technique, the interconnection between serratus anterior vessels and the intercostal perforator is clipped, granting the flap greater flexibility for the anatomical reconstruction of the affected area.

A third option is a flip over technique used for volume replacement without the need for the skin. These flaps are easier to harvest since the perforator may not be entirely skeletonised. The flap is de-epithelised and inserted directly into the breast deformity. This option is ideal for small to moderate lesions located right on the edge of the lateral breast footprint.

After the flap is safely moved into the breast defect and stabilised, drains are placed at the donor site, and then the wound is closed with three lines of suture. Afterwards, the patient is rotated to a fully supine position, and the flap is reviewed in its final place for refinements (Fig. 6.3).

Tips

- A SAAP flap can reach from 6 to 9 cm of pedicle length, giving it a good arch of rotation well towards the breast. As mentioned, the interconnection between the intercostal and the serratus anterior vessels can be clipped, and the SAAP flap would reach the inner parts of the breast area. In such cases, the serratus anterior pedicle can be dissected up to the thoracodorsal vessels, extending the length of the flap pedicle. The dissection is commonly performed, sparing the associated nerve. The thoracodorsal vessels can be released from the muscle with ligation of the main branches to combine length to the serratus anterior vessels. By preserving the LD muscle and its blood supply, one can still harvest a LD flap, if demanded, in the future.
- The connection grants a reliable blood supply to the SAAP flap. However, this connection diminishes the extension of the flap to fulfil central and medial breast defects. In addition, dissection of the intercostal perforator through the serratus anterior and intercostal muscles up to the exit from the costal notch provide an additional 3–4 cm of pedicle length to the LICAP flap. This harvesting is used when the surgeon plan to insert the flap in the breast defect using the propeller technique.

Pitfalls

- Despite the SAAP flap presenting several advantages, such as reliable vascularity and high-volume availability, it is not a simplistic dissection. From a technical point of view, adequate experience in dissecting perforators and the use of magnifying loupes are almost always required. For instance, the dissection of the intercostal perforator through the serratus anterior and intercostal muscles up to the exit from the costal notch provides an additional 3–4 cm of pedicle length. However, there is a considerable risk of pneumothorax.
- The surgeon must also be cautious with the lateral thoracic nerve, which confers function to the SAM. If the nerve is damaged, the patient will have a permanent dysfunctional arm movement termed the winged scapula.

After-Care

- The dressing is placed over the flap without pressure. Then, the perforator status is tested with an 8 MHz hand-held Doppler instantly after the surgery and repeated twice a day till the patient is discharged from the hospital. The patient recovers directly at the regular plastic surgery ward, with dedicated nurses that follow pre-established protocol.
- If a blood supply impairment is identified within the first 24 h after the surgery, the first treatment alternative is a take-back review in the operating theatre. Customarily, the flap's inadequate arterial and venous supply is resolved after the suture near the pedicle is released. Finally, the operation wound is closed without pressure on the pedicle, and the patient returns to a regular ward.

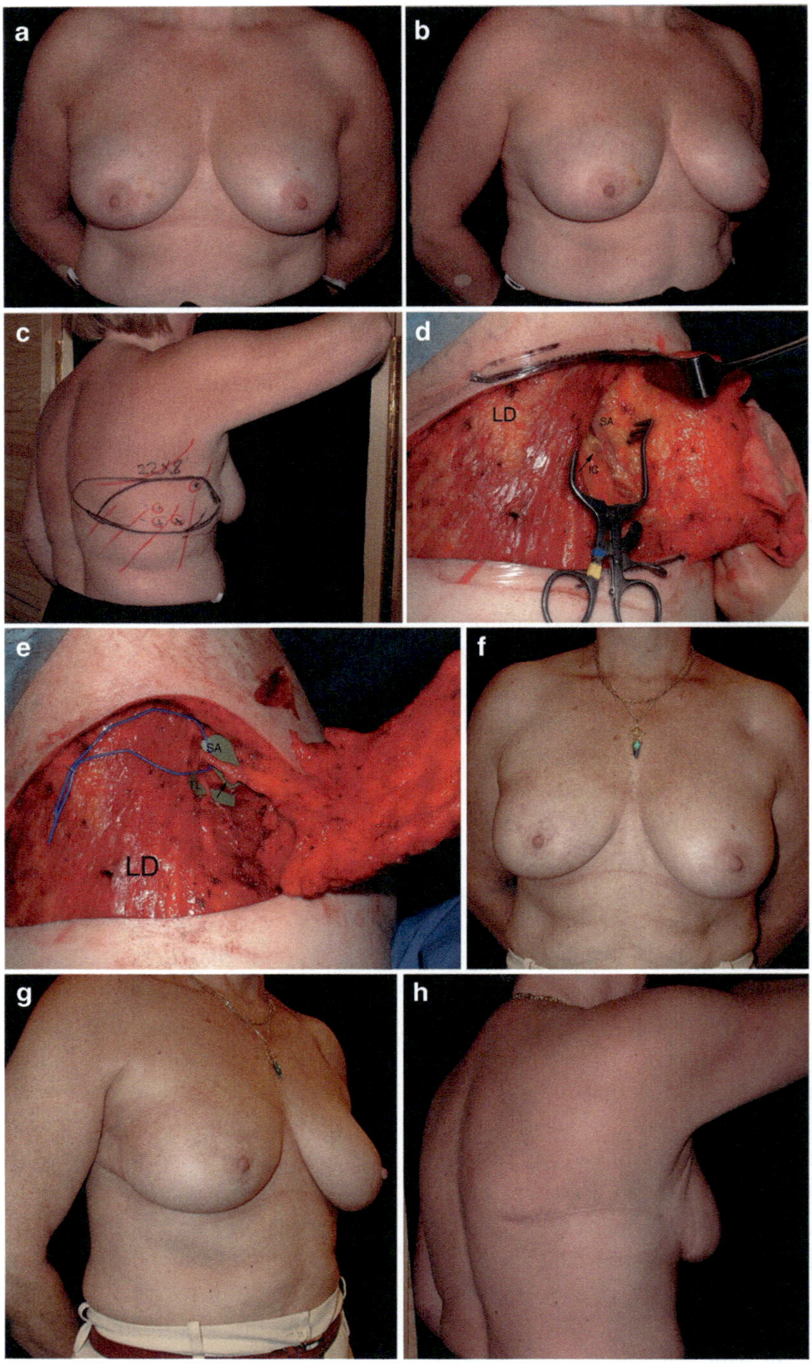

Fig. 6.3 (**a**) Preoperatory anterior view. (**b**) Oblique right-side view. (**c**) Oblique posterior view of the right side. A large flap of 22 × 8 cm^2 marked with a horizontal shape containing the identified hot spots of the perforators, which were identified with a handheld Doppler device. The overview demonstrates the marking for a possible TDAP, LICAP, or SAAP flap. (**d**) The illustration outlines the presence of the interconnection between the serratus anterior vessel (SA) and the intercostal perforator (IC), right anteriorly to the latissimus dorsi muscle (LD). (**e**) The communication between the SA and IC was clipped (arrow) to increase the flap range. (**f**) Anterior view presents an excellent cosmetic result. There is still a volume asymmetry between breasts which can be corrected with fat grafting of contralateral breast reduction. (**g**) Oblique right side view. (**h**) Oblique posterior right side view. A horizontal scar of the SAAP flap is positioned on the bra line

6.4 Conclusions

The area where the SAAP lies may also be part of several perforator flaps. The surgeon shall define the best technique to perform partial breast reconstruction, preserving the breast mound and symmetry. In some cases, the desired good or excellent final cosmetic result is not feasible with one procedure. Often patients require a contralateral breast reduction. It is mandatory to wait for the patient to be submitted to radiotherapy before final refinements can be safely performed. Therefore, every case must be reviewed and discussed between surgeon and patient to arrange an adequate second procedure for minor adjustments.

Fat grafting is a valuable tool in immediate and delayed settings. The use of fat grafting has been reported for other chest wall perforator flaps but not for SAAP flaps. However, it is common sense that a fat graft is an avascular tissue that requires a reliable nourished bed to survive. Therefore, possibly only a limited volume can be inserted. On the other hand, fat grafting can be used for delayed refinements of the breast contour and volume. Fat grafting also can improve the actinic effects on the skin [11].

6.5 Clinical Application

Case 1
A 65-year-old patient with a breast cancer diagnosis on the lateral quadrants of the right breast underwent partial breast reconstruction with a SAAP flap.

References

1. Pittet B, Mahajan AL, Alizadeh N, Schlaudraff KU, Fasel J, Montandon D. The free serratus anterior flap and its cutaneous component for reconstruction of the face: a series of 27 cases. Plast Reconstr Surg. 2006;117(4):1277–88. https://doi.org/10.1097/01.prs.0000208297.02556.a5.
2. Hamdi M, Spano A, Landuyt KV, D'Herde K, Blondeel P, Monstrey S. The lateral intercostal artery perforators: anatomical study and clinical application in breast surgery. Plast Reconstr Surg. 2008;121(2):389–96. https://doi.org/10.1097/01.prs.0000298317.65296.cf.
3. Tamburino S, Menez T, Laloze J, Michot A, Paillet P, Perrotta RE, Casoli V. Free serratus anterior artery perforator flap: a case report with an anatomic and radiological study. Surg Radiol Anat. 2017;39(8):837–42. https://doi.org/10.1007/s00276-017-1824-0.
4. Losken A, Hamdi M. Partial breast reconstruction: current perspectives. Plast Reconstr Surg. 2009;124(3):722–36. https://doi.org/10.1097/PRS.0b013e3181b179d2.
5. Soumian S, Parmeshwar R, Chandarana M, Marla S, Narayanan S, Shetty G. Chest wall perforator flaps for partial breast reconstruction: surgical outcomes from a multicenter study. Arch Plast Surg. 2020;47(2):153–9. https://doi.org/10.5999/aps.2019.01186.
6. Mecham E, Park J, Phillips L. TAP, LICAP, SAAP, and AICAP flaps. In: Klimberg V, Kovacs T, Rubio I, editors. Oncoplastic breast surgery techniques for the general surgeon. Cham: Springer; 2020. https://doi.org/10.1007/978-3-030-40196-2_29.
7. Nahabedian MY, Patel K. Autologous flap breast reconstruction: surgical algorithm and patient selection. J Surg Oncol. 2016;113(8):865–74. https://doi.org/10.1002/jso.24208.
8. Hamdi M, De Frene B. Pedicled perforator flaps in breast reconstruction. Semin Plast Surg. 2006;20(2):073–8. https://doi.org/10.1055/s-2006-941713.
9. Hamdi M. Oncoplastic and reconstructive surgery of the breast. Breast. 2013;22(Suppl 2):S100–5. https://doi.org/10.1016/j.breast.2013.07.019.
10. Quinn EM, O'Ceallaigh S, Highton L, Murphy J. The use of local perforator flaps in delayed or secondary breast reconstruction. Plast Reconstr Surg Glob Open. 2020;8(12):e3263. https://doi.org/10.1097/GOX.0000000000003263.
11. Gentilucci M, Mazzocchi M, Alfano C. Effects of prophylactic lipofilling after radiotherapy compared to non-fat injected breasts: a randomised, objective study. Aesthet Surg J. 2020;40(10):NP597–607. https://doi.org/10.1093/asj/sjaa182.

Lateral Thoracic Artery Perforator (LTAP) Flap

7

Amit Agrawal

Contents

7.1 Background

Oncoplastic surgery has expanded the remit of breast conserving surgery. For comparable size tumour, in larger breasts, displacement techniques are possible whilst in smaller breasts, replacement techniques [1, 2]. Replacement techniques include LD miniflap [3, 4] and chest wall perforator flap (CWPF). LD miniflap uses a strip of LD muscle based on LD pedicle and is rotated into the tumour defect. CWPF is based on small perforating vessels that perforate the muscle or fascia to supply the subcutaneous fat. This muscle-free fat pad is then harvested based on perforating vessels to design a flap that is then rotated or flipped into the tumour defect with no associated muscle-related morbidity.

There are multiple CWPF options that include well established lateral intercostal artery (LiCAP) [5] and thoracodorsal (TDAP) artery flaps [6]. Lateral thoracic artery perforator (LTAP) flap is a relatively recent innovation. This flap was initially used in head and neck surgery and other body sites as free flaps [7]. Later use extended to correcting defects following breast conserving surgery, BCS [8]. The major advantages of a CWPF based replacement procedure are low evident rates of complications (<2% flap loss) and extremely low need for symmetrising surgery (<2%) as noted in the world's largest multicentre study [9].

A. Agrawal (✉)
Oncoplastic Breast Surgery, Cambridge University Hospitals, Cambridge, UK
e-mail: amitagrawal@doctors.org.uk

M. Hamdi et al. (eds.), *Pedicled Flaps in Partial Breast Reconstruction*,
https://doi.org/10.1007/978-3-031-08483-6_7

7.2 Anatomy

It is based on perforators arising from the superficial longitudinal branch of the LTA that arises from axillary artery though a variable origin can be from subscapular or thoracodorsal artery [10]. It has been noted to be absent in 15–18% subjects. An accessory LTA may arise with similar origins and may be used for similar design flaps.

LTA runs longitudinally anteriorly to TDA; the proximal course (3–4 cm) lies posterior to the lateral edge of the pectoralis muscle whilst the distal course lies on the serratus anterior muscle (Fig. 7.1). Perforators arising from LTA lie at the level of the third to fifth intercostal spaces, best at third or fourth intercostal spaces and hence often a flap designed in the proximity can include LiCAP vessels increasing the perfusion robustness of the flap [8].

Koshima's group [11] studied the intricate anatomy of the LTA perforators in 27 patients and elaborated type and incidence of the following branches of the LTA:

- superficial branch, 48.1% (diameter—0.79 mm);
- medial branch, 14.8% (diameter—0.63 mm);
- deep branch, 81.5% (diameter—0.97 mm).

Although these branches are vital for assured vascularity of the flap, for practical purposes, a sensible approach to the preservation of the main trunk and delicate handling of the vascular supply suffices for oft-used horizontally oriented flaps along or parallel to bra-strap, 90 degrees to the main LTAP pedicle.

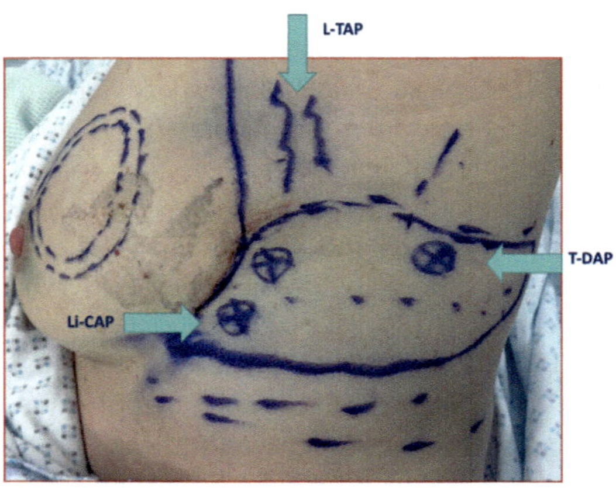

Fig. 7.1 Skin marking for LTAP flap and adjacent LiCAP and TDAP perforators with a flap design

7.3 Patient Selection

Assessment and planning for oncoplastic surgery is a complex process considering multiple factors [1]. Ideal patient factors include no previous surgery, no or minimal co-morbidity, non-smoker, regular physical work, or leisure activity. The average age is noted to be between 50 and 60 in most series with a body-mass index of around 25 [9, 12]. Since the LTAP flap is a pedicled flap, although smoking or diabetes may not be absolute contraindications, they are best avoided during early practice.

In general, relatively smaller breasts with a bra cup size of less than D cup with tumour located in the outer half of the breast and intended resection of less than a third volume of the breast are best suited. Extended indication may be for upper or lower inner tumours (Fig. 7.2) since the pedicle is long though TDAP is a more robust alternative. The key advantage of LTAP over TDAP is the obvious preservation of LD pedicle with preservation of muscle function. In addition, for any future recurrence that necessitates mastectomy (since radiotherapy following breast conserving surgery can be given only once), LD flap as an autologous-based option is not lost for full breast reconstruction.

7.4 Technique

New starters or early experience surgeons may wish to identify perforators before the date of surgery in the clinic; however, with experience, these perforators could be marked alongside flap on the day of surgery (Fig. 7.1). Design of the flap may not be different to the two other lower intercostal perforators, however, if a more medial reach needs to be achieved, given the length of the LTA, the flap may be designed away from the breast closer to LD flap territory. However, the size of the flap also depends on the laxity of the lateral chest wall skin.

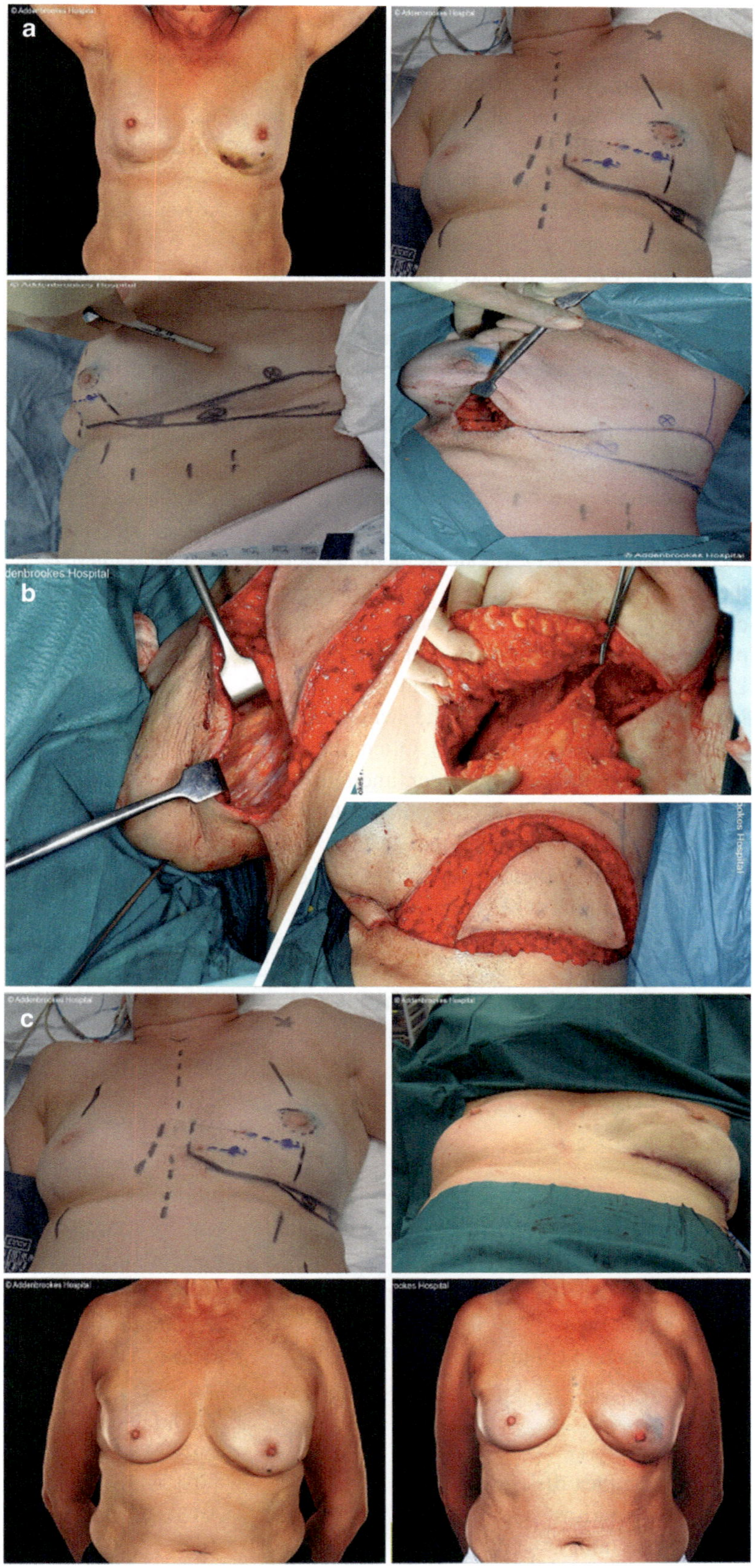

Fig. 7.2 Operative steps in an example of LTAP based partial breast reconstruction. (**a**) Pre-operative marking and intra-operative photo of 1st stage surgery (wide local excision). (**b**) 2nd stage showing WLE cavity, LTAP pedicle and dissected flap. (**c**) Pre-operative and post-operative photographs in supine and standing positions [1]

On the operating table, the patient can be positioned either in lateral (lying on the non-operating side) or supine with the ipsilateral side lifted either with a sandbag or an inflatable bag/cuff and the arm flexed towards the contralateral side across the patient's face supported by an L-bar or similar arm support. This is best decided with the patient on the operating table whilst awake since it depends on the length of the flap i.e., the distance of the distal end of the flap away from the perforators. Also, then it helps prevent hyper-abduction or over rotation of the shoulder to pre-empt post-operative shoulder joint issues or brachial plexopathy.

The LTA can be identified on pre-operative hand-held doppler (8Hz frequency suffices) closer to the breast border in the axillary space between the breast border and anterior border of the LD flap (Fig. 7.1). It can be identified along the superior edge of the flap lying deeper and closer to the chest wall. After that, dissection can proceed superiorly aiming to achieve a length of LTA that would allow the movement of the flap into the defect i.e., the longer the swing the more cranial the dissection (Fig. 7.2). Often, the sentinel note is identified within a centimetre of LTA at appropriate level assisted further with a dye technique. It should be noted that absolute skeletonization of the pedicle is unnecessary; a sheath of fascia helps minimise venous injury.

7.5 Comparison with Other Perforators

7.5.1 LTAP Vs. LiCAP

Advantages

- narrow pedicle so more flexible with paddle placement,
- propeller flap thus useful beyond the lateral half of the breast,
- can be used in conjunction with LiCAP.

Disadvantages

- more complex dissection,
- a flimsy narrow vessel at high risk of intra-operative injury,
- at increased risk during axillary node clearance.

7.5.2 LTAP Vs TDAP

Advantages

- less complex with no intra-muscular dissection,
- preserves LD pedicle so less donor site morbidity,
- narrower pedicle so more flexible with paddle replacement.

Disadvantages

- a flimsy narrow vessel at high risk of damage,
- at increased risk during axillary node clearance.

7.6 Outcomes

Oncologically, CWPF including LTAP enables higher tumour margin clearance rates regardless of tumour margin policy as shown in a study comparing 0- 1- and 2-mm margin widths [13]. Regardless of immediate surgical oncology outcomes, it could be extrapolated that recurrence rates will be non-inferior for each tumour stage when compared with non-CWPF surgery since the oncological principles remain the same.

Surgically, large series on LTAP-based PBR are lacking. However, two larger datasets in CWPF have been reported recently. A systematic review [14] including 432 patients revealed an overall complication rate of 9.25% and donor site morbidity of 3.7%. A more recent large UK multicentre dataset [9] of 504 patients across 15 centres revealed low rates of complications: major (3.4%) and minor (14.3%). Major complications were defined by those that needed to return to theatre. The flap loss rate was noted to be 0.8% (full—1, partial—3), haematoma (9%), seroma (4%), fat necrosis (3%) and delayed wound healing (3%). LTAP-only PBR was performed in 4.4% whilst combined with LiCAP (19.9%) and AiCAP, Anterior intercostal artery perforator flap (0.2%). A single stage when the confidence of achieving clear tumour margins is high was performed in 72.7% whilst two stages flap was performed in 25.7%, especially when there was the presence of DCIS or invasive lobular cancer with higher odds of positive margins. Overall, the re-excision of margins was less than 15% and mastectomy was less than 2% in the UK series.

7.7 Conclusions

LTAP flap adds to the repertoire of CWPF based PBR that include LiCAP and TDAP flaps. It allows for more flexibility and the length permits greater reach within the breast than LiCAP and is less complex in dissection than TDAP flap.

Ethical Statement Funding: No funding was provided by any source for this chapter.

Conflict of interest: There is no actual or potential conflict of interest in relation to this article. The author has no financial or personal relationship with other people or organisations that could inappropriately influence (bias) this work.

References

1. Agrawal A. Assessment and planning for oncoplastic and reconstructive breast surgery: a review and a proposed chart. Eur J Plast Surg. 2016;39(5):321. https://doi.org/10.1007/s00238-016-1221-7.
2. Clough KB, Lewis JS, Couturaud B, Fitoussi A, Nos C, Falcou MC. Oncoplastic techniques allow extensive resections for breast-conserving therapy of breast carcinomas. Ann Surg. 2003;237(1):26–34. https://doi.org/10.1097/01.SLA.0000041230.77663.22.
3. Navin C, Agrawal A, Kolar KM. The use of latissimus dorsi miniflap for reconstruction following breast-conserving surgery: experience of a small breast unit in a district hospital. World J Surg. 2007;31(1):46–50. https://doi.org/10.1007/s00268-006-0396-7.
4. Rainsbury RM. Breast-sparing reconstruction with latissimus dorsi miniflaps. Eur J Surg Oncol. 2002;28(8):891–5.
5. Hamdi M, Spano A, Van Landuyt K, D'Herde K, Blondeel P, Monstrey S. The lateral intercostal artery perforators: anatomical study and clinical application in breast surgery. Plast Reconstr Surg. 2008;121(2):389–96. https://doi.org/10.1097/01.prs.0000298317.65296.cf.
6. Holmström H, Lossing C. The lateral thoracodorsal flap in breast reconstruction. Plast Reconstr Surg. 1986;77(6):933–43. https://doi.org/10.1097/00006534-198606000-00010.
7. Kim JT, Ng SW, Naidu S, Kim JD, Kim YH. Lateral thoracic perforator flap: additional perforator flap option from the lateral thoracic region. J Plast Reconstr Aesthet Surg. 2011;64(12):1596–602. https://doi.org/10.1016/j.bjps.2011.06.048.
8. McCulley SJ, Schaverien MV, Tan VK, Macmillan RD. Lateral thoracic artery perforator (LTAP) flap in partial breast reconstruction. J Plast Reconstr Aesthet Surg. 2015;68(5):686–91. https://doi.org/10.1016/j.bjps.2015.01.008.
9. Agrawal A, Romics L, Thekkinkattil D, Kaushik M, Mortimer C, Courtney C-A, Goyal A, Garreffa E, Carmichael A, Hamad A, Lane R, Blackhall V, Rutherford C, Pitsinis V, Goh S, Ray B, Grover K, Mansell J, Vidya R, Murphy J. Partial breast reconstruction with chest wall perforator flaps - initial data from 'partbrerecon' collaborative. Eur J Surg Oncol. 2021;47:293. https://doi.org/10.1016/j.ejso.2021.03.220.
10. Harii K, Torii S, Sekiguchi J. The free lateral thoracic flap. Plast Reconstr Surg. 1978;62(2):212–22. https://doi.org/10.1097/00006534-197808000-00009.
11. Tashiro K, Harima M, Mito D, Shibata T, Furuya M, Kato M, Yamamoto T, Yamashita S, Narushima M, Iida T, Koshima I. Preoperative color Doppler ultrasound assessment of the lateral thoracic artery perforator flap and its branching pattern. J Plast Reconstr Aesthet Surg. 2015;68(6):120–5. https://doi.org/10.1016/j.bjps.2015.02.011.
12. Mangialardi ML, Baldelli I, Salgarello M, Raposio E. Breast reconstruction using the lateral thoracic, thoracodorsal, and intercostal arteries perforator flaps. Plast Reconstr Surg Glob Open. 2021;9(1):e3334. https://doi.org/10.1097/GOX.0000000000003334.
13. Bali R, Kankam HKN, Borkar N, Provenzano E, Agrawal A. Wide local excision versus oncoplastic breast surgery: differences in surgical outcome for an assumed margin (0, 1, or 2 mm) distance. Clin Breast Cancer. 2018;18(5):1053–7. https://doi.org/10.1016/j.clbc.2018.06.004.
14. Mangialardi ML, Baldelli I, Salgarello M, Raposio E. Thoracodorsal artery perforator flap in partial breast reconstruction: a systematic review. Plast Reconstr Surg Glob Open. 2020;8(10):e3104. https://doi.org/10.1097/GOX.0000000000003104.

Extended Thoracodorsal Artery Perforator (TDAP) Flap

8

Claudio Angrigiani and Guillermo Artero

Contents

8.1 Anatomy

The TDAP flap is irrigated by the proximal perforator of the descending branch of the thoracodorsal artery [1–5]. This branch is consistently present, according to several anatomical studies [6–8]. Therefore, the superior (scapular) and inferior (lumbar) fat compartments can be partially captured and irrigated by this proximal muscle perforator in the same manner as in the extended latissimus dorsi (LD) flap [9] when the additional volume is needed without the muscle. In our experience, the most common anatomical finding is shown in Fig. 8.1.

8.2 Applications

TDAP flaps are indicated for: (a) primary or additional volume for breast reconstruction; (b) salvage procedure for exposed implants; (c) primary surface (envelop) reconstruction; and combined implant autologous tissue reconstruction and d) additional surface in insufficient expanded reconstructions. Decision making process between conventional LD flap and TDAP should be done before designing the flap (and especially the skin island). The LD flap involves muscle

C. Angrigiani (✉)
Oncoplastic Surgery Program, University of Buenos Aires, Buenos Aires, Argentina

G. Artero
Microsurgery Unit, Trinidad and Anchorena Clinics, Buenos Aires, Argentina

M. Hamdi et al. (eds.), *Pedicled Flaps in Partial Breast Reconstruction*,
https://doi.org/10.1007/978-3-031-08483-6_8

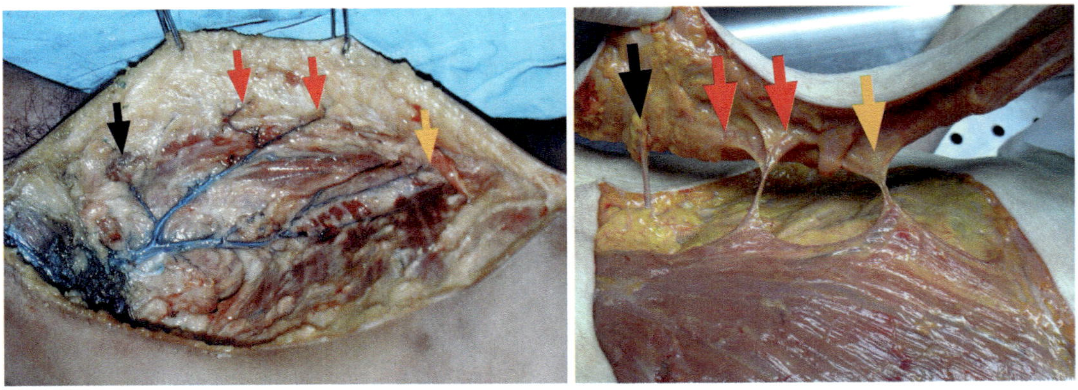

Fig. 8.1 Left side frontal view of an anatomical specimen injected with a coloured latex (dark green). The anterior lateral border of the LD muscle is observed. Some fibres of the edge have been resected to monitor the distribution of the descending branch of the thoracodorsal artery (TDA) inside the muscle. The black arrow indicates the most proximal branch of the TDA, which is frequently a direct branch of the trunk of the TDA. Before it divides into its two branches in horizontal and vertical. The red arrows indicate the proximal branch, which divides into two branches but, when it is dissected inside the muscle, they blend into one main branch. This is the pedicle of the TDAP. The yellow arrow indicates the distal perforator of the descending branch

harvesting, is easier to perform, and requires a shorter operating time. The TDAP flap involves a more complex technique but preserves the muscle and is associated with less seroma in the donor area. Skin island design in TDAP flaps must include the piercing point of the proximal perforator of the thoracodorsal artery vertical branch which is the main vascular source. Contrarily, skin island can be designed almost in any place over the muscle in conventional LD musculocutaneous flap

8.3 Steps

8.3.1 Planning

The first step for TDAP flap design is verification of active LD muscle contraction by voluntary adduction shoulder movement by the patient against resistance. The absence of this noticeable contraction in mastectomy sequelae cases is real evidence of nerve lesion which is most frequently associated with lesion of the muscle vascular pedicle. In this case TDAP flap procedure is contraindicated

A point "X" is marked on the anterolateral muscle line, 8 cm below the axillary fold and 2 cm lateral to that line . This point represents the most probable location of the first (or most proximal) skin perforator of the vertical branch of the thoracodorsal. A direct cutaneous branch from the descending branch of the thoracodorsal artery around the anterior border of the LD muscle is observed in 20% approximately. Thus, the design of the flap must exceed the edge of the muscle to assure the presence of this branch in the raised flap. A vascular Doppler is then applied for the accurate detection of the piercing point. If any doubt, ultrasound colour Doppler is definitive for perforator location.

The flap length reaches 22–23 cm approximately in a normal adult patient. Absolut dimensions may vary according to different sizes of thoracic cage. Clinical criterium is important for evaluation of flap vitality, especially the distal part. However, the possibility of evaluating flap viability intraoperatively with indocyanine green angiography is mandatory to discard underperfused tissue.

The longitudinal axis of the flap can be placed in any direction (Fig. 8.2). In the cases of breast reconstruction, the TDAP is used as an island, and the axis is directed towards the back. An ascending curved flap gives a better final scar of the donor area, as Hammond described for the latissimus dorsi flap [10]. Flap dimension is directly related to the perforator diameter and the

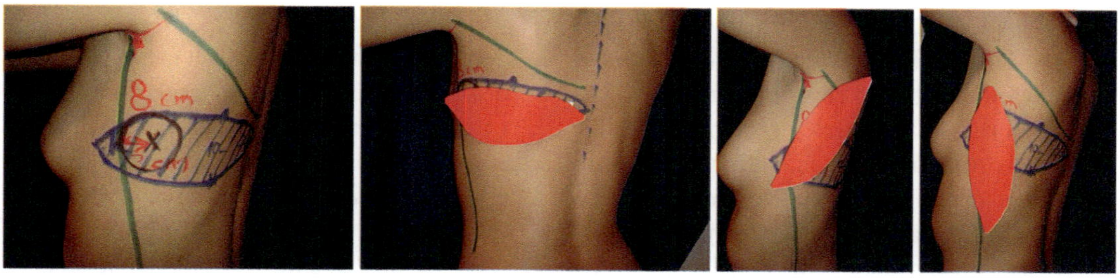

Fig. 8.2 Extended TDAP flap design. The X indicates where it is located, approximately the proximal branch of the descending branch of the TDAP. There are different possibilities for placement of the longitudinal axis of the TDAP

subcutaneous vascular network status. This network might be compromised in tobacco smokers, diabetes, vascular diseases, etc. The flap width is designed according to the possibility of direct closing of the donor site evaluated by pinch test. It is preferable to achieve a direct closure than skin grafting the donor area for patient satisfaction even if the surgeon would be benefited by a larger flap.

8.3.2 Harvesting

The patient is placed in lateral decubitus opposite to the flap side. The arm is draped free.

We elevate the flap from distal to proximal. Several authors reported the convenience of perforator location initially. However, this approach is unnecessary because once Doppler locates the proximal perforator, there is no doubt about its presence. The distal approach is more convenient, faster and equally safe. We dissected the deep fascia with low power cautery. Bipolar is used while the perforator area is approached. It is of utmost importance to have good anaesthesia to observe perforator vessels pulsating.

Once the perforator is visualized, a decision is made about how the procedure is continued according to these possibilities: 1—propeller type flap; 2—muscle-sparing; 3—flip over; 4—conventional TDAP.

1. Propeller: Once the perforator is observed there is no need for further dissection. The flap is rotated 180° to the breast mound area The procedure is quick and straightforward. A special dissection technique is not required. The main disadvantage is its shorter length compared to a complete intramuscular dissection A substantial portion of the flap remains in the subaxillary area, where it is not necessary for breast reconstruction while the medial portion of the breast does not receive adequate volume [11]. It is not advisable to harvest a longer flap for resolving this inconvenient because most probably distal tissue suffering and necrosis might occur. In cases of mastectomy sequelae, the scar is released and resulting gap is covered with the flap with a final continuous scar with the donor area.
2. In immediate reconstructions, when performing skin-sparing mastectomy or when no scar at the breast side is present, the flap is de-epithelialized and tunnelled, remaining under the skin below the tunnel. Donor site closure is performed in two planes. A suction drain is placed and removed 48–72 h after surgery.
3. Muscle sparing: Muscle-sparing flap. The flap is raised from distal to proximal direction until the perforator area is located. The muscle containing the perforators is sectioned-muscle sparing technique [12, 13]; the flap can be turned over or rotated to the breast area. The disadvantage of this technique is that it damages the muscle innervation and has a reduced reaching point. It is used for partial volume deficit reconstruction on the lateral aspect of the breast.
4. Flip over. This manoeuvre was proposed several years ago. It is a variation of the muscle sparing technique. Once the lateral border of the latissimus dorsi the flap is de-epithelialized and turned over for volume reconstruction without dissecting a determined perforator.

5. Conventional TDAP flap. In this procedure, the perforator is dissected free from the muscle (following the classic "perforator flap technique"), LD muscle is completely preserved. Although this is a somewhat more cumbersome and complex procedure, it affords the greatest pedicle length because the thoracodorsal pedicle is dissected up to its origin. The flap reaches the thoracic anterior midline, allowing better flap in-setting and positioning of the fat volume. The main disadvantage of this method is the necessity for magnification and specialized instruments. The flap may be deepithelialized for volume replacement or used as a skin subcutaneous flap (Fig. 8.3).

8.3.3 Transference

In unilateral cases, the flap is transferred directly. When there is no scars in the lateral part of the breast, the flap is tunnelized with the section under the tunnel deepithelialized. If the mastectomy scar is located in the lateral part of the breast, it is continued with the flap donor site. In bilateral cases, the flap is left without final in-setting; the back wound is covered, and the patient is turned to dorsal decubitus position, at which time the anterior area is prepared again.

Tips

The best way to evaluate the necessary volume to be replaces is to weigh or measure the resected tissue. Care must be taken not to underestimate the necessary volume in secondary or delayed reconstruction. Intraoperative evaluation after releasing the retractive scar is the best way to evaluate the actual volume deficit as well as a surface defect. Contralateral comparison, if possible, may provide a good approximation. We commonly use a wet gauze to fullfil the volume defect until simmetrization with the contralateral breast is obtained. By doing this maneouvre, we get a better and faster evaluation of the necessary volume (Fig. 8.4).

When an "extended TDAP" is planned, the subcutaneous tissues superior and inferior to the skin incision are harvested for obtaining a larger volume and a scaffold for lipofilling which is essential in lean patients [14]. Flap volume may be initially augmented by lipotransference or as a delay procedure. We usually add 150 cc.

Pitfalls

Careful evaluation of the distal part of the flap is of utmost importance to avoid steatonecrosis and distal tissue suffering which are the most common complications. Red active bleeding of the skin edges is a good tool. Indocyanine green test may be the best evaluating weapon whenever is possible to use. Medial breast volume reconstruction requires a conventional thoracodorsal perforator flap with complete dissection of the pedicle to reach the midline with well-irrigated tissue.

After-Care

Common gauze dressings are applied without covering the flap for direct visual. The patient is recovered in a regular ward If there is any blood supply impairment identified during the first 24 h, patient is returned to the operating room for revision. If there is normal evolution, the patient leaves the hospital at 48 h after surgery.

8.4 Conclusions

The incorporation of the TDAP flap, a derivation of the perforator flap era and which was initially described as "the LD flap without muscle", permits harvesting of the same skin and subcutaneous tissue area customarily obtained with the conventional LD flap without the muscle, thereby avoiding the possible morbidities of this procedure. The incidence of seroma is almost none in regular TDAP; it is slightly higher in extended TDAP due to the necessary undermining of the donor area but lower than the LD flap. In addition, it is not associated with any impairment of shoulder motion. No aesthetic sequelae at the anterolateral border of the muscle on the lateral side are evident in normal-weight women.

The presence of the muscle might be considered necessary considering the necessity of volume for the reconstruction. However, the most voluminous part of the muscle remains under the axilla after transferring the flap to the anterior area. The muscle transferred to the breast mound is relatively thin, with minimal volume contribution. Therefore, TDAP is a good election for lateral defects of the breast. It can be transferred as a propeller in a pretty fast procedure without "microsurgical dissection" of the pedicle. Medial defects often require complete pedicle dissection in the conventional way of a perforator flap for maximal flap reaching.

8.5 Clinical Application

Case 1

A 46-year-old female with a severe sequela of quadrantectomy. A lateral riding nipple is observed. A contralateral view is used for an approximative preoperative assessment of the amount of coverage needed in the affected side. A propeller TDAP was used for defect coverage after complete scar release.

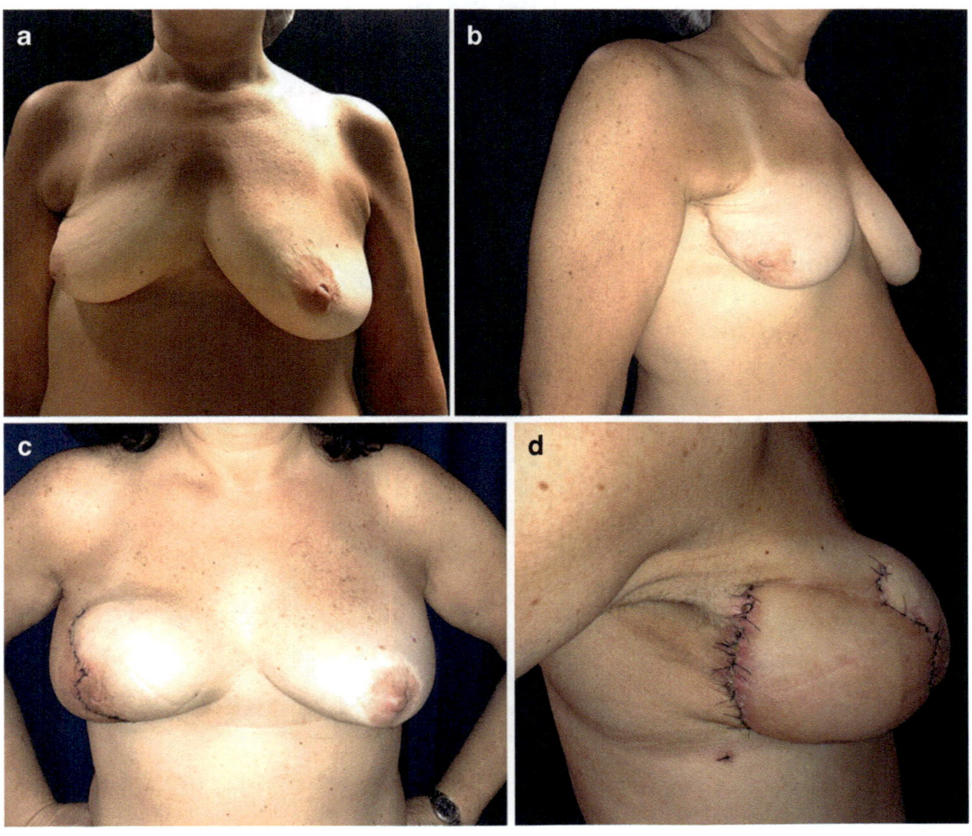

Fig. 8.3 (**a**, **b**) Laterally displaced nipple-areola complex after quadrantectomy. (**c**, **d**) Postoperative view after propeller TDAP flap

Case 2

A superolateral sequela of quadrantectomy plus radiotherapy in a 52-year-old female. Lateral high riding nipple produces disfigurement. Preoperative assessment of the actual defect is complex. First, the scar was released and the nipple was repositioned. Next, a wet gauze is placed in the defect until symmetry is obtained. Then the surface defect is evaluated as well as the volume defect.

An initial propeller TDAP was harvested, but it did not reach as medial as necessary. It can be observed that the flap does not reach the nipple area. The flap was converted into a conventional TDAP by complete dissection of the pedicle to get a more distal length. Then the flap could fulfil the medial part of the breast mound. The flap was partially de-epithelialized. The latissimus dorsi muscle was preserved entirely—the final result at two months postoperative. Radiotherapy defects usually are underestimated regarding the amount of volume to be repaired.

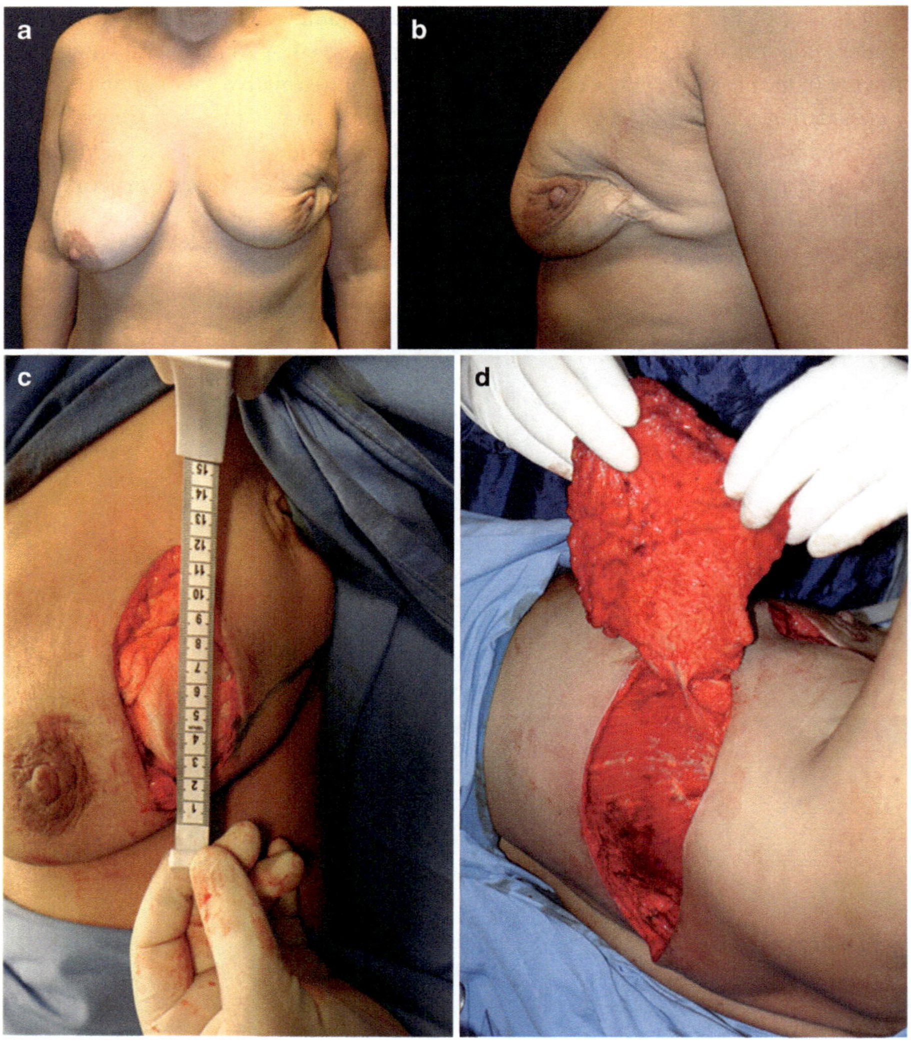

Fig. 8.4 (**a**, **b**) Lateral high riding nipple after quadrantectomy. (**c**) The scar was released and defect measured. The gauze gives an idea of the volume needed. (**d**, **e**) The TDAP flap is elevated as a propeller and transferred to the breast to see where it reaches. (**f**) The flap is "converted" in a "conventional" TDAP flap and is tunnelled under the anterior fibres of the LD muscle. (**g**, **h**) Postoperative view

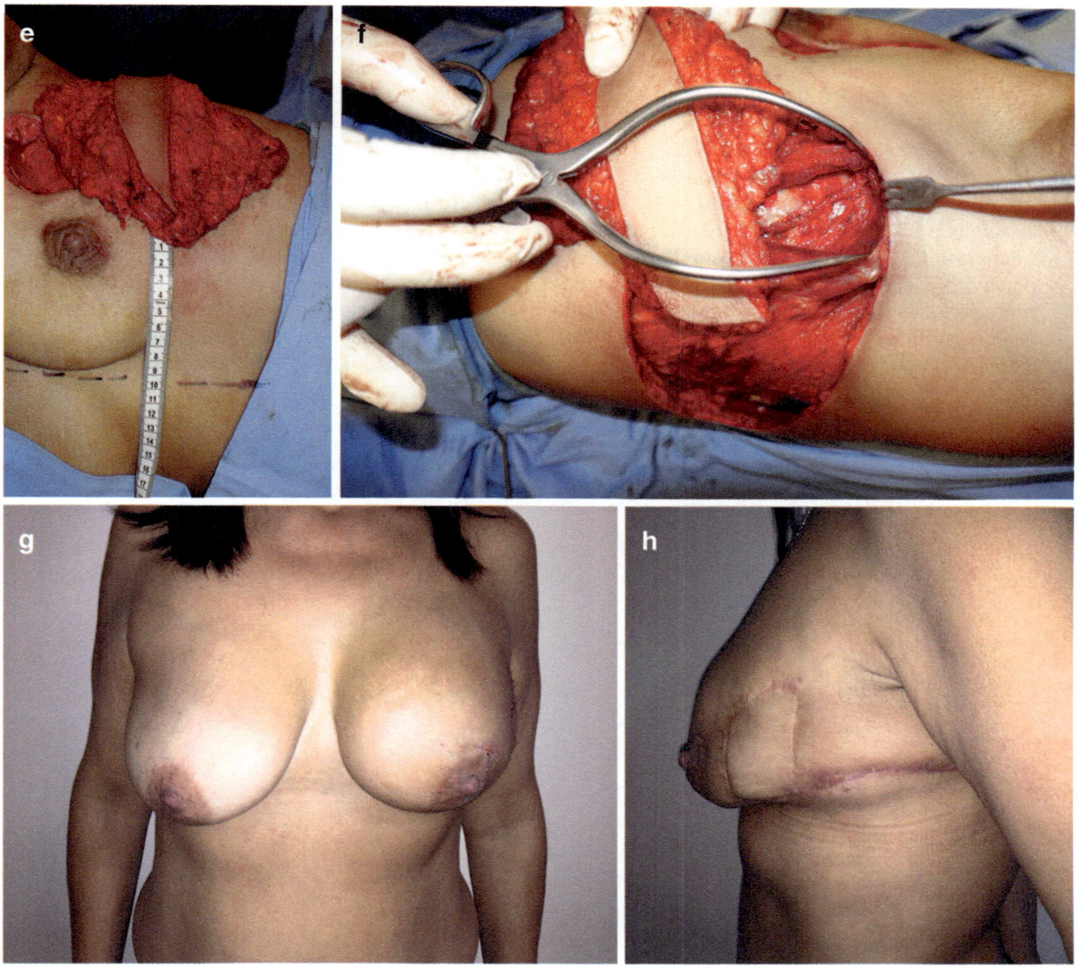

Fig. 8.4 (continued)

References

1. Angrigiani C, Grilli D, Siebert J. Latissimus dorsi musculocutaneous flap without muscle. Plast Reconstr Surg. 1995;96(7):1608–14. https://doi.org/10.1097/00006534-199512000-00014.
2. Hamdi M, Van Landuyt K, Monstrey S, Blondeel P. Pedicled perforator flaps in breast reconstruction: a new concept. Br J Plast Surg. 2004;57(6):531–9. https://doi.org/10.1016/j.bjps.2004.04.015.
3. Hamdi M, Salgarello M, Barone-Adesi L, Van Landuyt K. Use of the thoracodorsal artery perforator (TDAP) flap with implant in breast reconstruction. Ann Plast Surg. 2008;61(2):143–6. https://doi.org/10.1097/SAP.0b013e318158fd7b.
4. Schwabegger AH, Bodner G, Ninković M, Piza-Katzer H. Thoracodorsal artery perforator (TAP) flap: report of our experience and review of the literature. Br J Plast Surg. 2002;55(5):390–5. https://doi.org/10.1054/bjps.2002.3878.
5. Adler N, Seitz IA, Song DH. Pedicled thoracodorsal artery perforator flap in breast reconstruction: clinical experience. Eplasty. 2009;9:24.
6. Thomas BP, Geddes CR, Tang M, Williams J, Morris SF. The vascular basis of the thoracodorsal artery perforator flap. Plast Reconstr Surg. 2005;116(3):818–22. https://doi.org/10.1097/01.prs.0000176253.42394.7c.
7. Lin CT, Huang JS, Yang KC, Hsu KC, Chen JS, Chen LW. Reliability of anatomical landmarks for skin perforators of the thoracodorsal artery perforator flap. Plast Reconstr Surg. 2006;118(6):1376–86. https://doi.org/10.1097/01.prs.0000239525.44657.81.
8. Heitmann C, Guerra A, Metzinger SW, Levin LS, Allen RJ. The thoracodorsal artery perforator flap: anatomic basis and clinical application. Ann Plast

Surg. 2003;51(1):23–9. https://doi.org/10.1097/01.SAP.0000054189.14799.F3.
9. Germann G, Steinau HU. Breast reconstruction with the extended latissimus dorsi flap. Plast Reconstr Surg. 1996;97(3):519–26. https://doi.org/10.1097/00006534-199603000-00004.
10. Hammond DC. Latissimus dorsi flap breast reconstruction. Plast Reconstr Surg. 2009;124(4):1055–63. https://doi.org/10.1097/PRS.0b013e3181b6bf05.
11. Angrigiani C, Rancati A, Escudero E, Artero G, Gercovich G, Deza EG. Propeller thoracodorsal artery perforator flap for breast reconstruction. Gland Surg. 2014;3(3):174–80. https://doi.org/10.3978/j.issn.2227-684X.2014.06.04.
12. Saint-Cyr M, Nagarkar P, Schaverien M, Dauwe P, Wong C, Rohrich RJ. The pedicled descending branch muscle-sparing latissimus dorsi flap for breast reconstruction. Plast Reconstr Surg. 2009;123(1):13–24. https://doi.org/10.1097/PRS.0b013e3181934838.
13. Berry MG, Curnier A, Fitoussi AD, Couturaud B, Salmon RJ. The muscle-sparing latissimus dorsi flap for breast reconstruction. Plast Reconstr Surg. 2009;124(3):1000–1. https://doi.org/10.1097/PRS.0b013e3181b03940.
14. Coleman SR, Saboeiro AP. Fat grafting to the breast revisited: safety and efficacy. Plast Reconstr Surg. 2007;119(3):775–87. https://doi.org/10.1097/01.prs.0000252001.59162.c9.

Anterior Intercostal Artery Flap: AICAP FLAP

9

Cristian Carrasco Lopez and Raghavan Vidya

Contents

The first fascio-cutaneous flap was described by Badran and El-Helaly in 1984 followed by Hamdi in 2004 [1, 2]. Subsequently Hallock described the use of AICAP in 2009 [3]. Over the last decade the use of perforator flaps have gradually emerged as useful volume replacement technique in oncoplastic breast surgery [4].

Anterior intercostal artery flap is a versatile perforator local flap used in oncoplastic breast surgery. This flap extends from the inframammary crease superiorly to the costal margin inferiorly (depending on pinch test), to the midline medially and anterior axillary line laterally [5].

Supplementary Information The online version contains supplementary material available at [https://doi.org/10.1007/978-3-031-08483-6_9].

C. Carrasco Lopez (✉)
Department of Plastic Surgery, Germans Trias i Pujol Hospital, Badalona, Spain

Badalona, Spain
e-mail: ccarrasco.germanstrias@gencat.cat

R. Vidya
Department of Breast Surgery, The Royal Wolverhampton NHS Trust, Wolverhampton, UK
e-mail: Raghavan.Vidya@nhs.net

9.1 Anatomy

According to the anatomical study performed by Hamdi, LICAP is defined for perforators located between the latissimus dorsi and lateral pectoralis major muscles. For this reason, we defined the anterior intercostal perforator flap as those that are irrigated from perforators arising from the intercostal artery located between the anterior axillary line and the xyphoid process.

M. Hamdi et al. (eds.), *Pedicled Flaps in Partial Breast Reconstruction*,
https://doi.org/10.1007/978-3-031-08483-6_9

The blood supply is based on the anterior thoracic vessels such as intercostal or superior epigastric vessels. The superior epigastric artery (SEA) is a terminal branch of the internal mammary artery (musculophrenic artery being the other branch) and arises opposite the sixth costal cartilage. It then descends along the rectus abdominis muscle and penetrates the muscle and fascia below the xiphoid process to reach the skin. AICAP is mainly based on superficial epigastric artery perforators along the inferior aspect of the breast in the thoracoepigastric region. However, it can be modified to recruit lateral chest wall perforators.

Anatomic dissection reveals that the length of the perforator is usually about 3 cm and the diameter about 0.4 mm [3, 6]. The AICAP flap can vary in length between 9 and 14 cm depending on the length of the inframammary crease. The width of the flap varies between 3 and 5 cm depending on the patient body and can be confirmed on the pinch test or roll test.

For descriptive purposes, some divide the area of the chest wall beneath the inframammary fold (IMF) into three regions. A flap based on the internal segment called the internal AICAP (IAICAP) flap, based on the middle third the middle anterior ICAP (MAICAP) flap and based on the lateral third called the lateral anterior intercostal artery flap (LAICAP).

According to the recent anatomical publication [5], the mean distance (cm) of the intercostal perforators from the xiphoid process varied: internal (x, y: 2.57, 1.41), medial (x, y: 8.6, 0.82), and lateral (x, y: 13.37, −0.94) (Fig. 9.1). In all the dissected hemitrunk were found perforators for harvest AICAP flap.

Two or more perforators were found in the lateral, internal, and medial thirds in 30%, 6%, and 3%, respectively (Fig. 9.2). No dominant perforator was identified.

According to the anatomical study, the origin of the perforators was as follows: internal mammary (40%), intercostal artery (30%), and indeterminate (i.e., either internal mammary or intercostal artery) in the remaining 30% of cases because the origin is the connection of both arteries.

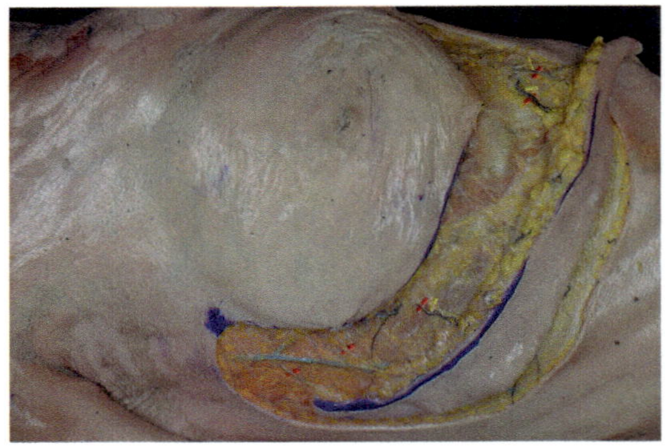

Fig. 9.1 Fresh hemitrunk with five perforators dissected (two internal, one medial, and two lateral). Vascular bundles are marked in red and nerves in yellow

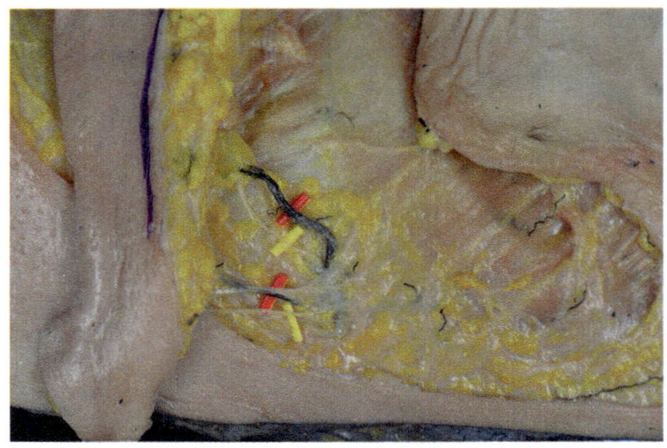

Fig. 9.2 Macroscopic focus over two vascular bundles (marked in red) and the nerves (in yellow)

9.2 Indications

- It can be used for defects in the inferior quadrant mainly, which could be infero medial, central, and lateral. Although not as usual in external quadrants (if you use AICAP based on lateral third perforators o MICAP) can be used as well.
- Immediate or delayed partial breast reconstruction following wide local excision or quadrantectomy [7].
- Salvage procedure after significant partial failure of free flap for breast reconstruction.
- Correction of congenital asymmetry.

9.3 Contraindications

- Previous radiotherapy to the breast can damage the perforators and hence need to be cautious [8].

Selection of Patients
The selection is mainly based on

- Patient choice,
- Estimated breast volume to be resected- excision volume of more than 20%,
- Tumour to breast ratio, and for any excision in the lower or external quadrant,
- The flap can be used in small to medium size breasts with or without ptosis. Now with the advancement of lipomodelling it can be used for large size breasts as the flap can act as scaffold and lipomodelling can be used to match the volume.

9.4 Planning and Preoperative Marking

Adequate preoperative planning is essential for the procedure. Preoperative clinical examination aided by radiological assessment is required. The tumour position, size (maximum dimension by imaging), and the amount of tissue that needs to be resected needs to be determined. Oncoplastic planning including skin marking or localisation of lesions is essential. Unifocal lesion can be marked using single wires and bracketing is essential for multi-focal lesions.

To flap is aligned horizontally along the inframammary crease and the scar is hidden by the submammary fold. To determine the amount of flap that can be harvested a pinch test or a roll test is a useful manoeuvre. This enables to assess the amount of skin and subcutaneous tissue that can be taken allowing adequate closure without tension. Hand held Doppler (8 Hz) can be used to assess the position of the perforator, ascertain surface marking and design the flap. Advanced imaging techniques such as Duplex and CT scan can be used to map the perforator anatomy in complex cases (Fig. 9.3).

Preoperative marking can be carried initially in the standing and then lying position. Patients need to stand straight with arms by their side. The limits of the breast are marked: midline, inframmary fold

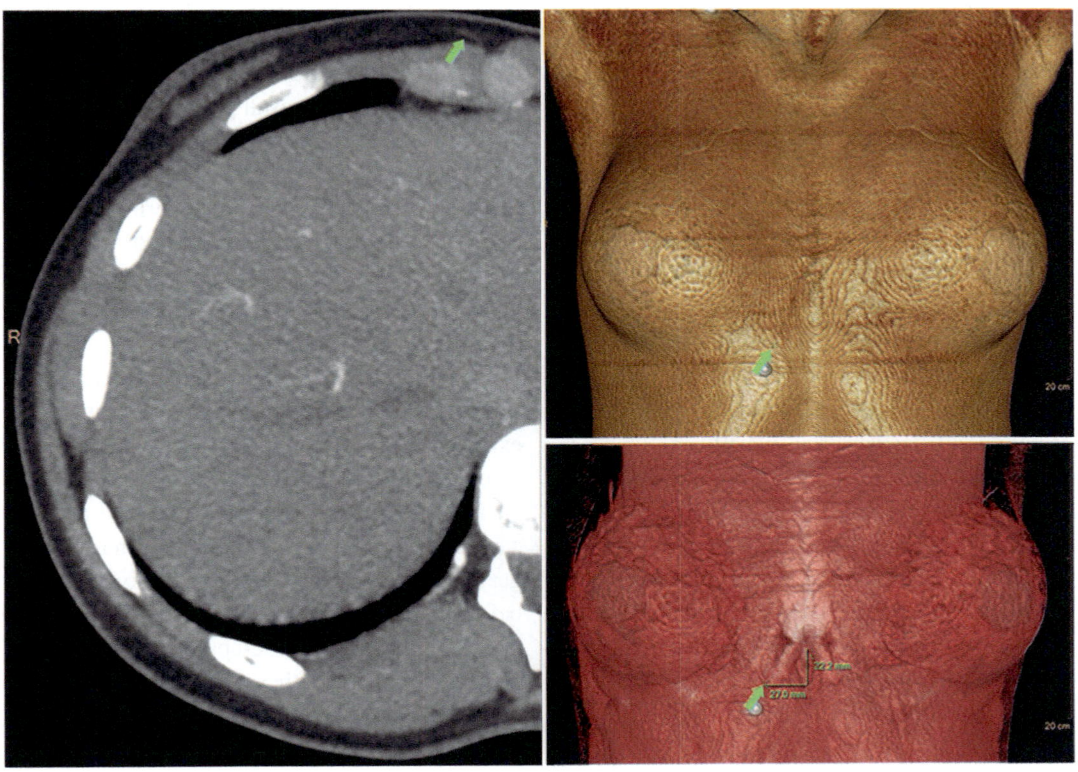

Fig. 9.3 Internal perforator (marked with green arrow) identified on CTA

and lateral extent. It is easier to mark the flap with the patient lying down as it enables to get a better visibility. The flap is marked with the base of the flap running horizontally along the inframammary fold extending from the medial aspect of the breast to the lateral fold. Usually, I recommend to mark and doing preoperative marking with the patient lying and with the arm in the same position which it will be during the surgery (for sentinel node biopsy).

The top of the ellipse can be determined by pinching the tissue below the inframammary fold so the tissue can be closed easily without undue tension. The incision can be adjusted according to the position of the most prominent perforator. Preoperatively the ability of the flap to cover the defect and reach the distance can be estimated while mapping and marking the perforator. In our experience the flap can be easily rotated around the pivot to reach the defect.

9.5 Intra Operative (Video 9.1)

Patient is usually supine and both arms are secured on an arm board. Both breasts are prepared and draped in an aseptic manner. Usually a single dose of antibiotic according to the local hospital policy is administered before incision. The preoperative marking needs to be checked using a pinch or roll test and ensure that the flap can be closed without undue tension. The hand held Doppler can be used to check the position of the perforators and to plan the surgery. It is important to ensure that the blood pressure (above 100 mmHg) is adequate to detect a Doppler signal.

The breast tumour is removed following the principles of oncosurgery (usually in our cases, we manage with the oncologic surgeon to use the inframammary incision to do the excision of the tumour and we remark to make the oblique incision to avoid the injure of perforators close to the inframammary fold). The dissection is carried out in the normal oncoplastic plane anteriorly, medially, and laterally, down to the pectoralis major muscle posteriorly preserving the pectoral fascia if possible. It is important that the dissection needs to adequate to ensure tumour free margin.

The breast specimen needs to be weighed and the weight noted. Intra operative specimen X-ray is routinely undertaken in most centres to determine the adequacy of margin resection. If needed further cavity shaves can be undertaken or bed biopsies carried out depending on the local practice. The breast cavity needs to be thoroughly washed with warm saline until clear. Clips needs are applied to the breast cavity according to the local protocol to facilitate radiotherapy planning at a later date.

The flap is then raised as an elliptical fasciocutaneous flap with the base extending from the medial to the lateral border of the breast. The dissection is performed in a subfascial plane (in our cases, we do suprafascial plane and when we find the perforator we dissected it under the fascia. In this way, the flap is more flexible to adapt to the breast) and the main perforators are identified and preserved. It is important to keep the blood pressure above 100 mg systolic to hear the Doppler sound. It is best to use the perforator close to the defect. Dissection is continued to the base of the flap and the ICAP flap is then totally isolated on this intercostal perforator.

The routine use of loops is not advocated but can be used depending on the local practice. It is possible to achieve an adequate perforator length to advance or rotate the almost 180°. The skin incisions are stapled temporarily and the patient is positioned upright to assess final flap position, moulding, and checked for symmetry. The flap can be secured in position using an anchoring suture (usually 2-0 vicryl) to the breast (in our experience, as few points as possible gets better results).

The flap needs to be de-epithelized and this can be performed during the initial phase of surgery as it is easier while some surgeons do it before insetting the flap. I usually leave a small island of skin which I de-epthelise at the end of surgery to confirm the vascularity of the flap (Fig. 9.4).

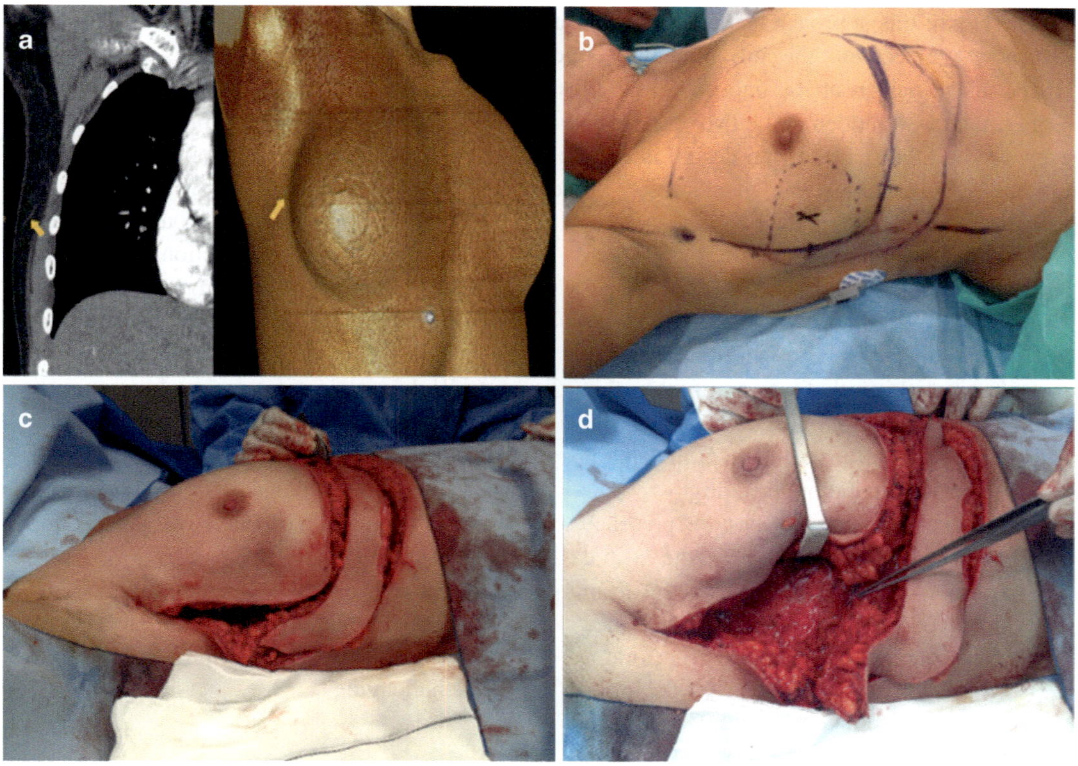

Fig. 9.4 Preoperative and surgical plan were shown. (**a**) Presurgical angio-CT technique. (**b**) Presurgical planification. (**c**, **d**) Show surgical technique

Axilla can be staged using the standard sentinel node biopsy in node negative disease or using axillary clearance or limited axillary staging in node positive disease depending on the local practice. A separate incision would be needed along the axilla to allow access.

A drain (we use penrose drain) is placed is the breast and closed primarily after ensuring adequate haemostasis. The wound is closed in two layers using 3–0 vicryl for subcutaneous layer and 4–0 monocryl for subcuticular layer. A separate drain can be placed in the axilla is needed particularly if axillary clearance is performed. Steri-strips or skin glue can be applied and simple dressings as per local practice. The drains are managed postoperatively as per institutional protocol. Drains are usually removed when less than 10–20 ml over two consecutive days (48 h). Patients can be discharged on the same day or next day as appropriate.

Some centres use frozen section to determine the adequacy of margins and it depends on the centre and the country. To process frozen section dedicated pathology team and laboratory is needed [9]. The advantages of frozen section includes immediate intra operative margin assessment and if needed further breast tissue can be removed to ensure complete oncological resection [10]. Disadvantage includes the possibility of false negative report, which needs to be addressed.

The procedure can be carried out as single stage or two-stage surgery [11]. The advantage of single stage surgery includes single operation, easy to replace the volume immediately as there is no scar tissue formation, better theatre utilisation, cost effective, and improved patient experience. However, a two-stage approach can be undertaken depending on the local practice, after neoadjuvant therapy, lobular cancers and if there is an uncertainty about margin adequacy. The time interval depends on the availability of the complete histology report and usually varies 2–4 weeks following surgery.

The key of this approach is the design of scar and how we recreate the inframammary fold (IMF). If the design of the flap is narrow, most scars can be well hidden in the IMF crease; however, on the other hand, if the design is wide, it can be resulting in downward displacement of the scar that is visible below the breast.

Tips

- During de-epithelisation of the flap leave a small triangle of skin at the distal end to check for perfusion at the end of the procedure before insetting
- Distal approach to observe the presence of the perforator. During the initial learning curve it is best to dissect from distal to proximal aspect of the flap. This enables to preserve the perforator which is usually 1–2 cm below the inframammary fold. It is the safest way to initially detect the presence and location of the perforator.
- Ensure that the systolic blood pressure is above 100 mmHg while checking for Doppler signal.
- Once the flap is completely elevated check flap vitality by de-epithelising the skin island and check for perfusion.
- The breast cavity should be irrigated and washed until clear before insetting of the flap.
- Remember that one-third of the flap will remain between the rotation point and the beginning of the breast. Hence it is important to plan the insetting and assess the degree of volume replacement needed.
- Posteriorly, the incision was closed with stitches marking the old mammary fold to avoid scar migration (only the inferior border of the scar are fixed to the closest rib to avoid deformation of inferior breast pole and at the same time avoiding scar migration).

Pitfalls

- Patients with a few skin laxity could be a problem to get appropriate tissue in our flap for wide excisions.
- Perforators far down away from the patient inframmary fold could worse the results of our reconstruction because not all the flap could be introduce inside the breast. So try to choose the closest perforator to the inframammary fold.
- Wide excision in superior breast quadrants is not a contraindication for this flap, but we should move breast tissue from inferior breast to upper breast and the flap will be used to cover the inferior breast.
- The internal third perforator could usually be smaller than the lateral third so the dissection could be more challenging.

After-Care

- No special care has to be followed after this kind of reconstruction.
- Pain could be managed with NSAID and acetaminophen every 4 h.
- In our experience, drainage as Penrose type are only used for the first 24 h.
- In this kind of reconstruction there is not needed to immobility. The patient could do her normal life.

9.6 Conclusions

Based on the published articles, we found that this flap has a consistent vascularization with good perforators. And moreover, it is really useful for partial breast reconstruction in A or B cup breasts with an unsightly scar, simply surgery and does not have any negative impact in the satisfaction of the patient. The results comparing with classical flaps are much better. A few patients need a scar revision or lipofilling due to the changes after radiotherapy. However, in general, the patients had a very high satisfaction with the results and the low morbidity.

References

1. Badran HA, El-Helaly MS, Safe I, Badran HA. The lateral intercostal neurovascular free flap. Plast Reconstr Surg. 1984;73:17–26.
2. Hamdi M, Van Landuyt K, Monstrey S, Blondeel P. Pedicled perforator flaps in breast reconstruction: a new concept. Br J Plast Surg. 2004;57:531–9.
3. Hallock GG. The island anterior intercostal artery perforator flap as another option for the difficult epigastric abdominal wound. Ann Plast Surg. 2009;63:414–7.
4. Losken A, Hamdi M. Partial breast reconstruction: current perspectives. Plast Reconstr Surg. 2009;124:722–36.
5. Carrasco-López C, Julian Ibañez JF, Vilà J, Rodriguez-Baeza A, Carrera-Burgaya A, Reina-de-la-Torre F, et al. The anterior intercostal artery flap: anatomical and radiologic study. Plast Reconstr Surg. 2017;139:613–9.
6. Carrasco-López C, Julian Ibañez JF, Vilà J, Luna Tomás MA, Navinés López J, Pascual Miguel I, et al. Anterior intercostal artery perforator flap in immediate breast reconstruction: anatomical study and clinical application. Microsurgery. 2017;37:603–10.
7. Persichetti P, Tenna S, Brunetti B, Aveta A, Segreto F, Marangi GF. Anterior intercostal artery perforator flap autologous augmentation in bariatric mastopexy. Plast Reconstr Surg. 2012;130:917–25.
8. Harris JR, Levene MB, Svensson G, Hellman S. Analysis of cosmetic results following primary radiation therapy for stages I and II carcinoma of the breast. Int J Radiat Oncol Biol Phys. 1979;5:257–61.
9. Jorns JM, Daignault S, Sabel MS, Wu AJ. Is intraoperative frozen section analysis of reexcision specimens of value in preventing reoperation in breast-conserving therapy? Am J Clin Pathol. 2014;142:601–8.
10. Gray RJ, Pockaj BA, Garvey E, Blair S. Intraoperative margin management in breast-conserving surgery: a systematic review of the literature. Ann Surg Oncol. 2018;25:18–27.
11. Roy PG, Tenovici AA. Staged approach to partial breast reconstruction to avoid mastectomy in women with breast cancer. Gland Surg. 2017;6:336–42.

10 Superior Epigastric Artery Perforator (SEAP) FLAP

Moustapha Hamdi
and Leonardo Pires Novais Dias

Contents

10.1 Anatomy

The perforators that nourish the SEAP flap originate from the superior epigastric artery (SEA), which arises from the internal mammary artery (IMA). The IMA bifurcates around the sixth costal cartilage into the musculophrenic artery and the SEA. The SEA continues inferiorly along the same vertical line as the IMA and pierces the posterior rectus sheath approximately 7 cm below the costal margin. At this point, the SEA often sends a large superficial branch through the origin of the rectus abdominis muscle (RAM) that pierces the anterior rectus sheath to enter the subcutaneous layer and proceeds caudally to supply the overlying skin. The main trunk of the SEA enters the posterior surface of the RAM. The main branch of the SEA subdivides into an average of two branches that arborise further to anastomose inferiorly with the deep inferior epigastric artery (DIEA) and laterally with terminal branches of the intercostal arteries (Fig. 10.1) [1–7].

The SEA has an average of four perforators below the costal margin up to the second tendinous intersection situated midway between

M. Hamdi (✉)
Head of the Plastic Surgery Department, Brussels University Hospital, Vrije Universiteit Brussel, Brussels, Belgium
e-mail: moustapha.hamdi@uzbrussel.be

L. P. N. Dias
Head of the Breast Surgery Department, Mater Dei Hospital, Salvador, Brazil
e-mail: leonardo.dias@materdei.com.br

M. Hamdi et al. (eds.), *Pedicled Flaps in Partial Breast Reconstruction*,
https://doi.org/10.1007/978-3-031-08483-6_10

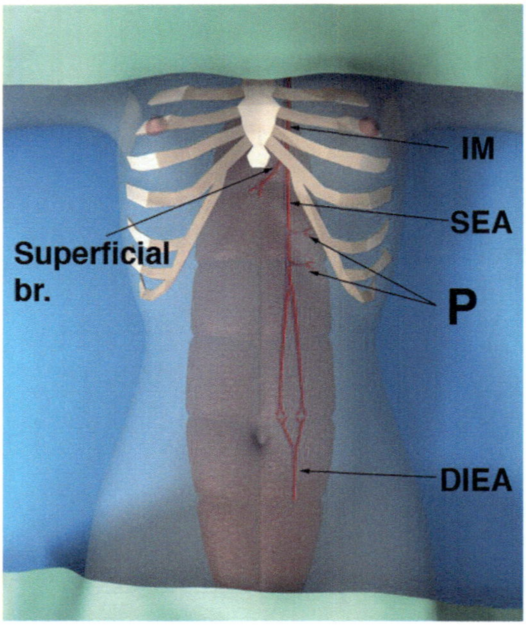

Fig. 10.1 Overview of the epigastric vascular system. *IM* internal mammary, *SEA* superior epigastric artery, *P* perforators, *DIEA* deep inferior epigastric artery. Note: Adapted from [7]. Copyright 2009 by Elsevier. Reprinted with permission

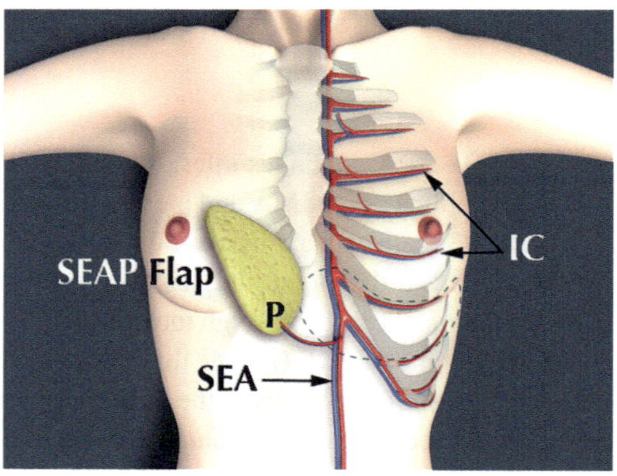

Fig. 10.2 Anatomy of the SEAP flap. *IC* intercostal vessels, *SEAP* superior epigastric artery perforator, *P* perforator, *SEA* superior epigastric artery

the xiphisternum and the umbilicus with an average diameter of 0.5–1.0 mm. These perforators pierce the RAM or occasionally enter the sheath beside the lateral border of the muscle. Emerging perforators with a calibre of >0.5 mm are most regularly found 2–6 cm from the midline and

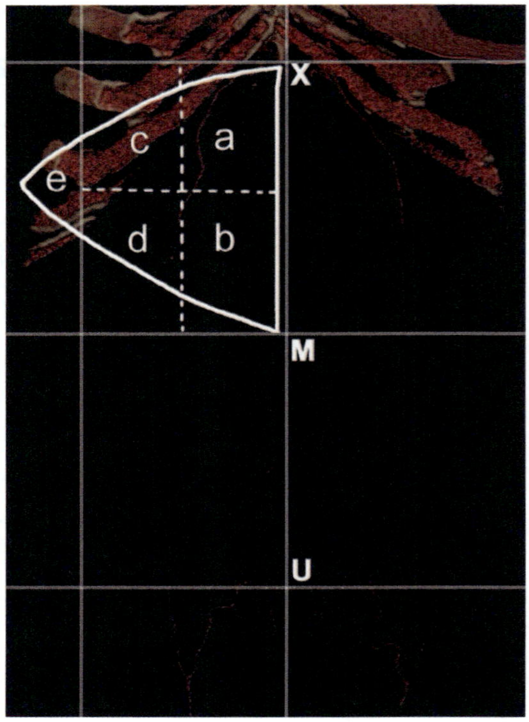

Fig. 10.3 Schematic of the abdominal wall demonstrating the area irrigated by the SEAPs. *X* xiphisternum, *U* umbilicus, *M* midway between *X* and *U*, Zones "*a, b, c*" and "*d*" are irrigated by the SEAPs. Zone "*e*" are irrigated by intercostal perforators. Note: Adapted from [9]. Copyright 2009 by Wolters Kluwer Health. Reprinted with permission

0–10 cm below the xiphoid process. At least one single vein follows each dissected perforator. In 11% of the patients, two accompanying veins are present with the SEA [8]. The SEAP flap is often based on the proximal perforator below the costal margin (Fig. 10.2). The suprafascial perforator length until arborisation has around 3.5 cm [7].

The territory irrigated by SEA perforators ranges from 21×12 cm^2 to 150×40 cm^2, according to the literature [8, 10, 11]. Nevertheless, anatomical studies identified the nourished limits for the SEAPs and established the lower edge around two fingers above the umbilicus with an oblique extension toward the breast axis [7, 9]. In conformity with the skin laxity and indication, SEAP flaps are designed vertically on the paramedian region or transversely under the inframammary fold [9]. Extending the flap design laterally towards the anterior axillary line or below the midpoint (M) has contributed to tip necrosis of the flap (Fig. 10.3) [7].

10.2 Applications

The SEAP flap is a valuable option for partial breast reconstruction of the inferior quadrants when a large volume or skin replacement is required. Another indication is breast augmentation after bariatric surgery or in aesthetics [12–14].

10.3 Steps

10.3.1 Planning

In case of indication of SEAP flap, the patient is oriented to perform a preoperative computed tomography angiography (CTA) to identify the vessels and plan the surgery. Before surgery, the perforator vessels from the SEA are identified with an 8 MHz acoustic handheld Doppler and marked over the upper abdomen. Then, the SEAP flap is designed elliptically with the patient in the supine position. The first draw of the flap is determined by the projected defect planned on the breast, which is finally measured after the demolition surgery is finished.

10.3.2 Harvesting

The perforators are approached under loupes magnification from the incision created by the defect on the breast. The harvesting starts in a supra fascial plane from the breast towards the midline in a diagonal direction. The SEA perforators usually have a supra fascial course above the deep fascia for 1–3 cm and are easily visualised a few centimetres after the medial insertion of the inframammary fold is raised. After the perforator is identified, the rectus abdominal fascia is opened around where the perforator pierces it. The perforator dissection follows through the RAM fibres while side branches are clipped or coagulated until the central pedicle is reached.

10.3.3 Transference

After that, the pedicle length is measured to check if the flap reaches the medial area of the defect in the breast. If the pedicle reaches the defect, the length and width of the gap are measured, and the flap design may follow the transversal elliptical fashion. Then, the skin ellipse is incised, and the flap elevated. Finally, the flap is transferred as a V–Y or rotated up to 180° into the defect. The primary closure of the deep fascia is arranged with a non-absorbable running suture. Later, one suction drain is installed on the donor site area. Finally, the donor site is closed primarily in layers after limited skin edge undermining (Figs. 10.4 and 10.5).

Tips

The rate of success with the SEAP flap is high, though some aspects must be underscored. Postoperative management is vital, and close monitoring of the flap by a well-trained plastic surgery team involving specialised and dedicated nurse care is necessary. The main postoperative feature of venous congestion is probably higher than in other pedicled perforator flaps, mainly if the propeller method is employed for flap transfer. The SEA perforating vessels calibre is sometimes tiny and associated with a short length of the pedicle. These anatomical particularities explain the great sensitivity of this flap to a pedicle twist. To limit this phenomenon, the perforating vessels must be dissected as far as conceivable to diminish the venous curve and consequent flap congestion. It is also necessary to avoid an excessively tight closure of the flap, to allow a compression-free during the flap's swelling, maximum at 72 h postoperative time.

Preoperative assessment of the perforators with CTA positively affects the SEAP flap surgical planning. Quality detailed information on position and course allows the reconstruction surgeon to select the most reliable perforator, which would reduce operating time and postoperative complications. Also, both unidirectional Doppler flowmetry and colour Duplex scanning have proved to be valuable tools in evaluating vascular anatomy preoperatively and can be combined with CTA. The CTA is mandatory in patients with the previous abdominoplasty, DIEAP flap or salvage cases where it is difficult to tell if perforators are still available.

Pitfalls

The flexibility to design the SEAP flap is due to the origins of the SEA perforators' axial vascular anatomy. The SEA integument irrigation seems to extend from the inferior breast crease up to just above the umbilicus area. Therefore, the best-vascularised site is closer to the breast, safely comprising horizontal flaps. On the other hand, the limit to the vertical flap is not constant since the territory near the umbilicus area is nourished by small calibre perforators originating from choke vessels. Therefore, the vertical flap design depends on the location of the SEA perforator. If the chosen one is the first perforator branch for partial breast reconstruction, safe vascularise support seems to end above the umbilicus area.

After-Care

The postoperative care following a SEAP flap procedure starts in the operative room. The wound is closed in layers to avoid pressure on the pedicle. Drains are often necessary. The dressing is placed without pressure, leaving easy access to the pedicle area, controlled immediately after surgery and twice a day during recovery. The patient is observed by a dedicated team of nurses at the regular ward and is stimulated to move out of bed on the first day after the procedure.

If the flap presents blood supply insufficiency within the first 24 hours, it is strongly advised to review the issue under direct view in the operating theatre. The problem is often related to excess pressure on the flap's pedicle, which can be easily solved by realising the regional sutures and resetting the wound closure to protect the flap's free nourish. Afterwards, the patient is redirected to the regular ward for vigilance under the institutional protocol for this sort of surgery.

10.4 Conclusions

The pedicled SEAP flap may prevent the need for a microscope, intensive care unit, and microvascular anastomosis risks while providing plastic surgeons with a safe method for breast reconstruction of the lower quadrants. However, in some cases, the amount of tissue transferred leads to a not ideal cosmetic result. For such cases, surgeons and patients must set the following plan to achieve an acceptable result aligned with the patient's expectations. In most cases, a contralateral breast reduction or fat grafting is sufficient to achieve the desired result. However, the shared decision-making process must consider the claim to complete the oncological treatment first with adjuvant radiotherapy. Afterwards, the cosmetic refinements can be arranged.

10.5 Clinical Application

Case 1

A 71-year-old female patient presented major fat necrosis after a pedicled latissimus dorsi flap used for partial breast reconstruction. A SEAP flap was planned based on the CTA exam.

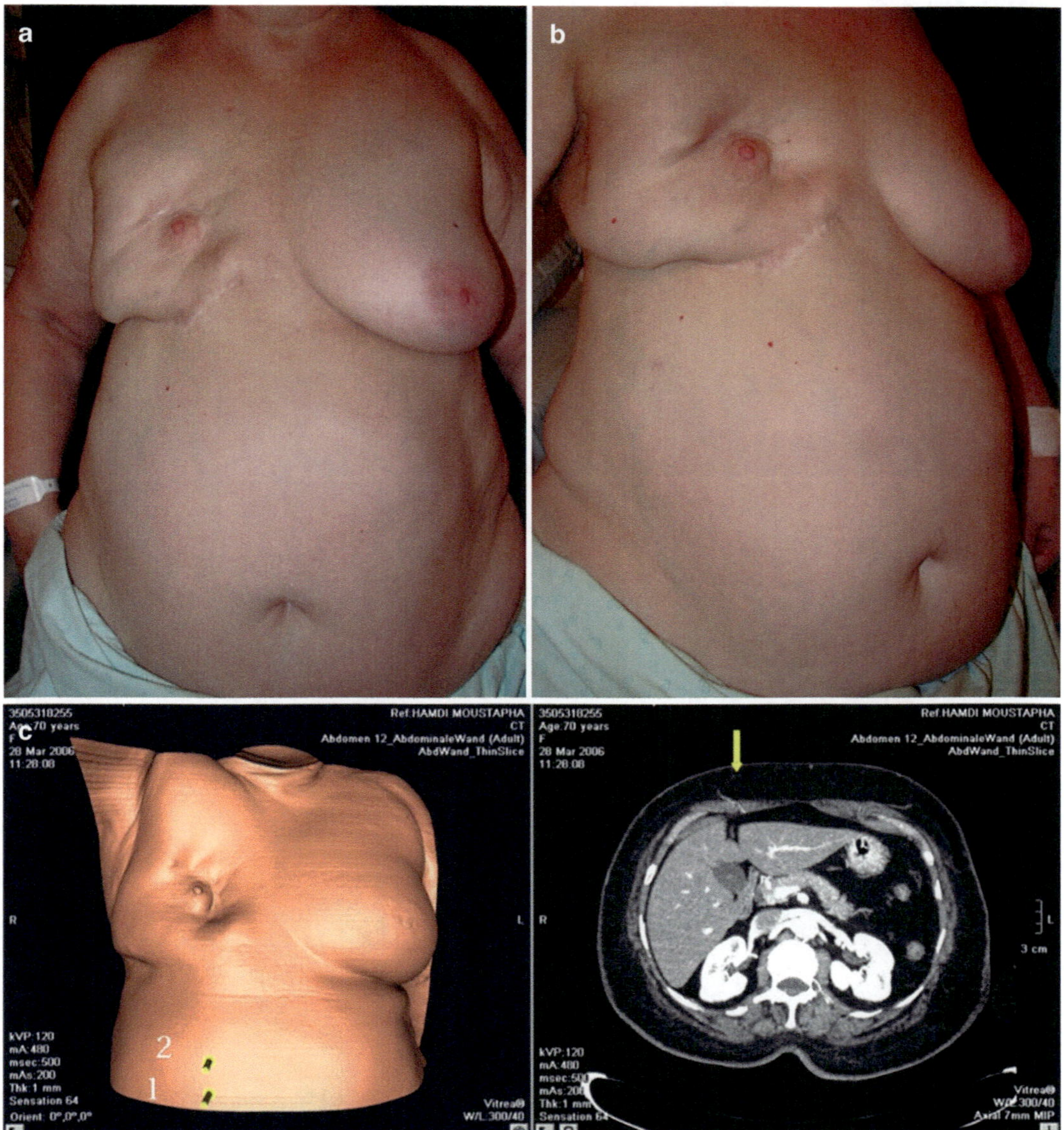

Fig. 10.4 (**a**) Preoperative anterior view. (**b**) Preoperative lateral right-side view. (**c**) Computed tomography reconstruction of the anterior trunk area with two yellow and black arrows pointing to the position of two large SEAPs. The axial image of the CTA of the upper abdomen area shows one large SEAP originating from the right pedicle (yellow arrow). (**d**) Sagittal image of the CTA shows the second large perforator (yellow arrow). (**e**) Preoperative markings of the vertical SEAP flap (27 × 7 cm^2). (**f**) The debridement of the fat necrosis within the right breast. (**g**) The more distal SEAP was dissected. (**h**) The flap was transferred to the defect with primary closure of the donor site. (**i**) The result at 1 year postoperatively with complete wound healing

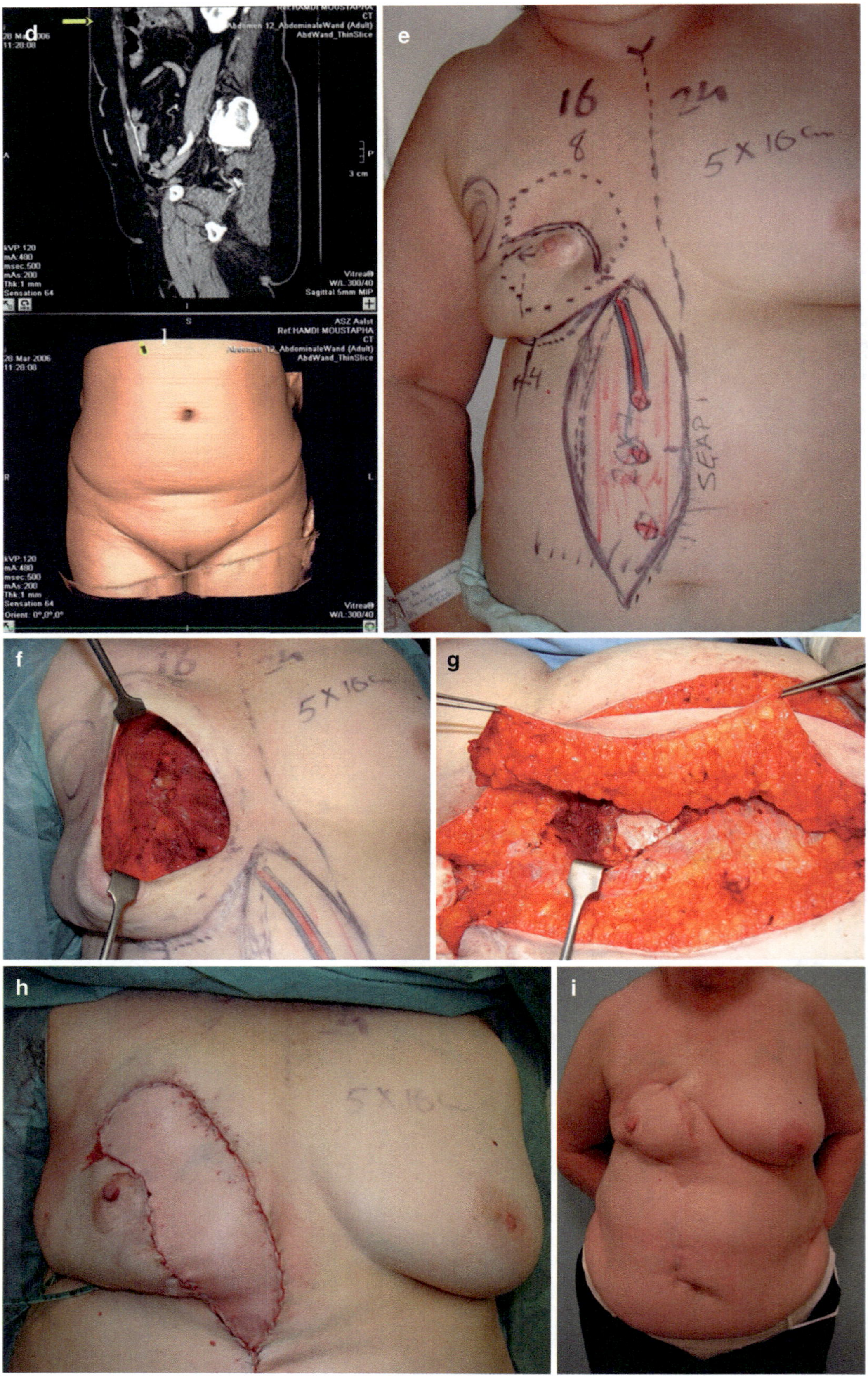

Fig. 10.4 (continued)

Case 2

A 52-year-old patient underwent considerable fat necrosis after a free DIEAP flap breast reconstruction over the superomedial quadrant of the right side. A pedicled SEAP flap was planned based on unidirectional Doppler.

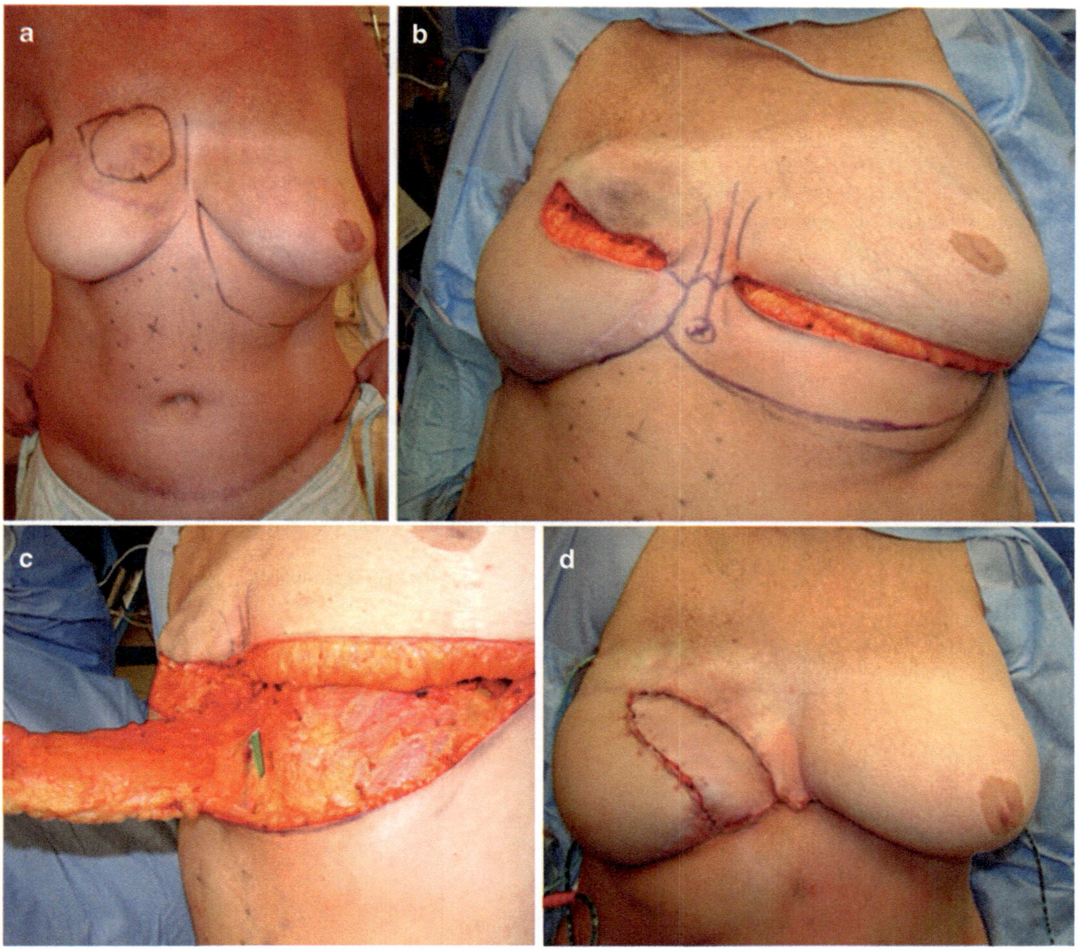

Fig. 10.5 (**a**) Preoperative marking of the transversal SEAP. The fat necrosis was outlined over the breast, and the SEAP flap was designed horizontal with an extension under the inframammary fold (IMF) of the contralateral breast. (**b**) Intraoperative view shows the debridement of the fat necrosis, but the breast skin was severely damaged due to the previous radiotherapy and the inflammatory reaction after fat necrosis. The Doppler perforator was explored through the IMF incision. (**c**) Overview shows the SEAP isolated and the harvested flap, ready to be placed in the defect. (**d**) Final result after SEAP flap positioning. The damaged breast was resected, and the SEAP flap was turned 150° to fit the defect

References

1. Hartrampf C, Scheflan M, Black P. Breast reconstruction with a transverse abdominal island flap. Plast Reconstr Surg. 1982;69(2):216–24.
2. Boyd JB, Taylor GI, Corlett R. The vascular territories of the superior epigastric and the deep inferior epigastric systems. Plast Reconstr Surg. 1984;73:1–16.
3. Schusterman MA, Kroll SS, Miller MJ, Reece GP, Baldwin BJ, Robb GL, Altmyer CS, Ames FC, Singletary SE, Ross MI. The free transverse rectus abdominis musculocutaneous flap for breast reconstruction: one center's experience with 211 consecutive cases. Ann Plast Surg. 1994;32(3):234–42. https://doi.org/10.1097/00000637-199403000-00002.
4. Koshima I, Soeda S. Inferior epigastric artery skin flaps without rectus abdominis muscle. Br J Plast Surg. 1989;42:645–8.
5. Hallock GG. The superior epigastric (RECTUS ABDOMINIS) muscle perforator flap. Ann Plast Surg. 2005;55:430.
6. Uemura T. Superior epigastric artery perforator flap: preliminary report. Plast Reconstr Surg. 2007;120(1):1–5. https://doi.org/10.1097/01.prs.0000263538.71343.b7.
7. Hamdi M, Van LK, Ulens S, Van HE, Roche N, Monstrey S. Clinical applications of the superior epigastric artery perforator (SEAP) flap: anatomical studies and preoperative perforator mapping with multidetector CT. J Plast Reconstr Aesthet Surg. 2009;62:1127–34.
8. Schmidt M, Tinhofer I, Duscher D, Huemer GM. Perforasomes of the upper abdomen: an anatomical study. J Plast Reconstr Aesthet Surg. 2014;67(1):42–7. https://doi.org/10.1016/j.bjps.2013.08.017.
9. Mah E, Rozen WM, Ashton MW, Flood S. Deep superior epigastric artery perforators: anatomical study and clinical application in sternal reconstruction. Plast Reconstr Surg. 2009;123(6):1719–23. https://doi.org/10.1097/PRS.0b013e3181a3f3cf.
10. Offman SL, Geddes CR, Tang M, Morris SF. The vascular basis of perforator flaps based on the source arteries of the lateral lumbar region. Plast Reconstr Surg. 2005;115(6):1651–9. https://doi.org/10.1097/01.prs.0000161464.11134.c1.
11. Ziegler K, Schmidt M, Huemer GM. A pedicled superior epigastric artery perforator (SEAP-) propeller flap for 2-cavity reconstruction after oncologic rib resection. Microsurgery. 2011;31(4):335–6. https://doi.org/10.1002/micr.20886.
12. Hamdi M, Craggs B, Stoel AM, Hendrickx B, Zeltzer A. Superior epigastric artery perforator flap: anatomy, clinical applications, and review of literature. J Reconstr Microsurg. 2014;30(7):475–82. https://doi.org/10.1055/s-0034-1376399.
13. Szychta P, Anderson WD. Islanded pedicled superior epigastric artery perforator flaps for bilateral breast augmentation with mastopexy after massive weight loss. J Plast Reconstr Aesthet Surg. 2011;64(12):1677–81. https://doi.org/10.1016/j.bjps.2011.04.025.
14. Zeltzer A, Dupont Y, De Baerdemaeker R, Hamdi M. Autologous islanded breast enhancement by reversed abdominoplasty (AIBERA) flap. Eur J Plast Surg. 2021;44(5):699. https://doi.org/10.1007/s00238-021-01781-w.

Subcostal Artery Perforator (SCAP) Flap: A New Application in Breast Reconstruction

11

Nathaniel Stroumza Escoffier and Maha Eid

Contents

11.1 Anatomy

11.1.1 General Information on the Anterolateral Abdominal Wall

Each anterolateral hemi-wall is formed by four muscles:

Three large muscles, from the surface to the depth:

- The external oblique muscle
- The internal oblique muscle
- The transverse muscle

Placed in three layers, they form a muscular webbing whose great solidity is reinforced by the different direction of the fibers of each muscle.

- The rectus abdominis muscle: superficial, anterior and vertical, located on either side of the midline, is contained in an inextensible aponeurotic sheath.

The sheath of the rectus abdominis muscle is an inextensible aponeurotic sheath formed by the aponeuroses of the lateral muscles (Fig. 11.1).

N. Stroumza Escoffier (✉)
Private Practice, Paris, France

M. Eid
Department of Obstetrics and Gynecologic Surgery, Bichat University Hospital, Paris, France

M. Hamdi et al. (eds.), *Pedicled Flaps in Partial Breast Reconstruction*,
https://doi.org/10.1007/978-3-031-08483-6_11

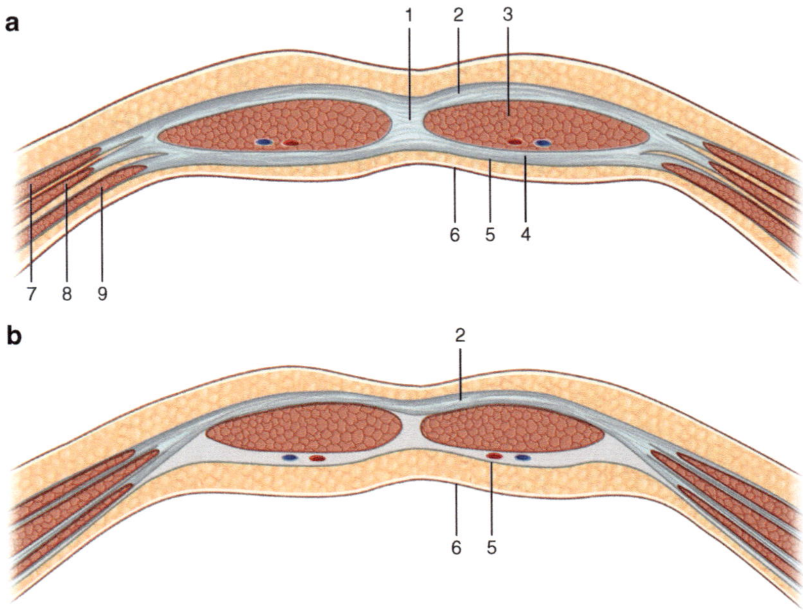

Fig. 11.1 Axial section of the rectus abdominis muscle sheath. (1) linea alba, (2) anterior aponeurosis, (3) rectus abdominis, (4) posterior aponeurosis, (5) fascia transversalis, (6) peritoneum, (7) external oblique muscle, (8) internal oblique muscle, (9) transverse abdominis. (**a**) Above arcuate line. (**b**) Below arcuate line

- Above the arcuate line, i.e. in the upper 2/3 of the rectus muscle, this sheath is formed by:
  - In front: the two sheets of the aponeurosis of the external oblique muscle associated with the anterior sheet of the aponeurosis of the internal oblique muscle.
  - At the back: the combination of the posterior sheet of the internal oblique muscle fascia and the two sheets of the transverse muscle fascia
- Below the arcuate line:
  - Anteriorly: the anterior aponeurosis is formed by the aponeuroses of the three broad muscles.
  - Posteriorly: there is no longer a posterior sheet of the rectus sheath but only the transversalis fascia and the peritoneum.

11.1.2 General Information on the Vascularization of the Anterolateral Abdominal Wall

11.1.2.1 Arterial Vascularization

The anterolateral abdominal wall is richly vascularized by vessels of various origins, widely anastomosed and represented by two longitudinal axes: internal mammary (or internal thoracic) and inferior epigastric, joined by transverse vessels, recalling the primitive metamerism of the trunk.

On the midline (Fig. 11.2), located on the posterior aspect of the rectus abdominis, the wall receives:

- from above, the branches of the internal mammary artery,
- and from the bottom, those of the inferior epigastric.

The internal mammary artery is a collateral of the subclavian artery. It divides opposite the sternal extremity, at the level of the 6th intercostal space, into two branches:

- an external or musculo-phrenic branch which travels obliquely downwards and outwards, behind the costal margin. It feeds the intercostal branches and the subcostal branch, which run obliquely downward and forward to anastomose with the superior epigastric artery.
- an internal or superior epigastric branch which travels on the posterior surface of the rectus muscle in its sheath and anastomoses with the inferior epigastric artery at the level of the

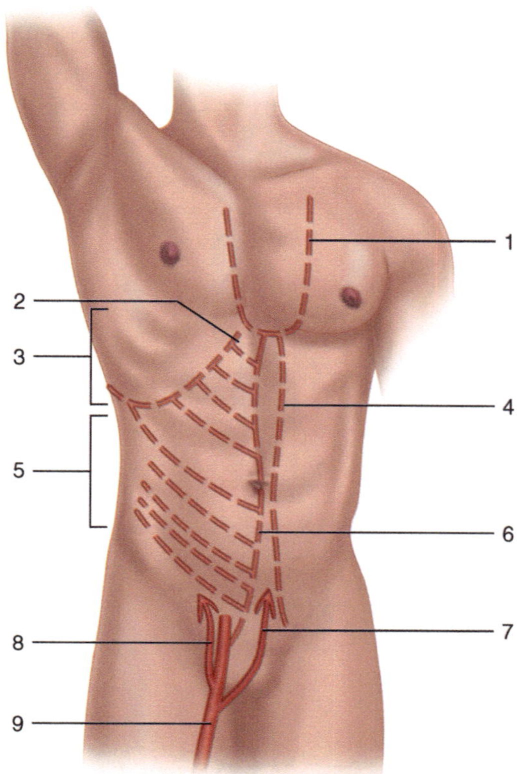

Fig. 11.2 Arterial supply to anterolateral abdominal wall. (1) internal thoracic artery, (2) musculo-phrenic artery, (3) intercostal arteries, (4) superior epigastric artery, (5) lumbar arteries, (6) inferior epigastric artery, (7) superficial epigastric artery, (8) superior circumflex iliac artery, (9) femoral artery

umbilicus. Note: the superior epigastric artery rapidly gives a retro-xiphoid branch which anastomoses with the retro-xiphoid branch of the contralateral epigastric artery.

The inferior epigastric artery arises from the external iliac artery and travels upward medially to the umbilicus where it anastomoses with the superior epigastric artery. It has a deep, subperitoneal course to the arcuate line where it enters the rectus sheath. It terminates in numerous branches anastomosing with the inferior intercostal arteries, branches of the inferior epigastric artery or perforating branches penetrating the rectus muscle and subcutaneous tissue.

Laterally, the wall receives:

- The intercostal arteries and the subcostal artery arise from collateral branches of the thoracic aorta (Fig. 11.3).
- The lumbar arteries: there are 4 on each side and they arise from the posterolateral aspect of the aorta. They run anterior to the psoas and follow the curve of the abdominal wall to reach the lateral border of the rectus muscle where they perforate the sheath and give branches to the skin, muscle branches and others anastomosing with branches of the inferior epigastric, iliac circumflex and iliolumbar.
- The iliolumbar artery: arises from the internal iliac artery and divides into a posterior lumbar branch and a transverse iliac branch giving a superficial and a deep branch.
- The superficial and deep iliac arteries.

11.1.2.2 Venous Vascularization

The veins have, on the whole, the same layout as the arteries with longitudinal currents anastomosing with transverse metameric vessels. Note: the presence of two veins for one artery. It is also necessary to distinguish two planes:

- A superficial plane.
- A deep plane.

The superficial plane is represented by the superficial subcutaneous epigastric veins and the superficial circumflexes that follow the course of the corresponding arteries. It also includes a large venous arcade: the thoracoepigastric vein, connecting the axillary vein to the common femoral vein. Next to this, there is a rich collateral venous network, which is widely anastomosed.

In the deep plane, the venous network follows very exactly the arterial pattern (Fig. 11.4)

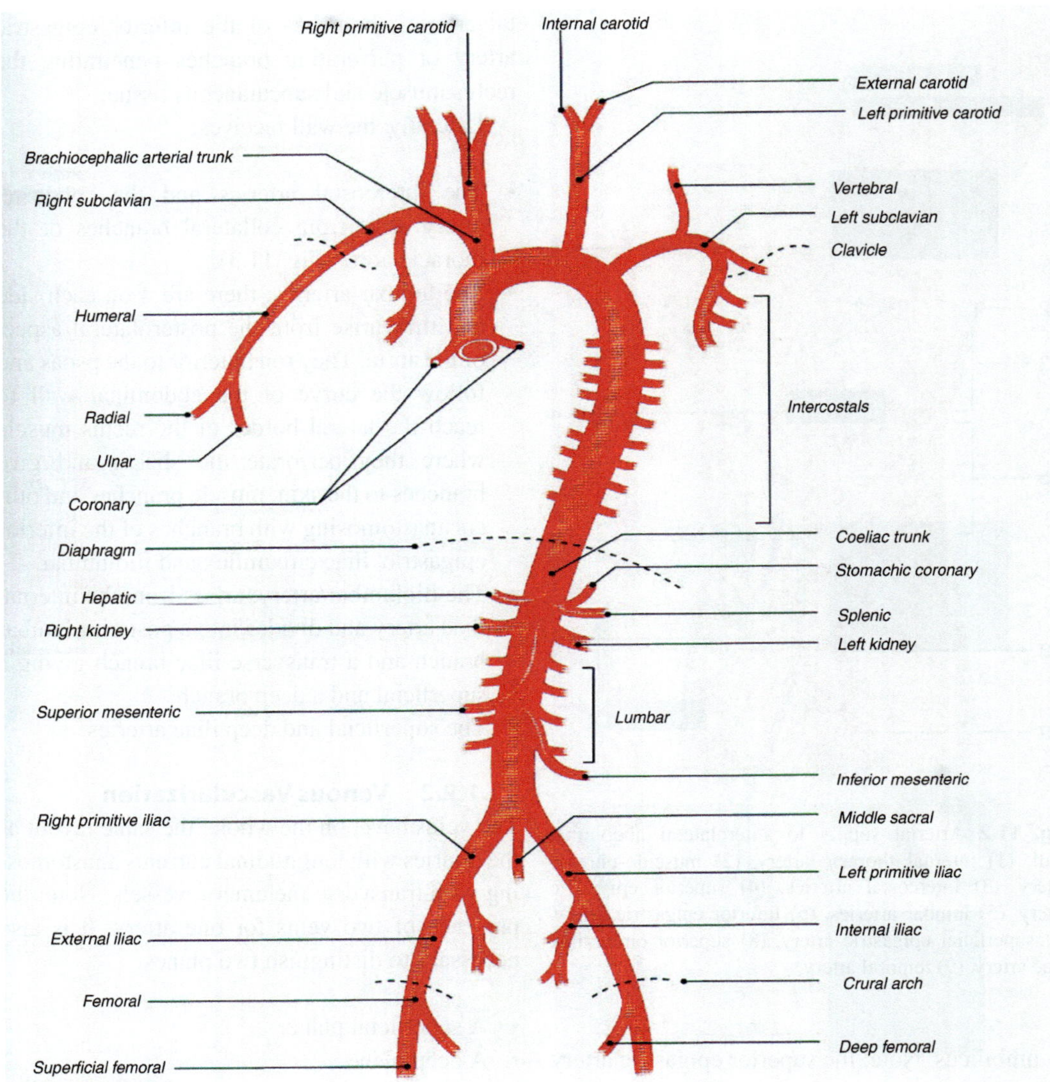

Fig. 11.3 Illustration of the collateral branches of the thoracic aorta

11.1.3 Anatomy of the Subcostal Pedicle

It is in this space (Fig. 11.5) that the vascular-nervous pedicle travels including:

- An intercostal artery: which originates at the posterior aspect of the thoracic aorta (at each stage), and passes below the azygos system. It is also supplied anteriorly (supplementary network) by the musculo-phrenic branch from the internal thoracic artery.
- An intercostal vein: which will drain into the azygos venous system but also by satellite veins of the thoracic artery in front.
- The intercostal nerve: which exits from the foramen magnum and terminates anteriorly in sensory branches for the skin.

11.1.3.1 The Subcostal Artery

The 12th intercostal or subcostal artery originates, like the subcostal arteries, from the thoracic aorta of which it is the last collateral branch. It passes below the lateral border of the 12th rib and extends in an integral fashion in the antero-

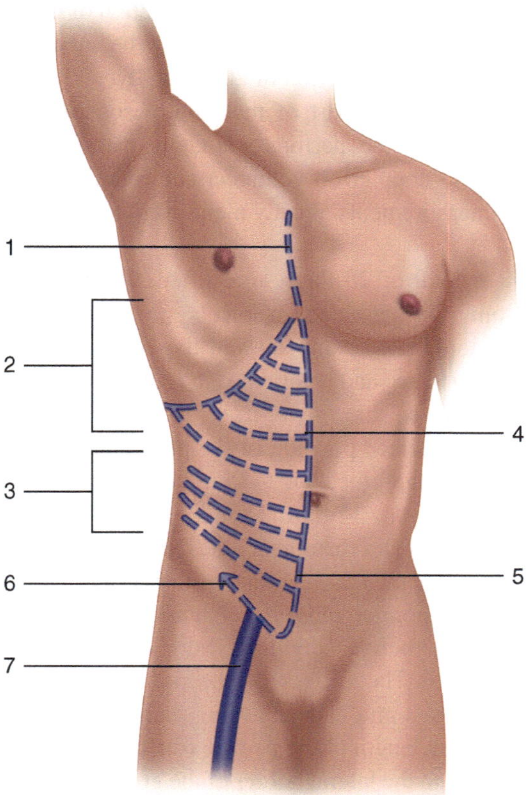

Fig. 11.4 Venous supply to anterolateral abdominal wall. (1) internal thoracic vein, (2) anterior intercostal veins, (3) lumbar veins, (4) superior epigastric vein, (5) deep circumflex iliac vein, (6) femoral vein

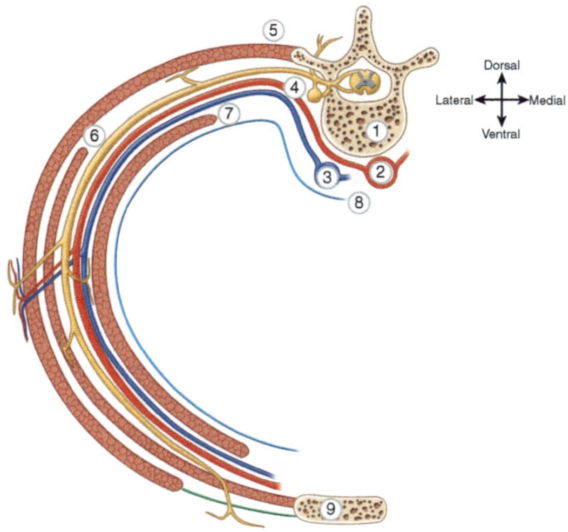

Fig. 11.5 The intercostal space. Longitudinal section. (1) Vertebral body, (2) thoracic artery that supplies the intercostal artery, (3) Azygos vein that supplies the intercostal vein, (4) intercostal nerve, (5) external intercostal muscle

lateral abdominal wall. It travels into the abdominal wall passing under the lateral arch ligament, in front of the quadratus lumborum muscle, and insinuates itself between the transverse and internal oblique muscles and then continues its oblique course downward and forward to anastomose with the epigastric artery.

It is also supplied, like the subcostal arteries of the 7th, 8th, 9th, 10th, and 11th ribs, by the musculo-phrenic artery, a branch of the internal mammary artery. It distributes itself integrally to the anterolateral abdominal wall.

11.1.3.2 The Subcutaneous Vein

The subcutaneous vein belongs to the deep venous network of the abdominal wall. Its anatomy is similar to that of the corresponding artery: anastomosing with the epigastric vein, it travels obliquely upward and backward. Unlike the subcostal veins, which drain into the musculophrenic vein (branch of the internal thoracic), the subcostal vein does not relay to the internal thoracic vein and drains directly into the azygos system.

11.1.3.3 The Nerves

The abdominal wall is essentially innervated by the last six intercostal nerves and the abdomino-genital nerves coming from L1 which have retained their metameric arrangement. Among the intercostal nerves, only the 12th belongs entirely to the abdominal wall, the others are thoracoabdominal.

The subcostal nerve runs initially under the 12th rib and then between the transverse and internal oblique muscles to the outer edge of the rectus sheath.

The subcostal nerves divide into richly anastomosing threads before reaching the lateral border of the rectus muscle. Their branches travel along the posterior aspect of the rectus before entering the rectus to cross it and give sensory terminal branches innervating the skin and the sheath.

11.1.4 Anatomical Study of the SCAP Flap

Feinendegen et al. published an anatomical study of a subcostal artery perforator-vascularized [1]. Based on a case report in which a subcostal artery perforator-vascularized pedicle flap was used to fill a lumbar skin defect, the authors concluded that the flap was a good choice [2]. Based on a case report in which a pedicled flap vascularized by a subcostal artery perforator was used to fill a lumbar skin defect, their objective was to evaluate the anatomic variability regarding the size and location of the perforating artery and its flap (Fig. 11.6).

- The first part of their study involved the dissection of anatomic subjects. The location of the perforating artery of the subcostal artery was calculated in relation to other anatomical landmarks: distance from the spinous processes, distance from the termination of the 12th rib, distance from the lateral border of the greater dorsalis muscle. The following measurements were systematically reported: caliber, length, number of terminal branches of the perforating artery, and maximum length of the pedicle after dissection to the lateral border of the erector spinae muscles. The surface of the flap was evaluated by injection of methylene blue after cannulation of the subcostal artery and injection of 20 mL of dye.
- The second part of their study consisted of locating the perforator and its pathway via echo-doppler on volunteer subjects using the measurements already mentioned.

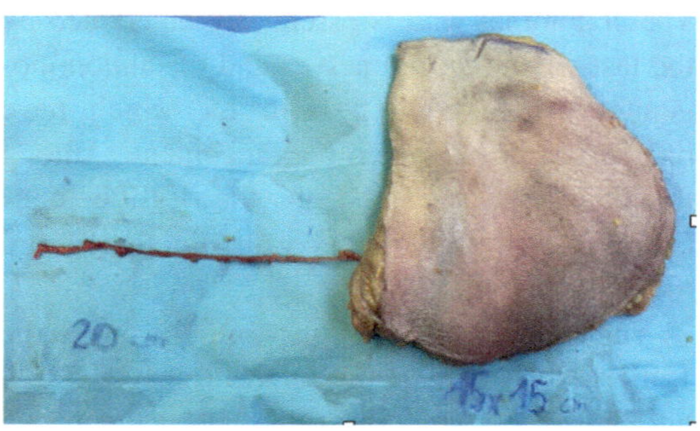

Fig. 11.6 Subcostal artery perforator (SCAP) flap. Size of the flap 15 × 15 cm with a 20 cm pedicle

A total of 28 flaps were lifted, 26 analyzed, from 14 anatomical subjects (7 men and 7 women). The results showed the consistency of the existence and position of the subcostal perforating vessels.

The surface position of the perforating artery was constant, located: 1–3 cm lateral and downward from the 12th rib, at an average distance of 13.75 cm from the dorsal midline. The subcostal perforator then traveled along the surface of the external oblique muscle for an average length of 3.6 cm before dividing into 2–4 terminal branches. The caliber of the perforator varied from 1 to 3 mm with an average caliber of 2 mm. The total length of the pedicle (distance from the surface to the lateral border of the greater dorsalis muscle) varied from 7 to 14 cm with an average length of 10.5 cm.

Regarding the surface of the flap, the areas removed varied from a minimum of 9 × 12 cm to a maximum of 11 × 16 cm with an average paddle of 10 × 14 cm.

The results were similar to the results of the study on anatomical subjects, showing the constancy of the location of the exit point of the perforator of the subcostal artery and also the symmetrical character of the perforators in the same subject. However, there was no intra-individual correlation between the caliber of the right and left perforators.

Finally, it is interesting from an anatomical point of view to note that the authors did not find any nerve branches accompanying the perforating vessels.

11.2 Applications

We therefore conducted a study on anatomical subjects in order to assess whether it was possible to consider breast reconstruction using a perforating pedicled cutaneous-fatty flap of the “love handles” supplied by a perforating artery of the subcostal artery or SCAP flap (Fig. 11.7). Three dissection sessions were performed at the Fer à Moulin surgical school in Paris. A total of 12 flaps were obtained from 6 anatomical subjects.

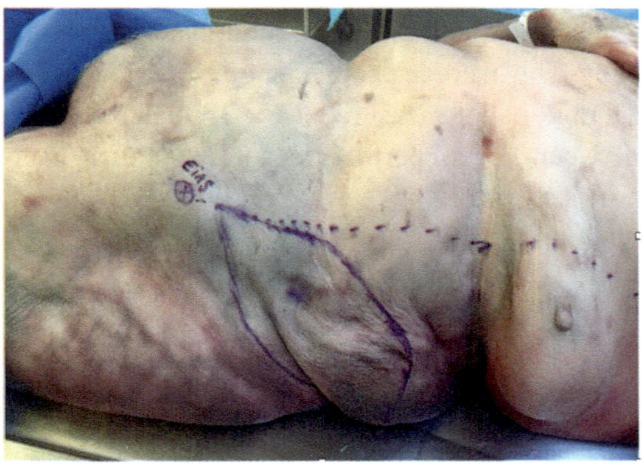

Fig. 11.7 Illustration of the subcostal artery perforator flap drawing on a cadaveric model. Note: Adapted from Delchet et al. [3], p. 1301, fig. 1A. Copyright 2019 by Elsevier. Reprinted with permission

11.3 Steps

First, the lower incision of the paddle was made down to the fascia of the external oblique muscle, followed by a careful dissection in search of the perforator of the subcutaneous artery, which runs from its exit point to the surface of the external oblique muscle. In order not to damage the perforator and its terminal branches, the dissection was performed from the bottom up, from the medial edge to the lateral edge.

Once the pedicle was located, it was dissected down to the last rib to obtain the longest possible pedicle length. The course of the subcutaneous pedicle was oblique superiorly and medially towards the lateral end of the last rib, and ran along the lower part of the rib to its posterior portion. The pedicle was systematically measured.

Once the pedicle was well individualized, the final skin incisions were made in order to raise our flap into a total vascular island (Fig 11.8).

The tunneling path, upward and inward on the anterolateral wall of the homolateral hemithorax, was dissected to be as direct as possible and to facilitate positioning of the paddle without plication of the pedicle. It was performed by finger dissection, in the subcutaneous fat, in front of the chest wall muscles. The flap was then tunneled and positioned in the breast area.

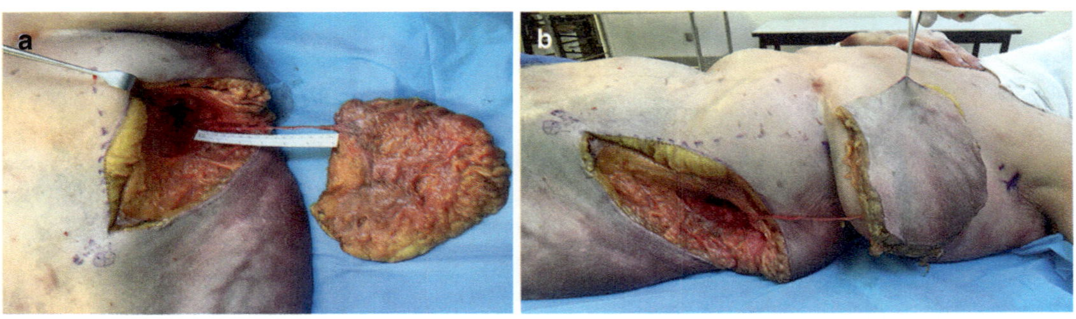

Fig. 11.8 Subcostal artery perforator flap with the dissected long pedicle. The flap was not lifted until the pedicle was perfectly individualized in order to not damage the subcostal pedicle. The second part of the operation consisted of tunneling the flap and positioning it at breast level. Note: Adapted from Delchet et al. [3], p. 1301, fig. 1B and 1C. (**a**) Pedicled SCAP flap dissected as a pure vascular block. Measurement of the pedicle length. (**b**) Pedicled SCAP flap located on the recipient site for a breast reconstruction. Copyright 2019 by Elsevier. Reprinted with permission

The pedicle was checked for tension, and for the absence of torsion or kinks that could hinder proper vascularization (Fig. 11.9).

Then the flap is partially de-epithelialized to be buried, while leaving a visible skin paddle, in order to facilitate postoperative monitoring (Fig. 11.10).

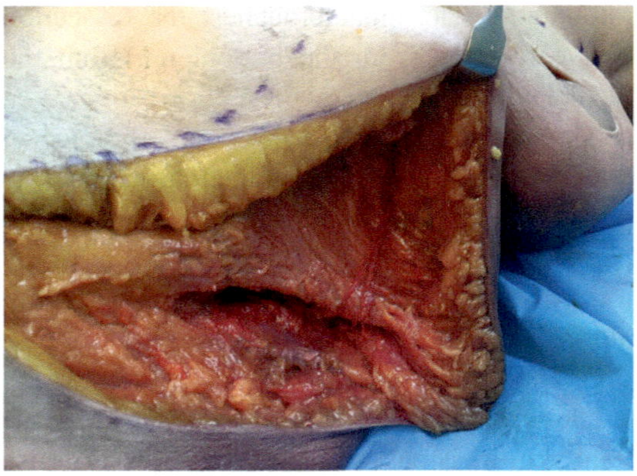

Fig. 11.9 Harvested tunnel for flap transference. Pedicle without tension

11.3.1 Regarding the Closure

The donor site was closed directly, plane by plane, leaving a scar on the flanks. The deep plane was closed with separate strands of Vicryl® 0, the subcutaneous plane with separate inverting strands of Vicryl®3/0, and the skin with an intradermal suture of Vicryl® 3/0 fast.

At the recipient site: closure of the flap at the level of the mammary region in two planes by absorbable sutures of the Vicryl® 3/0 type for the subcutaneous plane and the cutaneous plane by an intradermal suture of Vicryl rapide® 4/0.

During our study, the subcostal pedicle was constant: systematically found, and symmetrically. The average pedicle length was 17 cm. The average pallet measured 13 × 18 cm. We found between 1 and 3 perforators per flap with an average of 2 perforators per pallet.

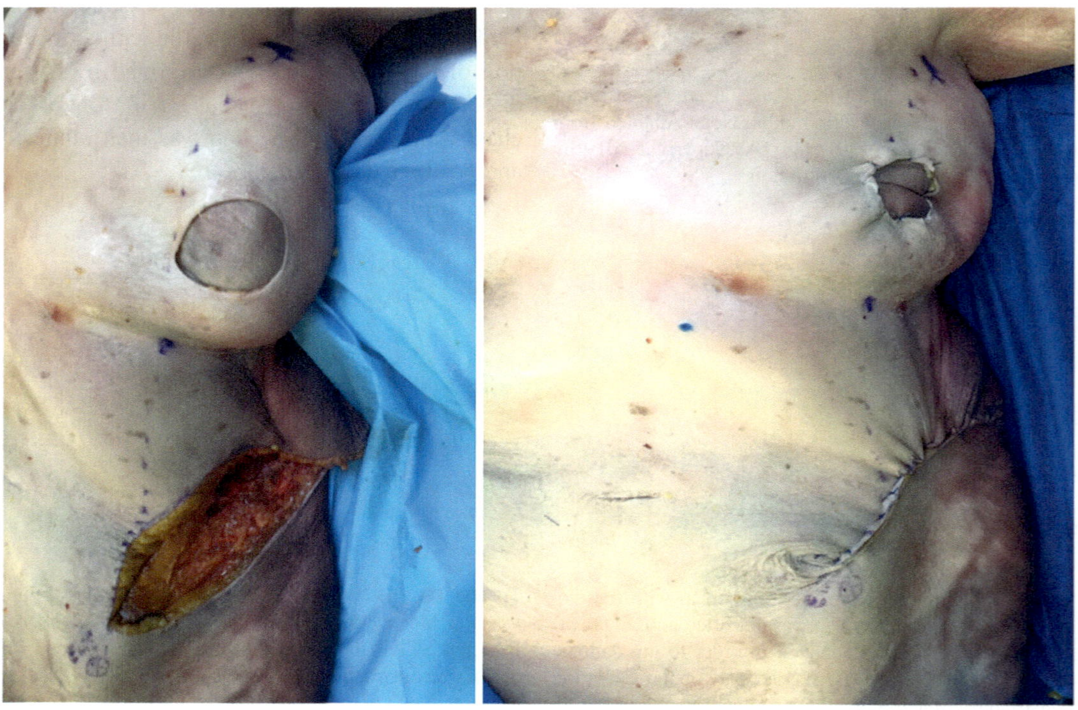

Fig. 11.10 Result after tunnelling and partial removal of the dermis. Skin flap is visible in order to allow monitoring of the flap and to enable areolar reconstruction at the same time. Note: Adapted from Delchet et al. [3], p. 1302, fig. 3B. Copyright 2019 by Elsevier. Reprinted with permission

Tips

In this study, we did not mention the need to perform para-clinical examinations. Nevertheless, preoperatively, an angioscan should be performed to ensure the integrity of the subcutaneous pedicle, to evaluate its caliber, and to identify the topography of the perforating vessels on the skin paddle of the flanks. In addition, the use of Doppler ultrasound, which has been previously described as a good means of accurately locating and marking vessels preoperatively will decrease the risk of pedicle injury. Postoperatively, the Doppler will allow monitoring of the flap.

In our case, the contralateral flap was systematically removed for the study. In the case of a living patient, in the event of unilateral reconstruction, we can achieve symmetrization of the "love handles" during the same operation or at a later date, by means of liposuction or by skin excision.

Among the limitations to the use of the SCAP flap, the main one is aesthetic with a donor site scar located in the flank region. However, the aesthetic sequelae of the SCAP flap remain limited because it will be more discreet than the scar of a dorsalis major flap and that of a DIEP flap. The SCAP scar can easily be camouflaged in daily life by an undergarment and will be shorter than a TRAM or DIEP flap donor site scar. Finally, the use of the excess cutaneous fat of the "love handles" gives the patient the satisfaction of a harmonious silhouette.

As in all breast reconstruction techniques using a flap, it will be necessary to remodel the flap if needed and/or to perform symmetrization, but also to reconstruct the areolar-mammary palette. Lipofilling will increase the volume of the reconstructed breast by autologous fat injection when the size of the breast is not satisfactory. It is also possible to intervene on the contralateral breast in order to reduce its volume while intervening on age-related breast ptosis.

Pitfalls

Care should be taken in patients with a history of abdominoplasty to ensure that the SCAP perforating arteries have not been damaged.

Tunneling of the flap should be very careful to avoid stripping of the pedicle. In addition, the pre-facial subcutaneous detachment should be wide to reduce the risk of pedicle compression.

After-Care

Doppler identification of the perforating artery in the preoperative phase may allow the flap to be monitored with a Doppler in the postoperative phase [4, 5].

A circular skin paddle can be left at the level of the future areola-nipple plate in order to allow monitoring of the flap (heat, staining, time of skin recoloration). In addition, this paddle can be used to prepare the reconstruction of the future nippleareolar complex.

11.4 Conclusion

In this experimental study on anatomical subjects, we have shown that breast reconstruction using a pedicled cutaneous-fat perforator flap of the "love handles" vascularized by a perforating artery of the subcutaneous artery or SCAP flap was feasible and reproducible.

We believe that this technique applied in breast reconstruction, can present a less invasive surgical alternative to DIEP or any other free flap in women with excess skin-fat of the flanks, and an interesting choice in women who have already benefited from an abdominoplasty, or who have undergone a failed DIEP flap [6].

A clinical application seems important to confirm the feasibility of this flap in breast reconstruction.

References

1. Feinendegen DL, Niederhäuser T, Herrmann G, Abderhalden S, Vögelin E, Banic A, Constantinescu MA. The subcostal artery perforator flap; an anatomical study. J Plast Reconstr Aesthet Surg. 2008;61(12):1496–502.
2. Feinendegen DL, Klos D. A subcostal artery perforator flap for a lumbar defect. Plast Reconstr Surg. 2002;109(7):2446.
3. Delchet O, et al. Experimental study of pedicled subcostal artery perforator (SCAP) flap: a new application in breast reconstruction. J Plast Reconstr Aesthet Surg. 2019;72(8):1301.
4. Blondeel P, Beyens G, Verhaeghe R, Van Landuyt K, Tonnard P, Monstrey SJ, Matton G. Doppler flowmetry in the planning of perforator flaps. Br J Plast Surg. 1998;51(3):202–9.
5. Blondeel PN, Van Landuyt KHI, Monstrey SJM, Hamdi M, Matton GE, Allen RJ, Dupin C, et al. The "gent" consensus on perforator flap terminology: preliminary definitions. Plast Reconstr Surg. 2003;112(5):1378.
6. Colebunders B, Depypere B, Van Landuyt K. The dog-ear flap as an alternative for breast reconstruction in patients who have already undergone a DIEAP flap. J Plast Reconstr Aesthet Surg. 2016;69(5):594–7.

The Latisimus Dorsi Miniflap

12

Richard Rainsbury

Contents

12.1 Introduction

Latissimus dorsi (LD) reconstruction was first described by Tansini in 1906 [1], and was used to reconstruct the large soft tissue defects following radical mastectomy. In the 1970s it was 'rediscovered' and has become a popular choice for breast reconstruction, with significant advantages over implant-only reconstruction in many patients. The use of the latissiumus dorsi muscle for volume replacement after breast-conserving surgery was first described in Japan in 1990 [2], and a new modification of this technique—the LD miniflap, or 'miniflap'—was described and introduced by Rainsbury into the UK in 1994 [3, 4]. Since then, the ability of miniflaps to reconstruct large resection defects after partial mastectomy has been confirmed, avoiding the need for full mastectomy in increasing numbers of patients [5].

R. Rainsbury (✉)
Breast Unit, Royal Hampshire County Hospital, Winchester, UK
e-mail: rrainsbury@aol.com

M. Hamdi et al. (eds.), *Pedicled Flaps in Partial Breast Reconstruction*,
https://doi.org/10.1007/978-3-031-08483-6_12

12.2 Indications

The main indications for considering a miniflap today are summarized in Table 12.1. Patient and tumour factors are equally important when selecting this approach, and very often the presence of several of these factors taken together will influence a decision to go ahead.

Volume replacement with a miniflap provides an increasingly useful third alternative to wide excision or mastectomy for a patient with a bulky tumour in a small- to medium-sized breast who wants to avoid more major surgery or an ugly deformity after conservation. The chance of a poor cosmetic outcome becomes very significant once more than 15% of the breast has been resected, particularly from the medial and lower poles [6]. Perforator flaps are becoming an increasingly popular method of volume replacement, as they require less extensive surgery, often carried out as a day case. The main indication for a perforator flap is for those patients with tumours in the outer half of the breast, with a predicted volume loss <100 g. By contrast, the miniflap can be used to reconstruct defects in any quadrant of the breast, following resections of up <450 g [5]. The technique is particularly useful following the resection of bulky tumours in the medial, upper central and lower parts of the breast, as perforator flaps don't have sufficient 'reach' and volume to reconstruct these areas.

A full evaluation of the type of patient and extent of a tumour is an essential part of the preoperative workup (Table 12.1). This is true for tumours in any location, both for in situ and invasive disease. Complete local excision with tumour-free margins is the fundamental goal, whether the tumour is located in a single breast quadrant, or spans two of more quadrants. Conservation using miniflaps is also oncologically safe when resecting either unifocal or multifocal lesions providing that clear pathological margins are confirmed [5]. The minimum preoperative workup should therefore include mammography and ultrasound, together with MRI if a lobular carcinoma or multifocal disease is suspected or in patients with dense breasts (BIRADS 5).

Table 12.1 Main indications for breast conservation with miniflaps

Patient factors	Tumour factors
Breast <500 g	Any quadrant
15–70% volume loss	In situ disease
Mastectomy declined	Invasive disease
Contralateral surgery declined	Unifocal or multifocal tumours
Radiotherapy planned	<T4 tumours
Good performance status	<400 g resections
Intact LD muscle	Clear margins

12.3 Deciding on the Suitability of a Miniflap

Three key questions need to be considered when assessing your patient's suitability for volume replacement with a miniflap:

Firstly, is this procedure an appropriate option? Indications include a predicted volume loss of 15–70%, tumours in any part of the breast, particularly the central, upper central, upper inner and lower pole of the breast, and a patient who's fully informed the procedure and prepared to accept the risks. Is she aware that if a total mastectomy is needed in the future, she will have 'used up' one of her options for reconstruction?

Secondly, is this a better option than a therapeutic mammoplasty? Does your patient have moderate to small-sized breasts (<500 cc), is she happy with her breast size, and would she prefer to avoid the contralateral surgery that may be necessary to achieve symmetry after therapeutic mammoplasty?

Lastly, should the procedure be carried out as a one-stage or a two-stage procedure? If simultaneous resection and reconstruction is planned, is your pathology department willing and able to provide a rapid frozen section report on resection margins? Will your theatre schedule accommodate the extra time required, and does your patient understand the implications of a false negative result? A two-stage approach is indicated if your pathologists aren't able to provide intraoperative margin analysis, or if the partial mastectomy is for DCIS, lobular cancer or after neoadjuvant treatment, when frozen section margin analysis is unreliable.

12.4 Operative Technique

A careful preoperative mark-up is key to achieving a successful outcome. This should be carried out with the patient on a couch or bed, propped up with pillows at 45°. The borders of the tumour and the resection margin needs to be carefully marked in the skin, together with an 'access tunnel' of breast tissue between the tumour and the lateral incision (Fig. 12.1). This is resected along with the tumour and will eventually accommodate the proximal part of the miniflap as it passes into the resection defect, preventing an ugly lateral bulge.

12.4.1 Incisions

The incision chosen will depend on the position of the tumour, and whether the procedure requires removal of skin. There are two main choices:

1. *The 'classical' miniflap operation:* this is carried out through a single lateral 'lazy S' incision. This runs down from the apex of the axilla, along the lateral border of the breast to the outer limit of the inframammary fold. The whole operation, including tumour resection, axillary procedure (sentinel node or clearance), harvesting a myofascial LD miniflap, and reconstruction of the resection defect is performed through this incision. This approach is best for tumours in the upper outer, upper inner, medial and central zones of the breast (Fig. 12.2).
2. *The 'myocutaneous' miniflap operation:* when skin needs to be resected to achieve clearance over the tumour (e.g., the nipple areolar complex for subareolar tumours) or to provide additional volume replacement (e.g., for lower pole tumours), a myocutaneous miniflap is the best choice. When reconstructing lower pole tumours, the limited 'reach' of a myofascial flap without a skin island prevents the transposition of sufficient volume to this more remote location. This problem can be over-

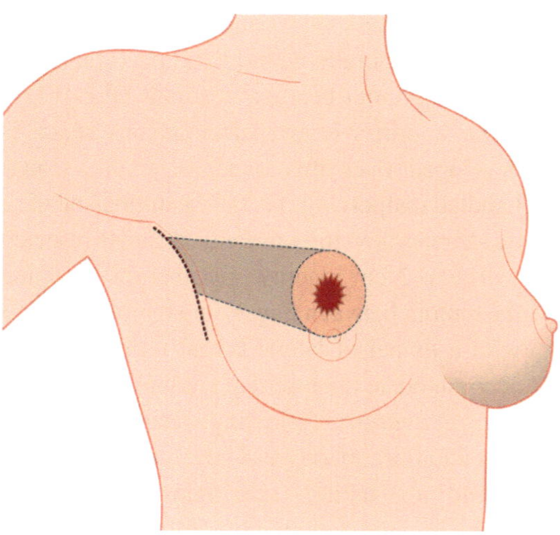

Fig. 12.1 Mark-up outlining tumour, resection margin, access tunnel and incision

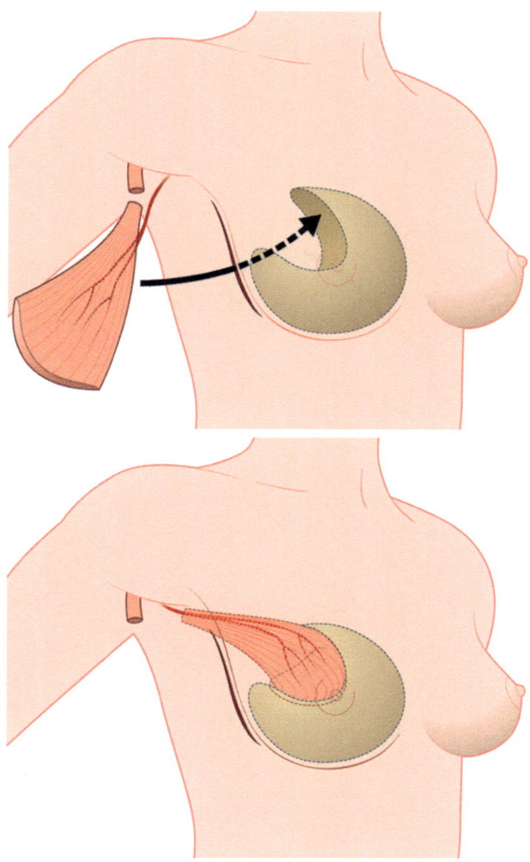

Fig. 12.2 The 'classical' miniflap operation

come by harvesting a skin island through a dorsal incision positioned more distally on the miniflap (Fig. 12.3).

12.4.2 The 'Classical' Miniflap Operation

1. *Patient position:* the patient is fixed in the lateral decubitus position, and the use of straps across the flexed hips and knees separated by pillows, helps to protect pressure points, and to maintain this position throughout the procedure. The uppermost shoulder is fixed carefully at 90° of abduction in an adjustable padded right-angled armrest. These key steps help to prevent a brachial plexus traction injury as a result of over-abduction and distraction of the shoulder joint in the anaesthetized patient (Fig. 12.4).

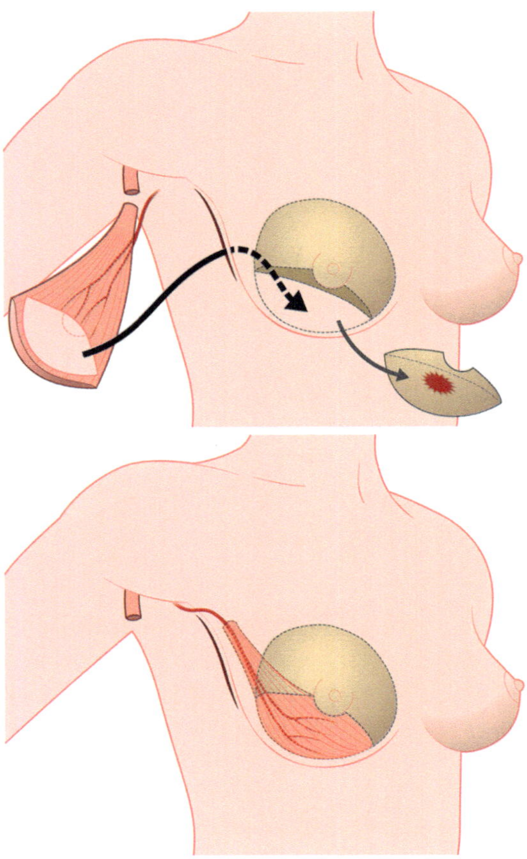

Fig. 12.3 The 'myocutaneous' miniflap

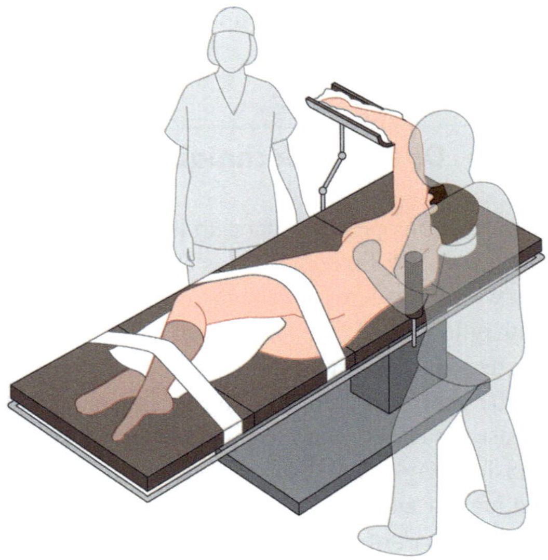

Fig. 12.4 Patient position and fixation

2. *Incision:* subcutaneous infiltration of the whole operative field with a dilute adrenalin/saline solution (1:250,000) helps to prevent bleeding and keeps the tissues well-hydrated. Infiltration runs anteriorly from the incision over the tumour-bearing quadrant, and posteriorly over the surface of the miniflap. The incision is now extended from the axilla to the inframammary fold, and the lateral edge of the pectoralis major muscle is identified lying deeply in the incision (Fig. 12.5).
3. *Partial mastectomy:* a retromammary space is then developed, dissecting medially from the edge of pectoralis deep to the pectoral fascia and the tumour-bearing quadrant (Fig. 12.6). Next, a mirror-image subcutaneous space is developed over this quadrant with a long-handled scalpel (Fig. 12.7). The tumour-bearing quadrant is now fully mobilized, and is resected with a 1–2 cm macroscopic margin, grasping the tumour between fingers and thumb, together with a tunnel of lateral breast tissue that will accommodate the miniflap tendon.
4. *Margin analysis:* following specimen orientation and intraoperative X-ray, attention is now turned to taking specimens for margin analysis. This may involve intraoperative frozen section analysis if facilities are available, or subsequent paraffin section examination.

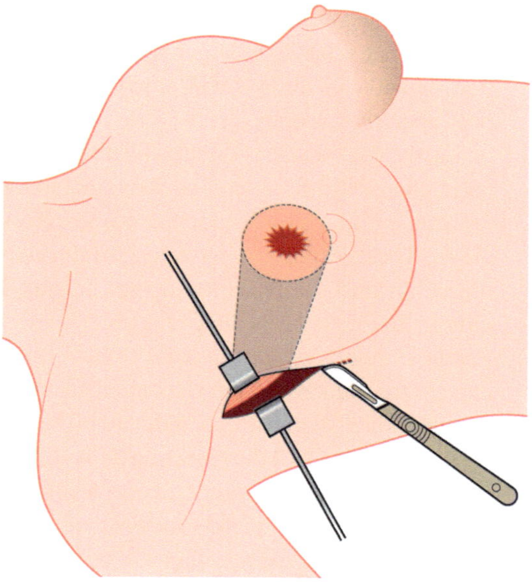

Fig. 12.5 Deepening the incision to reveal lateral border of pectoralis major

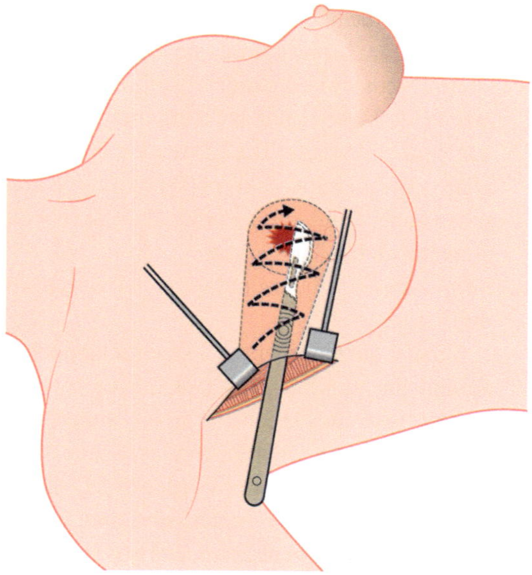

Fig. 12.7 Development of subcutaneous space over tumour by sharp dissection

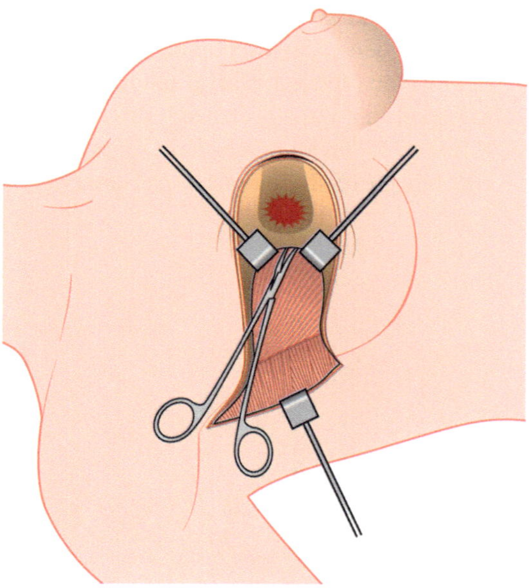

Fig. 12.6 Developing retromammary space behind tumour-bearing quadrant

Either way, bed biopsies are taken from the medial, lateral, superior and inferior aspects of the wall of the resection cavity. Any areas suspicious of residual tumour are also targeted, and all bed biopsies are sent for frozen or paraffin section analysis.

The entire cavity wall is then inked in situ with methylene blue, helping to identify the surface adjacent to the specimen. The whole cavity wall is excised as two continuous 'shavings', from the lower and upper aspects. Each of these specimens is stained blue on the inner surface to help subsequent orientation. If tumour is detected in any of the bed biopsies, a second biopsy is taken from the same position on the new cavity wall created by cavity shaving. If this is positive, the process may be repeated. In the rare situation where multiple bed biopsies remain positive, the procedure is normally terminated, awaiting a formal pathology report. Some patients give preoperative consent to proceed to mastectomy with or without immediate reconstruction if this situation arises.

5. *Axillary procedure:* if a decision has been made to perform a one-stage procedure with a sentinel node biopsy, intraoperative examination of the nodes simplifies the procedure, as a positive result may indicate immediate clearance. This is much easier than performing delayed clearance for positive nodes, after the flap has been harvested and the transposed pedicle crosses a recently dissected axilla.

Normally the axillary vessels are collapsed and appear to lie more superficially in a laterally-positioned patient. Failure to recognize a collapsed axillary vein may lead to inadvertent damage. The LD tendon is divided after identification and preservation of the subscapular and thoracodorsal vessels, in preparation for flap harvest.

6. *Flap harvest:* the miniflap is harvested in three steps.

   Firstly, development of a superficial pocket around the muscle. This is achieved by dissecting just underneath Scarpa's superficial fascia to create a rectangular space that extends from the anterior border of LD to the level of the scapula posteriorly, and to the level of the costal margin inferiorly (Fig. 12.8). To reconstruct larger resection defects, the volume of this flap can be increased by extending the posterior and inferior limits of the dissection.

   Secondly, a mirror-image pocket is developed deep to the flap, between LD and serratus anterior. The level of dissection of both the superficial and deep pockets aims to leave a layer of fat attached to both surfaces of the flap, increasing the overall volume available for transfer. Aiming to harvest a flap with a volume that's 10–20% larger than the resection defect will allow for a small degree of post-operative atrophy.

   Lastly, the muscle is divided all around the perimeter of the dissection pockets, including division of all fascial attachments to terres major. The miniflap is now delivered through the axilla into the resection defect, attached only by the vascular pedicle (Fig. 12.9).

7. *Reconstruction of the partial mastectomy defect:* the 'reach' of the flap is checked to confirm that there is enough mobility to ensure that it will fill the resection defect. *This is a really key step*, as failure to divide all fascial attachments completely means that a significant volume of the miniflap will be wasted, and will come to sit in the axilla, rather than in the defect. Two steps will help to overcome this problem. Firstly, check that *all* fascial attachments are divided completely, including the full thickness of the tendon and the entire layer of dense fascia running between the miniflap and terres major. If the reach is still too short, an extra 3–5cm of 'reach' can be achieved by dividing the main serratus anterior branch of the thoracodorsal artery. The

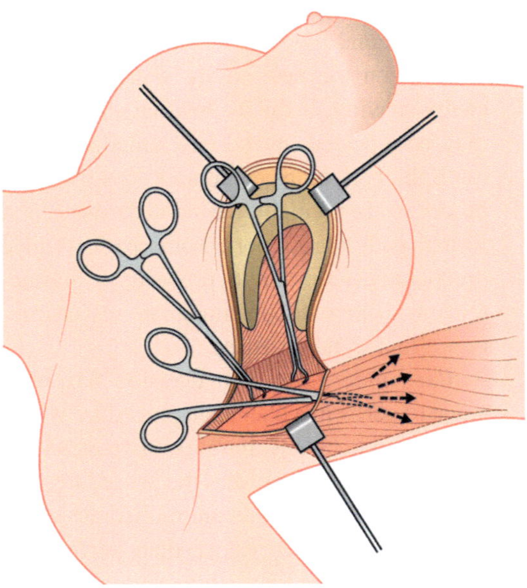

Fig. 12.8 Developing superficial pocket over miniflap, deep to Scarpa's fascia

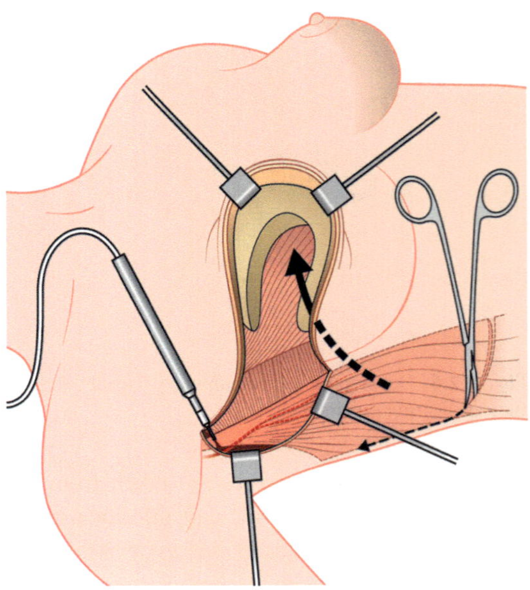

Fig. 12.9 Mobilization of miniflap by division of muscle and tendon

overall distance between the proximal and distal cut ends of the tendon should be between 7 and 10 cm in a fully mobilized miniflap (Fig. 12.10).

The miniflap tendon is now sutured to the lateral border of pectoralis major without tension. This prevents the flap subsequently retracting back into the axilla, and protects the vascular pedicle from twisting and traction injury. The flap is modelled with a few interrupted sutures into a shape that matches the resection defect, before being sutured loosely to the walls of the defect (Fig. 12.10).

8. *Closure and post-operative management:* the operative site is closed over at least 1 suction drain, positioned so that the tip lies along the inferior margin of the donor cavity (Fig. 12.11). A 'quilted' closure of this sizeable cavity with interrupted sutures helps to reduce the size and duration of post-operative seroma. Two specific complications may occur in the first 24 h, and need to be excluded.

   Firstly, flap viability should be confirmed by asking the patient to actively adduct her shoulder, pushing down with her hand onto her hip. This will cause contraction of the flap where it lies in the resection defect, and the contraction should be clearly visible through the skin. Contraction may be difficult to demonstrate in the first 2–4 h due to transient neuropraxia of the thoracodorsal nerve, but should have returned by 6–8 h. If there is any doubt about viability, the patient should be re-explored without delay to exclude and relieve any venous congestion—the most common reason for flap loss.

   Secondly, check for early bleeding into the breast and donor cavity. An expanding haematoma in either site demands early exploration, evacuation and control. Haematomas in the donor site may go undetected unless the patient is examined from behind in the sitting position.

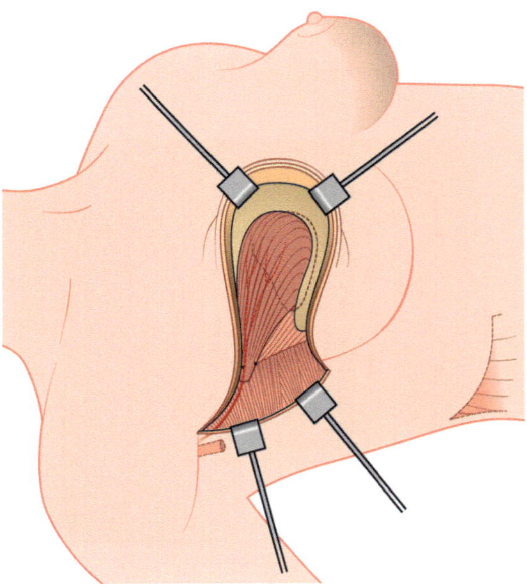

Fig. 12.10 Position of miniflap in resection defect after division of all fascial attachments

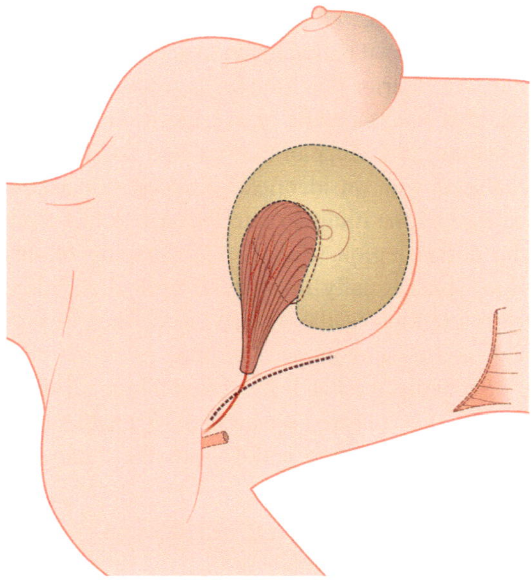

Fig. 12.11 Appearance after closure

12.4.3 The Myocutaneous Miniflap Operation

This variation of the 'classical' miniflap operation differs in two main aspects.

Firstly, the tumour-bearing quadrant is approached directly, rather than via the retromammary approach. A subareolar tumour is resected together with the nipple and areola via a circumareolar incision. This allows excellent access together with an 'en bloc' excision of a tunnel of breast parenchyma to accommodate the flap. An inferior pole tumour is resected directly together with a paddle or overlying skin. In both situations, the shape of the resected skin island is replaced with an identically-shaped skin island carried by the miniflap into the skin defect from the dorsal region (Fig. 12.12). Shaping of this skin island usually involves de-epithelialisation, with retention of the underlying dermis, to provide additional volume replacement.

Secondly, the flap is harvested through a small dorsal skin ellipse, positioned to enable easy transfer of the skin paddle into the cutaneous defect. The elliptical skin island needs to be positioned more distally on the flap when reconstructing defects in the remote lower inner quadrant, to enable transposition to this quadrant without tension (Fig. 12.3). Central defects are usually replaced with a miniflap carrying circular skin paddle matching the circular defect, ready for nipple reconstruction (Fig. 12.13a, b).

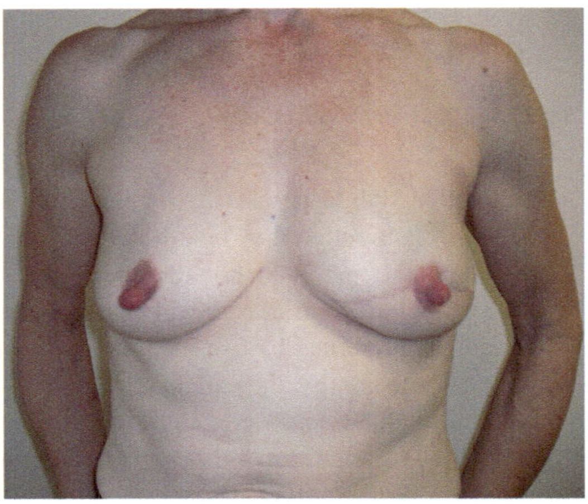

Fig. 12.12 Myocutaneous minflap reconstruction after lower pole resection of 75 mm DCIS

The rest of the operation is much the same as the 'classical' myofascial miniflap procedure. Sometimes final positioning and shaping of the flap is made easier by turning the patient into the supine position.

12.4.4 Tips for a Successful Result

- Develop skills in latissimus dorsi reconstruction after total mastectomy first.
- Select patients with bulky tumours normally treated by mastectomy.
- Take time to mark-up and position the patient carefully.
- Use high intensity directional lighting, infiltration and haemostatic dissection equipment that greatly simplify the procedure.
- Develop confidence in a 2-stage approach before considering a 1-stage operation with intra-operative margin analysis,
- Remember that the division of all the fascial attachments including the tendon will enable

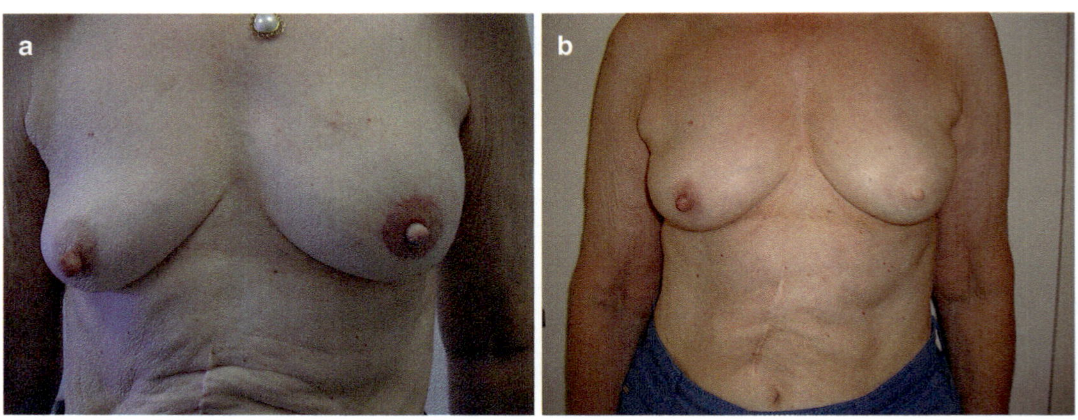

Fig. 12.13 (**a**) Myocutaneous miniflap and nipple-areola reconstruction after upper pole resection for 40 mm cancer. (**b**) Same patient 10 year after surgery and radiotherapy

the whole miniflap to be moved into the resection defect.

- Over-replace the resected volume by around 10–15% to allow for a small amount of irradiation-induced flap atrophy.

12.5 Outcomes

The outcomes of miniflap procedures are currently based on small retrospective studies from single centres (level 3 evidence). It is hoped that the rising popularity of a range of new volume replacement techniques will encourage coordinated prospective data collection, enabling more objective outcome reporting. The outcomes most important to patients include early and later clinical complications, oncological outcomes and the impact of these procedures on cosmesis, quality of life and well-being.

12.5.1 Complications

1. *Early complications:* 28/284 patients (10%) undergoing miniflap procedures on our unit developed complications requiring intervention by 30 days. These included one total flap loss, and skin necrosis (<1%), infection (<2%), haematoma and seroma (<3% each) and 2 cases of brachial plexopathy with full recovery. These rates compare very favourably with large prospective audits of implant reconstruction after total mastectomy, reporting infection rates as high as 25%, and major complications in 15% [7] (www.ic.nhs.uk/mbr).
2. *Late complications:* 85/284 patients (30%) of our patients required subsequent procedures (95 months mean follow-up). Two thirds of these involved reduction, augmentation or lipomodelling, to achieve symmetry or to correct deformity, with the remainder requesting nipple reconstruction or scar revision. This compares favourably with implant reconstruction, with 78% of our patients following implant-assisted latissimus dorsi reconstruction requiring an unplanned surgical procedure by 60 months mean follow-up [8]. These patients also experienced sensory loss over a significantly greater surface area (65%) of the reconstructed breast compared with only 10% of the surface area after miniflap reconstruction ($p = <0.05$).

12.5.2 Oncological Outcomes

The oncological effectiveness of miniflaps can be measured in the short term by recording rates of complete local excision as judged by margin positivity, and in the longer-term by rates of local recurrence and control.

1. *Completeness of local excision:* in a recent study of 'extreme' resections (tumour span ≥50 mm) carried out on our unit, the liberal use of intra-operative frozen section margin analysis resulted in a very low re-excision rate of 5% [5]. The ability to resect bulky tumours without fear of residual disease or major local deformity is a major strength of miniflaps as well as other oncoplastic techniques. Typically, resected specimens weigh 150–200 g (Table 12.2), but multi-quadrant resections may weigh >450g when resecting large tumours with spans >100mm [5]. A recent meta-analysis compared outcomes in >3000 patients following oncoplastic conservation with >5000 following conventional breast-conserving surgery [9]. Although there are limitations with this approach, women treated by oncoplastic techniques had significantly fewer re-excisions for positive resection margins.
2. *Local recurrence and control:* low annual local recurrence rates have been reported by six authors after miniflap procedures (Table 12.2), with one study from our own unit reporting an estimated 10 years local recurrence-free survival of 1.1% after extensive local resections [5]. Significantly lower local recurrence rates were reported following volume replacement compared with standard breast-conserving surgery (3.6 versus 7.0, $p < 0.0001$) in a meta-analysis of 8000 patients

Table 12.2 Studies including resection details and local recurrence rates

Author	Number	T size (mm)	Weight (g)	LR/FU (mo)
Raja et al. [4]	20	25	57% >150	NS
Gendy et al. [8]	49	22	NS	2/53
Nano et al. [14]	18	33	130	0/24
Navin et al. [15]	51	20	217	0/33
Rusby et al. [16]	110	34	207	1/41
Hernanz et al. [17]	41	22	167	1/54
Pearce et al. [5]	62	68	222	5/91

NS not stated

[9]. These impressive results have been achieved in spite of performing conservation for patients with more extensive disease normally treated by mastectomy [10–13]

12.6 Cosmesis, Quality of Life and Well-Being

There is a strong relationship between the physical outcomes of breast conservation and levels of overall satisfaction as judged by quality of life (QoL) and well-being. These can be assessed either by investigating patient-reported outcomes or by direct comparison of a range of outcomes with an established alternative such as a skin-sparing mastectomy and immediate breast reconstruction.

1. *Patient-reported outcomes after miniflaps:* the use of the Breast-Q self-administered questionnaire is a popular, validated method for the assessment of QoL after oncoplastic and reconstructive surgery [18]. It has been used in some 50 studies, and in many more with minor modifications [19]. We investigated patient-reported outcomes after miniflap procedures by distributing the Breast-Q questionnaire to 221 patients (age 49 [30–70] years, follow-up 112 [6–281] months, tumour diameter 32.5 [5–100] mm). Scores for breast appearance, and physical, emotional and sexual well-being were generated [20].

An excellent or good overall experience was reported by 78% respondents, with 80% reporting satisfaction with the physical outcomes of surgery (Figs. 12.12, 12.13, and 12.14). Eighty-eight percent felt that a miniflap procedure was definitely preferable to a mastectomy, and 76% had no regrets. Functional disturbance was uncommon at 7 years, with <7% reporting back or shoulder problems and <1% experiencing any impact on daily living. Mean outcome scores for breast appearance, physical and emotional appearance were high, and increased with length of follow-up, beyond 15 years. Similar high scores were returned by a subgroup of 15 patients following 'extreme resections' (≥50 mm) [5]. Finally, the overall scores compared favourably with those returned by patients following mastectomy and immediate autologous latissimus dorsi reconstruction (www.ic.nhs.uk/mbr).

Few other authors have investigated the long-term impact of volume replacement on overall satisfaction. QoL and self-esteem scores following volume replacement has been shown to be higher following volume replacement, compared with standard breast-conserving surgery, using the SF-36 questionnaire [21].

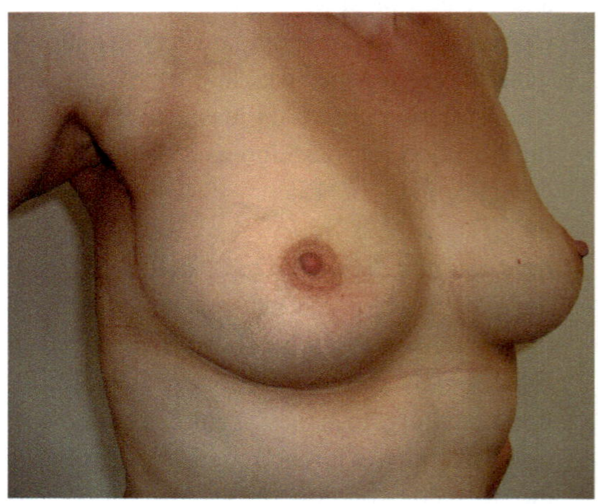

Fig. 12.14 Classical miniflap 2 years after resection of 177 mm multicentric DCIS from upper pole and radiotherapy

2. *Comparative studies:* three studies have compared outcomes after miniflaps with those after skin-sparing mastectomy with immediate reconstruction. The first study reported post-operative complications, further surgical interventions, nipple sensory loss, restricted activities and cosmetic outcome assessed by panel assessment [8]. These were all better in the miniflap group than in the group of patients undergoing mastectomy and immediate breast reconstruction. Anxiety about residual cancer and ease of breast self-examination were similar in both groups.

   A second study compared women undergoing miniflap reconstruction with those having standard breast-conserving surgery or mastectomy and immediate whole breast reconstruction. Patients with miniflaps reported better shape, symmetry and less self-consciousness [22].

   Finally, patients undergoing conservation with immediate volume replacement have been compared with those undergoing nipple-sparing mastectomy and immediate reconstruction with a latissimus dorsi flap. Evaluation by patient questionnaires and objective scoring of photographs using the Harris scale reported no significant difference in aesthetic results in the two groups [23].

12.7 Summary

- Our experience of using miniflaps to reconstruct partial mastectomy defects in almost 300 patients has confirmed good long-term clinical, oncological and cosmetic outcomes.
- These favourable results depend on appropriate patient and tumour selection, careful preoperative mark-up combined with meticulous intraoperative technique, and above all, efforts to achieve complete local excision.
- Complication and revision rates are low compared with more major alternatives including mastectomy and implant-based reconstruction.
- Unlike other types of volume replacement, miniflaps have sufficient volume and 'reach' to reconstruct bulky defects in any quadrant-including the difficult medial and lower quadrants.
- Indications for miniflaps have been extended to include large multicentric and multiquadrant tumours.
- These 'extreme' procedures can resect up to 70% of breast volume.
- Clear-margin resection results in good long-term local control in a group of patients traditionally treated by mastectomy.
- Patients in our series report long-lasting satisfaction and well-being up to 15 years and beyond.

References

1. Tanzini I. Spora il mio nuova processo di amputazione della mammilla. Riforma Med. 1906;22:757–62.
2. Noguchi M, Taniya T, Miyasaki I, et al. Immediate transposition of a latissumus dorsi muscle for correcting a postquadrantectomy breast deformity in Japanese patients. Int Surg. 1990;75:166–70.
3. Rainsbury R. Breast conservation with latissimus dorsi miniflap: a new technique. Eur J Surg Oncol. 1994;20:102–3.
4. Raja M, Straker V, Rainsbury R. Extending the role of breast-conserving surgery by immediate volume replacement. Br J Surg. 1997;84:101–5.
5. Pearce B, Fiddes R, Paramanathan N, et al. Extreme oncoplastic conservation is a safe new alternative to mastectomy. Eur J Surg Oncol. 2020;46:71–6.
6. Cochrane R, Valasiaou P, Wilson A, et al. Cosmesis and satisfaction after breast-conserving surgery correlates with the percentage of breast volume excised. Br J Surg. 2003;90:1505–9.
7. Potter S, Conroy E, Cutress R, et al. Short-term safety and outcomes of mastectomy and immediate implant-based breast reconstruction with and without mesh (iBRA): a multicenter, prospective cohort study. Lancet Oncol. 2019;20:254–66.
8. Gendy R, Abel J, Rainsbury R. Impact of skin-sparing mastectomy with immediate reconstruction and breast-sparing reconstruction with miniflaps on the outcomes of oncoplastic breast surgery. Br J Surg. 2003;90:433–9.
9. Losken A, Dugal C, Styblo T, et al. A meta-analysis comparing breast conservation therapy alone to the oncoplastic technique. Ann Plast Surg. 2014;72:145–9.
10. Asgeirsson K, Rasheed T, McCulley S, et al. Oncological and cosmetic outcomes of oncoplastic breast conserving surgery. Eur J Surg Oncol. 2005;31:817–23.

11. Chakravorty A, Shrestha A, Sanmugalingam A, et al. How safe is oncoplastic breast conservation? Comparative analysis with standard breast conserving surgery. Eur J Surg Oncol. 2012;38:395–8.
12. Clough K, Lewis J, Couturaud B, et al. Oncoplastic techniques allow extensive resections for breast-conserving therapy of breast carcinomas. Ann Surg. 2003;237:26–34.
13. Rietjens M, Urban C, Rey P, et al. Long-term oncological results of breast conservative treatment with oncoplastic surgery. Breast. 2007;16:387–95.
14. Nano M, Gill P, Kollias L, et al. Breast volume replacement using the latissimus dorsi miniflap. ANZ J Surg. 2004;74:98–104.
15. Navin C, Agrawal A, Kolar A. The use of latissimus dorsi miniflap for reconstruction following breast-conserving surgery: experience of a small breast unit in a district hospital. World J Surg. 2007;31:46–50.
16. Rusby J, Paramanathan N, Laws S, et al. Immediate latissimus dorsi miniflap volume replacement for partial mastectomy: use of intra-operative frozen sections to confirm negative margins. Am J Surg. 2008;196:512–8.
17. Hemanz F, Sanchez S, Cerdeira M, et al. Long-term results of breast conservation and immediate volume replacement with myocutaneous latissimus dorsi flap. World J Surg Oncol. 2011;9:159–66.
18. Pusic A, Klassen A, Scott A, et al. Development of a new patient-reported outcome measure for breast surgery: the BREAST-Q. Plast Reconstr Surg. 2009;124:345–53.
19. Cohen W, Mundy L, Ballard T, et al. The BREAST-Q in surgical research: a review of the literature 2009-2015. J Plast Reconstr Aesthet Surg. 2016;69:149–62.
20. Chand N, Browne V, Paramanathan P, et al. Patient-reported outcomes are better after oncoplastic breast conservation than after mastectomy and autologous reconstruction. Plast Reconstr Surg Glob Open. 2017;5:1–9.
21. Veiga D, Veiga-Filho J, Ribeiro L, et al. Quality-of-life and self-esteem outcomes after oncoplastic breast-conserving surgery. Plast Reconstr Surg. 2010;125:811–7.
22. Dixon J, Venizelos B, Chan P. Latissimus dorsi miniflap: a technique for extending breast conservation. Breast. 2002;11:58–65.
23. Bassiouny M, et al. Quadrantectomy and nipple saving mastectomy in treatment of early breast cancer: feasibility and aesthetic results of adjunctive latissmus dorsi breast reconstruction. J Egypt Natl Canc Inst. 2005;17:149–5.

13 Pedicle Perforator Flaps with "Invisible" Scar

Andrii Zhygulin

Contents

13.1 Introduction

Modern breast cancer (BC) treatment should take into consideration the quality of life of the patient during all stages of the treatment. Hence the treatment paradigm shifts towards less aggressive and traumatic approach. Obviously, breast preservation is better for the quality of the patient's life than breast removal in radical cancer surgery if it is technically and oncologically possible. However, the preservation of the breast is not the aim in itself; the goal is to achieve the good quality of life for each patient. Modern breast cancer surgery is based on the principle of minimizing glandular deformity caused by the oncological procedure. But we believe that oncoplastic surgery has to achieve the best aesthetic and also functional results. Therefore, new terminology was coined: "oncocosmetic" or "oncoesthetic" surgery, which emphasizes the importance of aesthetic outcomes. From this point of view, the surgeon and the patient should choose one of the two approaches: one where the breast does not change, or another, which improves the appearance of the breast. If the patient does not want to change the breasts, the first approach should be chosen. It is especially important when operating younger patients with smaller breast. Following the proposed logic, the results of the operation, ideally, should be invisible. Thus, we would like to share our concept of "invisible surgery." It is the combination of certain techniques that allows for complete restoration of the original shape and size of the breast after tumor removal, while avoiding scars on the breast. These techniques are based on certain principles:

A. Zhygulin (✉)
Breast Center, LISOD Hospital of Israeli Oncology, Kyiv, Ukraine
e-mail: zhygulin@lisod.ua

M. Hamdi et al. (eds.), *Pedicled Flaps in Partial Breast Reconstruction*,
https://doi.org/10.1007/978-3-031-08483-6_13

1. No scars on the breast. The incision is made in the lateral, lower-lateral, or lower contour of the breast in the submammary fold, with adoption to natural shape and measures of the breast and axillary region—we call it "contour access." The location of the incisions should be planned in such a way that they are as hidden as possible. All surgical actions are performed under the skin. It needs extensive mobilization of the skin and parenchyma within the breast.
2. Complete restoration of the breast shape and volume. To achieve this, we use the wide mobilization of the parenchyma with redistribution to close the defect if it is small or use flaps from surrounding regions (axillary and epigastric) if it is large.
3. Oncological safety through the intraoperative margin control. Due to the principle of "no inked margin" every millimeter does matter. To minimize the rate of re-excisions the lesion and the specimen's margins should be marked and assessed. The surgeon should carefully control it and closely cooperate with the radiologist and pathologist. In our practice, the pathologist always evaluates the specimen in the operating room after the surgeon's color marking of the margins. It is significantly simplifying the pathological examination and, if needed, the location of intraoperative re-excision. This also increases the surgeon's responsibility for the final oncological result.

However, during surgery, an extension of the resection margins may be required and the defect can become larger than planned. Therefore, when planning the surgery, the surgeon must anticipate, consider, and plan for possible changes in the surgical plan in advance. It is crucial to do this in such a way that each stage of the surgery does not complicate the following potential surgical scenarios. The operation is divided into stages, and the final cascade of stages has to be chosen according to the final size and geometry of the defect. It should be done only after confirmation of the free resection margins by the radiologist and pathologist in the operating theatre. We call it the "scenario strategy." Each of these scenarios should be carefully planned, prepared for, and most importantly discussed with the patient before surgery, since the final option is selected in the operating theatre. Thus, a combination of the tactical principle of "invisible surgery" (number of techniques that completely restore the breast without visible scars), and a strategic "scenario principle" that provides the optimal consistency and interrelation of these techniques is proposed. The purpose of this concept is to preserve the initial appearance of the breast after oncological surgery to the maximum extent, regardless of the chosen technique. Regional flaps are an important part of this concept. Some other techniques using the breast parenchyma and parenchymal flaps as well as nipple-sparing mastectomy with immediate reconstruction are also discussed.

13.2 Anatomy

The anatomy of the vessels in the axillary region is already well-presented in the previous chapters. This network includes many blood vessels that feed the tissues that can be used for breast restoration both in the breast itself and in the surrounding areas. These are the branches and perforators from Lateral Thoracic Artery (LTAP), Lateral Intercostal Artery (LICAP), and Superficial Epigastric Artery (SEAP). The important issue is the location of the main branches of a. thoracica interna, a. thoracica lateralis, and a. thoracoacromialis coming to the breast closer to the skin of the breast. It is used in clinical practice. Corduff and Taylor (2004) investigated the breast blood supply and proposed a reduction mammoplasty technique based on this principle. It allows for performing significant planar resections and parenchyma incisions in the basal area of the breast without compromising the breast parenchyma and skin blood supply, which could be effectively used in oncoplastic surgery for tumor removal.

13.3 Application

The main paradigm of the proposed concept is an extreme personalization of oncoplastic surgery aiming at the maximal aesthetic result. We tried

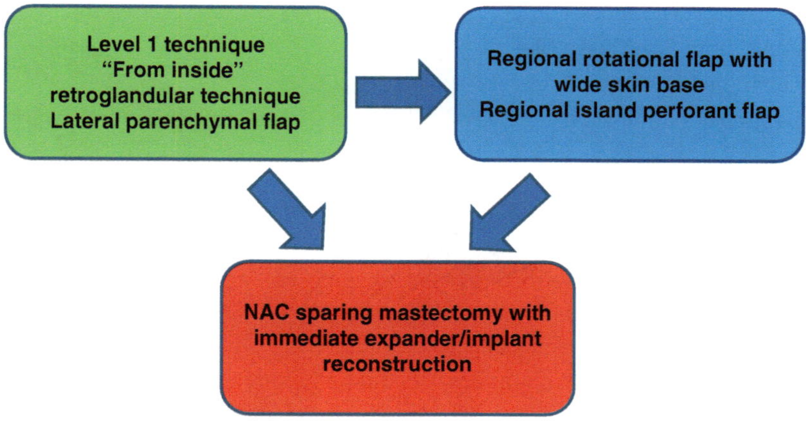

Fig. 13.1 The scheme of scenario strategy. The procedure should be planned in such a way when one technique can move into another without compromising technical aspects

to combine techniques which can completely restore the breast without scars on the breast skin. The hiding surgical approach, adapted to natural borders of the breast, wide mobilization of skin and parenchyma, hiding the tumor's excision under the intact breast skin, and utilization of regional flaps are the key points of these techniques. The concept will be presented by a sequence of techniques that can move from one to another without compromising the final aesthetic result. If the tumor is small and located close to the breast border the classical level 1 technique within the Krishna Clough classification of oncoplastic operations with contour access can be used. If the tumor is located medially and close to the chest wall the retroglandular "from inside" technique is effective. In case of re-excision of the tumor bed margins and increasing the size of the defect or in case of an initially big tumor, the first choice is a regional flap with a wide skin base or island perforant flaps. If the extensive intraductal carcinoma was unexpectedly found, the surgeon moves to NSM with immediate reconstruction (Fig. 13.1).

13.4 Techniques

"Level 1 technique" with contour approach The skin is mobilized above the tumor, with the preservation of the subdermal plexus. Then the tumor is removed. Surgeon proceeds from the anterior to the posterior surface of the breast. A wide mobilization of the parenchyma is performed around the defect in the retromammary space, and the defect is closed by the redistribution and suturing of the tissue (Fig. 13.2).

The main idea is to do this within the intact skin of the breast to hide the area of the surgery and to avoid creating a depression in the wound area. It is important to close the residual cavities in the wound. The area of the surgery is usually drained with vacuum drainage. Then the wound is closed along the contour of the breast. After healing, the area of the surgery and the scar should become inconspicuous (Fig. 13.3).

"From inside" retroglandular technique If the tumor is small and located close to the chest wall, the contour access is used, usually lower-lateral, hiding in the submammary fold. Then an extensive mobilization of the parenchyma over the retromammary space is carried out. The tumor is removed from the posterior surface of the breast, "from inside" (Fig. 13.4).

Here we go from the posterior to the anterior surface of the breast. The same approach was proposed and successfully used by Mátrai et al. (2019). In our practice to close the defect, the fascia covering the posterior surface of the parenchyma, and, if needed, the parenchyma is partially dissected to a depth of up to 5 mm. This allows for "releasing," straightening, and the redistributing of the tissue of the breast with the closure of the tumor bed (Fig. 13.5).

The wound is sutured with the approximation of the parenchyma with the patient in a sitting

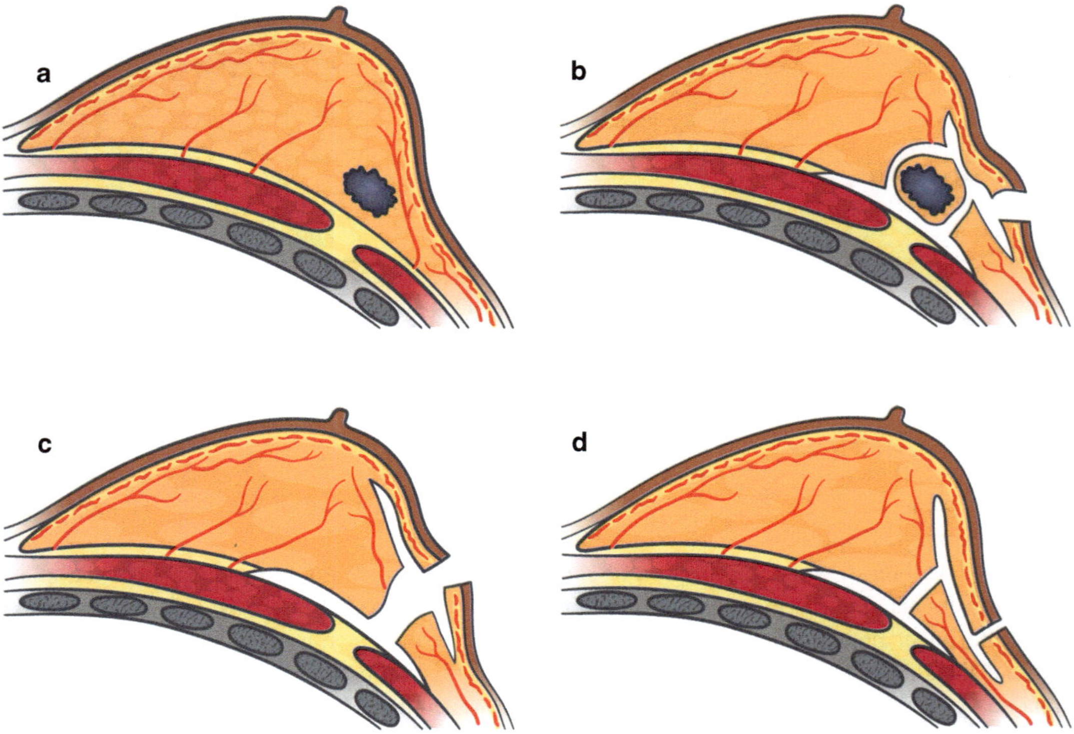

Fig. 13.2 The scheme of the level 1 technique. (**a**) location of the tumor; (**b**) contour access along the lateral border of the breast with mobilization of the tumor area and surrounding tissues along with the subcutaneous and retromammary space; (**c**) tumor area is excised, parenchyma is mobilized; (**d**) the wound is closed with the redistribution of the parenchyma by moving the lateral part of breast tissue and axillary adipo-fascial tissue under the skin

position to avoid the distortion of deformation of the breast (Fig. 13.6). This method is effective when the anterior surface of the defect does not reach the skin.

Lateral parenchymal flap This technique can be used when the tumor is located in the upper medial quadrant in patients with small and non-ptotic breasts. The surgical access is achieved along the lateral contour of the breast and the parenchyma of the upper sector is widely mobilized under the skin and above the muscle to the level medially of the tumor. Lumpectomy is performed with an orientation on the longitudinal axis of the body with the preservation of the lateral part of the parenchyma like a "tissue bridge," with its maximum vascularization (Fig. 13.7).

The branches of a. thoracica lateralis and intercostal perforants should be preserved according to the location of the tumor and the geometry of the wound. Later on, this lateral parenchymal bridge moves medially to close the defect (Fig. 13.8).

If required, the axillary subcutaneous adipo-fascial tissue can be used to fill and repair the lateral contour of the breast, which completely restores its shape (Fig. 13.9).

Rotational lateral thoracic flap In those cases, where the tumor is large and when more tissue is required to close the defect, the rotational flap with a wide skin base can be planned in the axillary area with lower (Fig. 13.10) or upper base (Fig. 13.11).

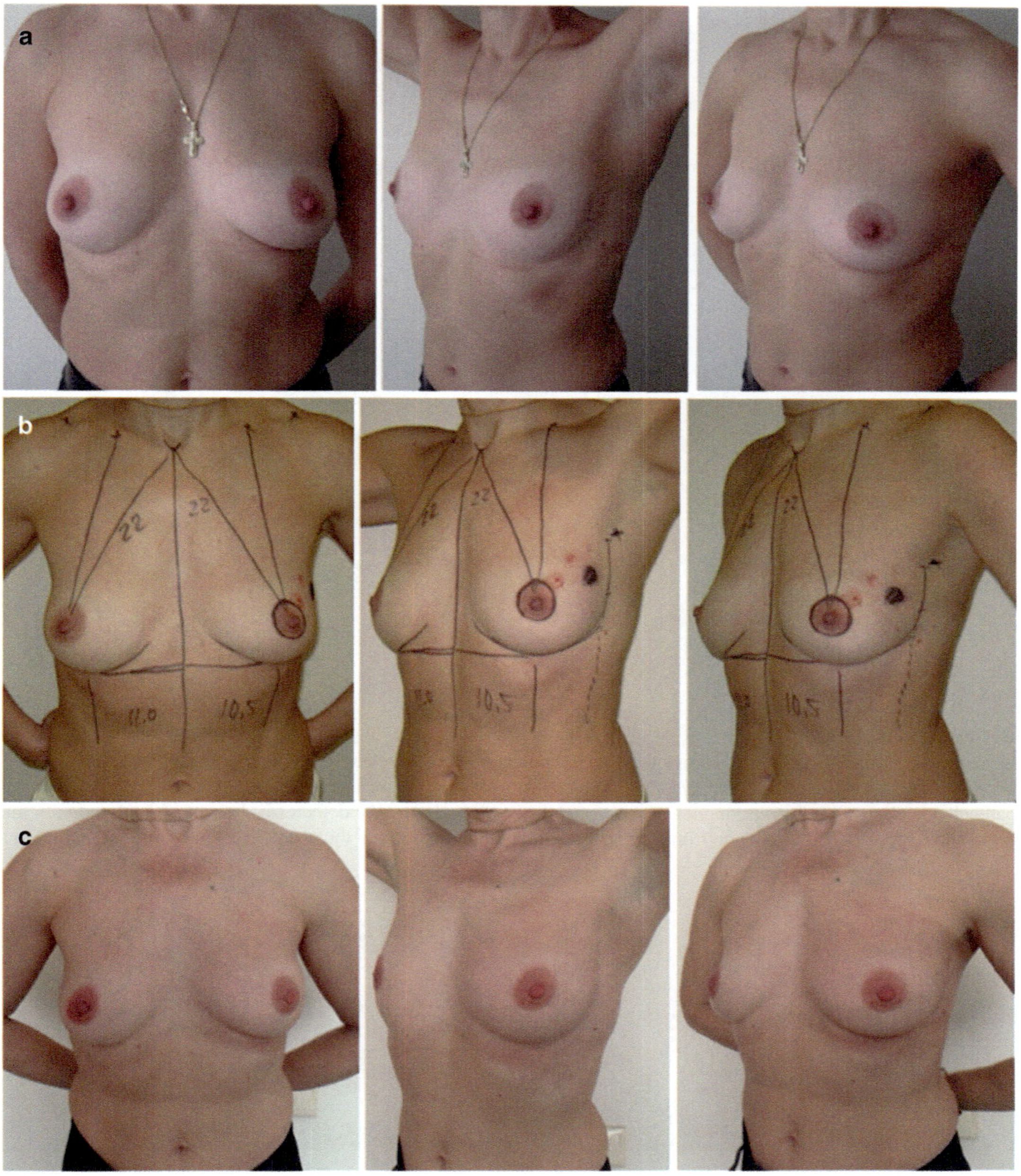

Fig. 13.3 Level 1 technique. (**a**) presurgery view; (**b**) presurgery markings with the position of the tumor; (**c**) postsurgeryview after 36 months, after radiotherapy. The weight of the specimen was 17 g

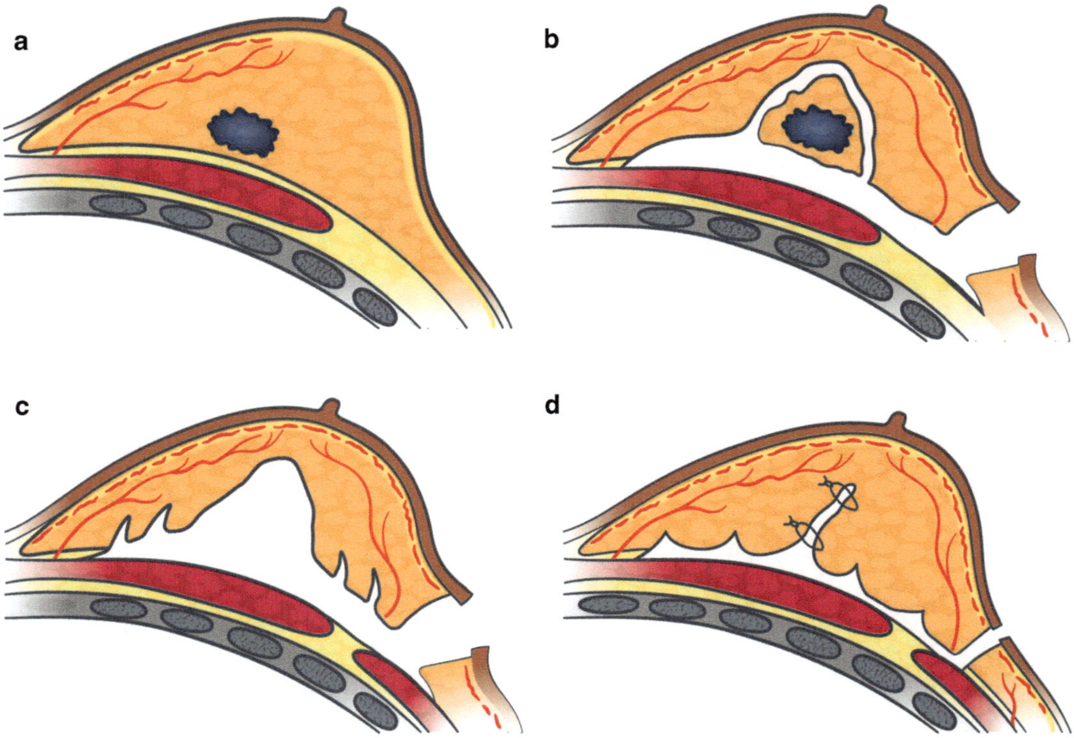

Fig. 13.4 The scheme of the "from inside" technique. (**a**) location of the tumor; (**b**) contour access along the lateral border of the breast with wide mobilization of the breast parenchyma along with the retromammary space and retroglandular excision of the tumor from the base of the gland—from inside; (**c**) tumor area is excised with incisions of the deep fascia and breast parenchyma superficially. It helps to release and redistribute the breast tissue with closing the defect; (**d**) the wound is closed with the redistribution of the parenchyma and suturing the defect

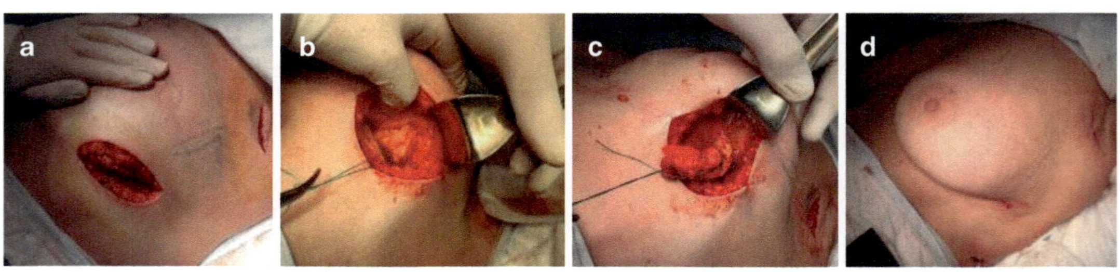

Fig. 13.5 Retroglandular "from inside" lumpectomy, intraoperative photos. (**a**) contour access along the inferior-lateral border of the breast; (**b**) breast parenchyma is mobilized widely along with the retromammary space and the tumor is fixed by suture; (**c**) the tumor is mobilized; (**d**) tumor bed is sutured and the wound is closed. Final view on the table

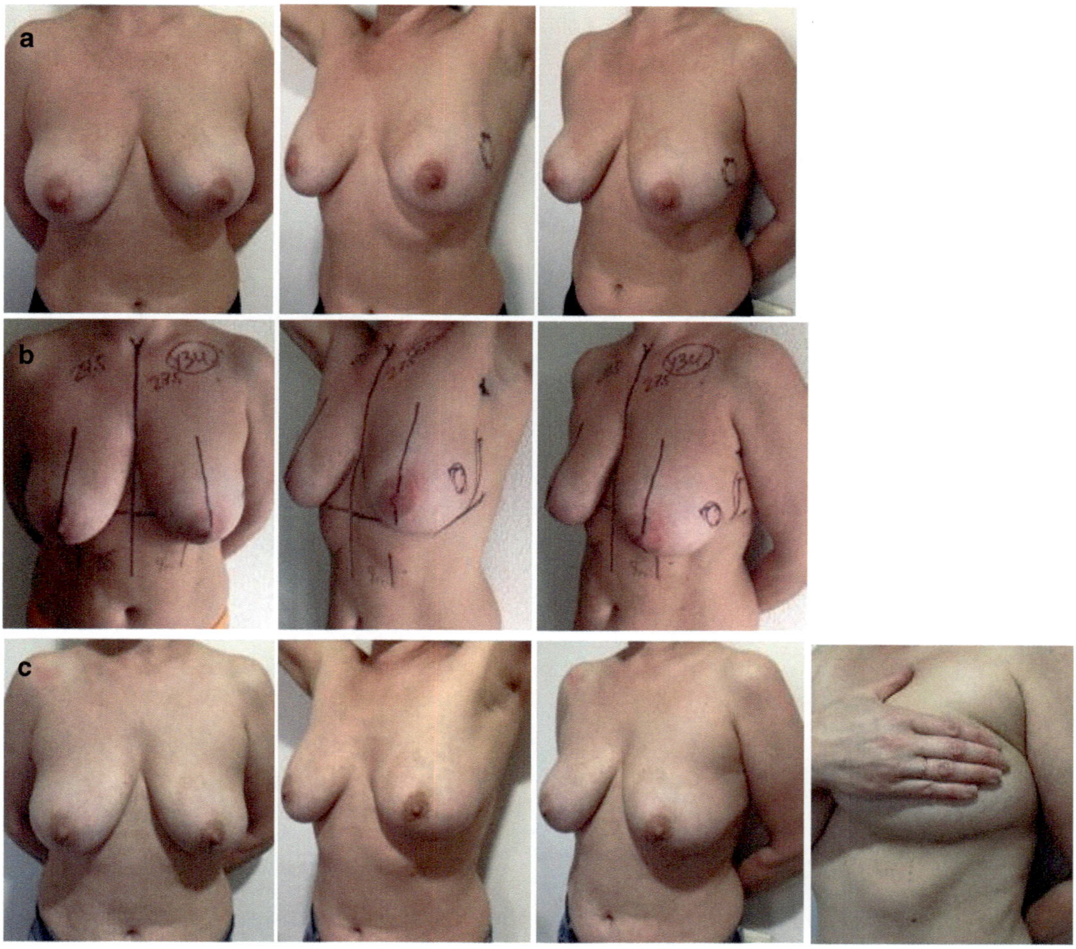

Fig. 13.6 Retroglandular "from inside" technique. (**a**) presurgery view with the position of the tumor; (**b**) presurgery markings; (**c**) postsurgery view after 7 months, after radiotherapy. The weight of the specimen was 28 g. The same patient as in Fig. 13.5

The same lateral contour access is performed, the skin over the tumor is widely mobilized and the tumor is removed. Then the rotational flap is prepared with the preservation of perforant vessels at the base. Its anterior border coincides with the contour incision. The flap is de-epidermized and moved to the defect under the skin of the breast (Fig. 13.12).

Its base is fixed along the lateral contour of the breast and the tip is fixed to the parenchyma in the tumor bed. Following this approach, the defect is completely covered by the skin of the

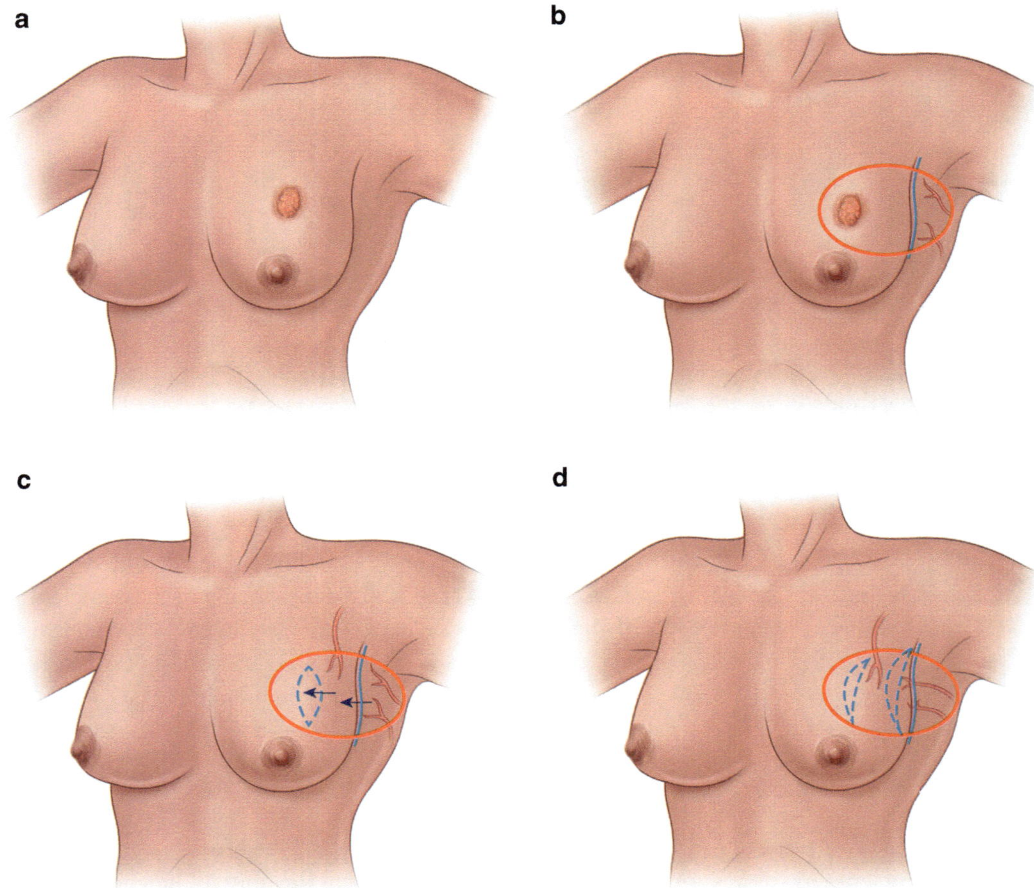

Fig. 13.7 The scheme of the lateral parenchymal flap technique. (**a**) location of the tumor; (**b**) contour access along with the lateral border of the breast (blue line) with wide mobilization of the breast parenchyma along the subcutaneous layer and retromammary space (red line); (**c**) tumor area is excised (dotted blue line) with preservation of lateral parenchymal bridge-like part of the breast tissue with feeding vessel; (**d**) the defect is closed by moving medially the lateral parenchymal flap with feeding vessel. The breast contour is restored by moving the mobilized axillary adipo-fascial tissue under the skin (lateral dotted blue line). The skin wound (blue line) is closed along the lateral border of the breast

breast and becomes "invisible" (Fig. 13.13). This technique in our practice is used less frequently, however, it could be like the first step in oncoplastic surgery for young surgeons on the way to the island perforant flaps which usually are more effective.

Regional island perforant flaps (Lateral intercostal arteria perforant (LICAP)/Lateral thoracic artery perforant (LTAP)/Anterior intercostal arteria perforant (AICAP)/Medial intercostal arteria perforant (MICAP)/Superior epigastric artery perforant (SEAP)) The use of regional perforant flaps from the axillary area (on the perforants of the intercostal and lateral thoracic arteries) and the epigastric area (on the perforants of the intercostal and superficial epigastric arteria) is very effective in closing significant defects in the upper-lateral, lower-lateral, lower and central sectors of the breast with minimal ptosis. The same contour access and extensive breast mobilization are used, with subsequent tumor removal "from

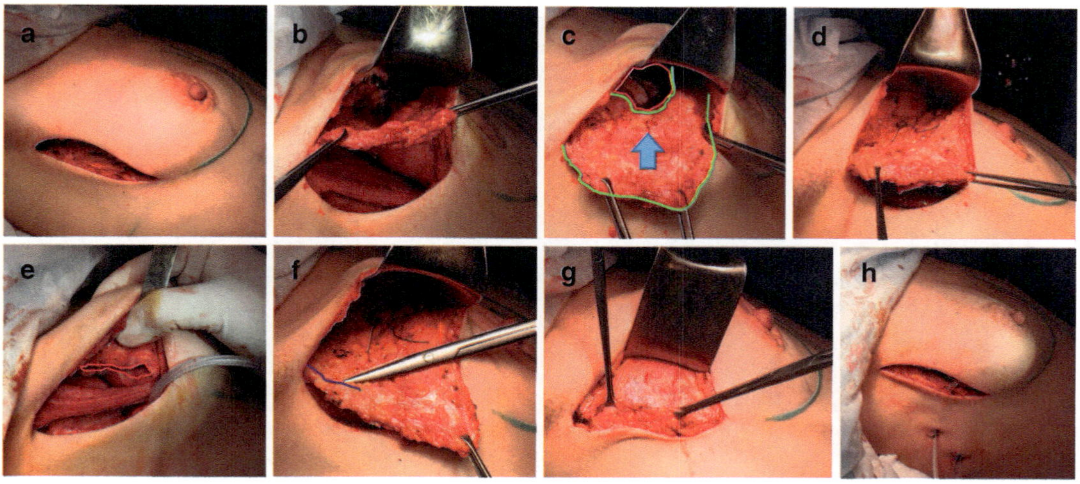

Fig. 13.8 Lateral parenchymal flap technique, intraoperative photos. (**a**) contour access along the lateral border of the breast; (**b**) breast parenchyma is mobilized widely along with the retromammary space and subcutaneously at the level medially to the tumor; (**c**) the tumor is excised (tumor bed marked by the red line) with preservation of lateral parenchymal bridge-like flap (green lines); (**d**) tumor bed is closed by moving the bridge-like lateral parenchymal flap medially and sutured; (**e**) view of the sutured tumor bed (red line) from inside, from the base of the gland; (**f**) scissors point to the branch of the lateral thoracic artery (marked by violet line) feeding the lateral part of the parenchyma; (**g**) the lateral breast appearance is restored by subcutaneous axillary adipo-fascial tissue mobilized under the skin and above the muscles; (**h**) final view on the table

inside"—from the base of the gland without skin mobilization. It helps to preserve the vascularity of the skin and parenchyma because the vessels are coming superficially, closer to the skin. It also helps to achieve better aesthetic results due to the minimizing of the trauma of the dermal plexus and skin which minimizes the postsurgical and post-radiotherapy fibrosis. Then the flap is formed according to the location and size of the defect and is moved on to the tumor bed. It is possible to plan the flap shape in different manners by using two curvilinear lines with adaptation to the border of the breast (Fig. 13.14) which allows for minimizing the deformation in the axillary region after wound closure and makes the scar less visible.

The final decision about the shape and size of the flap should be made after the confirmation of free margins by the pathologist and determination of the defect's shape. We start the flap mobilization from the distal part in the axillary region due to the absence of important vessels coming to the flap in this region, except thoraco-dorsal perforant which is not used in these techniques and could be ligated. The feeding vessels located medially should be identified and mobilized. Doppler ultrasound with mini-probe is useful for the identification of the vessels and final confirmation of adequate blood flow. It is better to provide some sources of blood supply of the flap—intercostal perforants and branches of a. thoracica lateralis. It is especially important for those cases when the size, shape, and position of the defect need more tissue, and a "combined" flap should be planned and prepared (Figs. 13.15 and 13.16).

The surgeon does not need to skeletonize every vessel, but the flap should be mobilized enough—it should "lie freely" in the tumor bed in the sitting position of the patient, without any tension and distortion. It is very important to

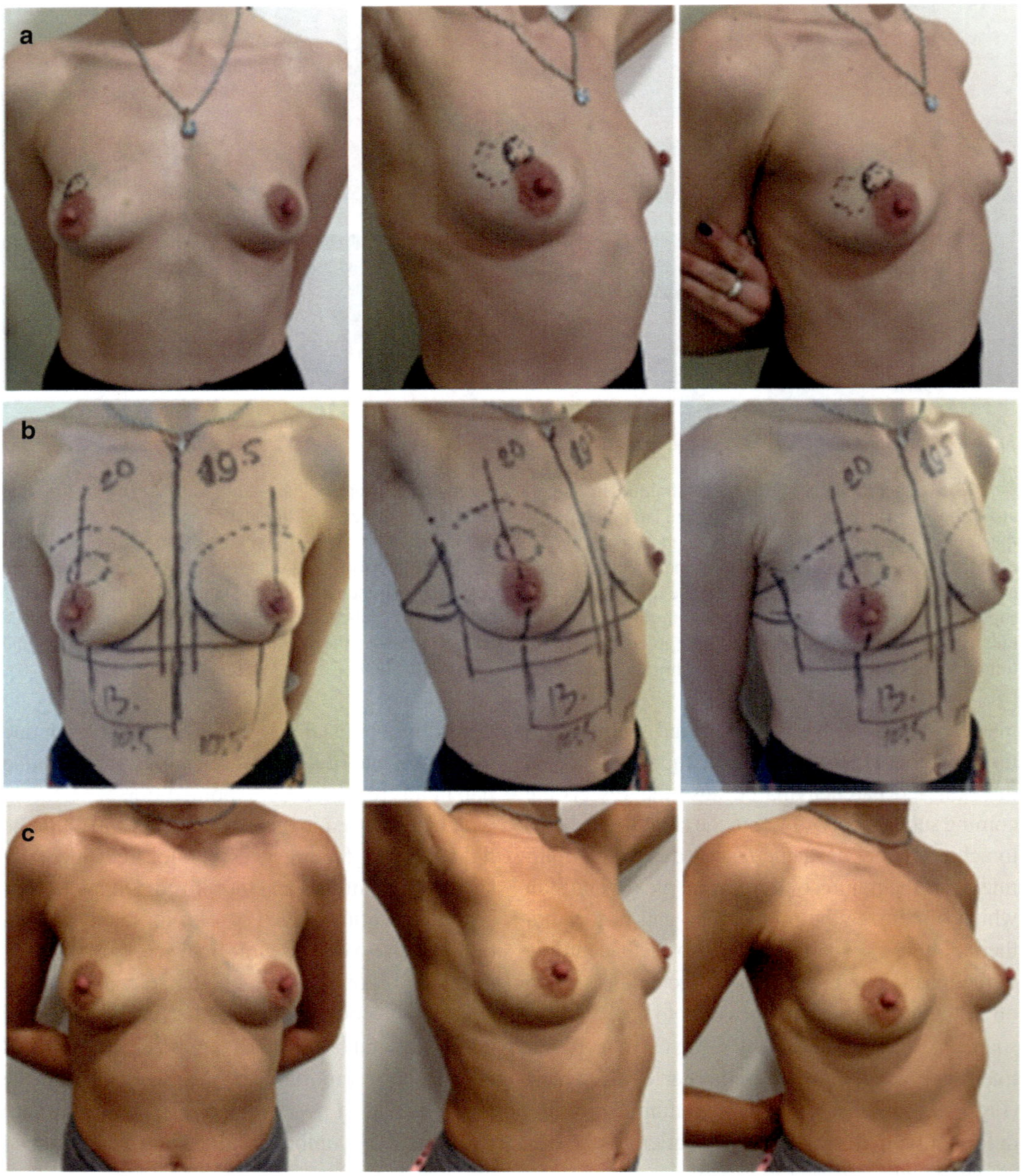

Fig. 13.9 Lateral parenchymal flap technique. (**a**) presurgery view with the position of the tumor; (**b**) presurgery markings with taking into account different scenarios (lateral parenchymal flap, LTAP/LICAP flap, NAC-sparing mastectomy); (**c**) postsurgery view after 22 months, after radiotherapy. Weight of the specimen was 20 g. The same patient as in Fig. 13.8

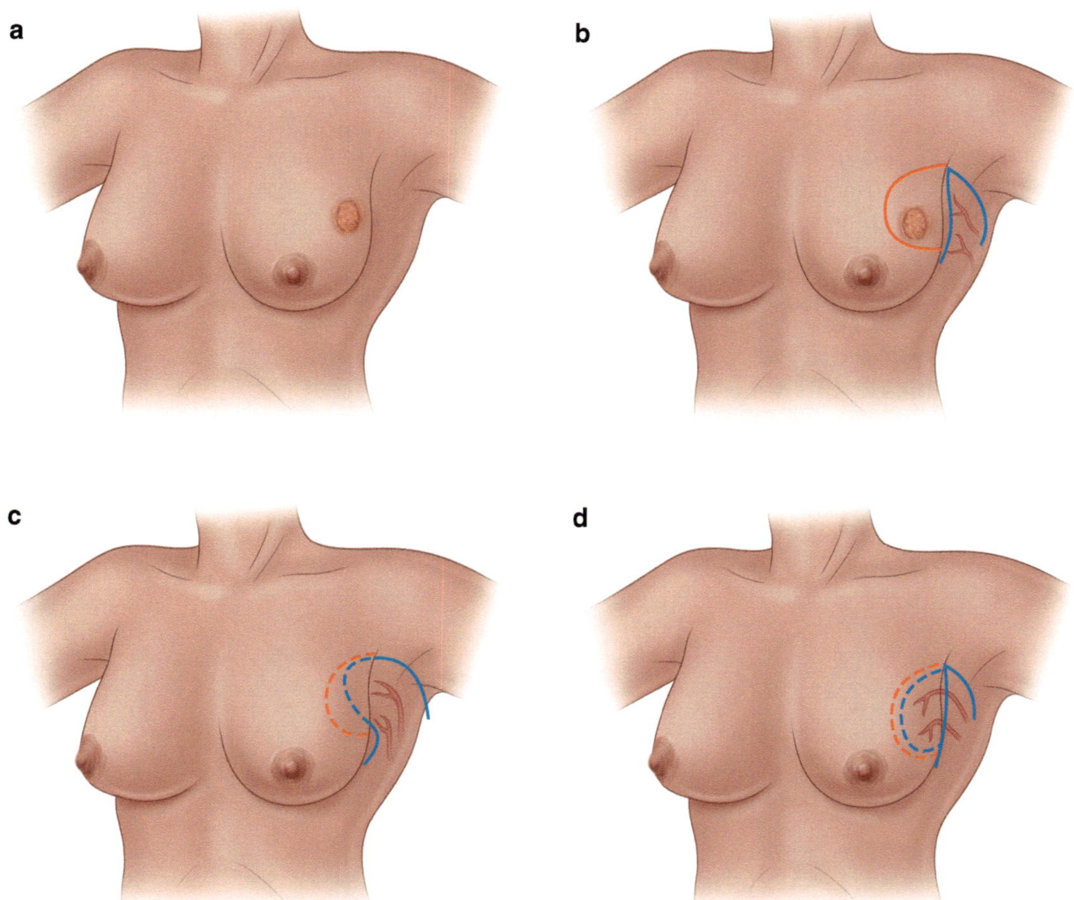

Fig. 13.10 The scheme of the lateral thoracic flap with lower base. (**a**) location of the tumor; (**b**) surgical markings of the flap (blue line) which medial border coincide the lateral contour of the breast—the location of surgical access; red line point at the level of skin and parenchyma mobilization around the tumor (**c**) tumor area is excised under the skin (dotted red line). The flap is mobilized with the preservation of feeding perforant vessels and is moved to the defect under the skin; (**d**) the deepidermized flap has filled the defect. The wound is closed along the lateral border of the breast (blue line)

check the final position of the flap in the sitting position of the patient on the operation table. Therefore, the vessels in the pedicle should be checked and in case of several sources of blood flow, the decision should be made about what vessels should be preserved and what should be sacrificed to avoid tension. The flap can be moved from the axillary or epigastric region to the defect by linear movement, flipping like a book page, or with a propeller rotation (Fig. 13.17).

It depends on the location, and size of the defect, location, and length of the vessel pedicle. If the defect is located centrally or medially and the lateral part of breast parenchyma is preserved, or if the vessel pedicle is short, usually there is no need to make the "tunnel" in the breast and excise the healthy tissue. It is suitable to make the "window" in m. pectoralis major along the fibers and to move the flap into the defect through this window (Fig. 13.18). This

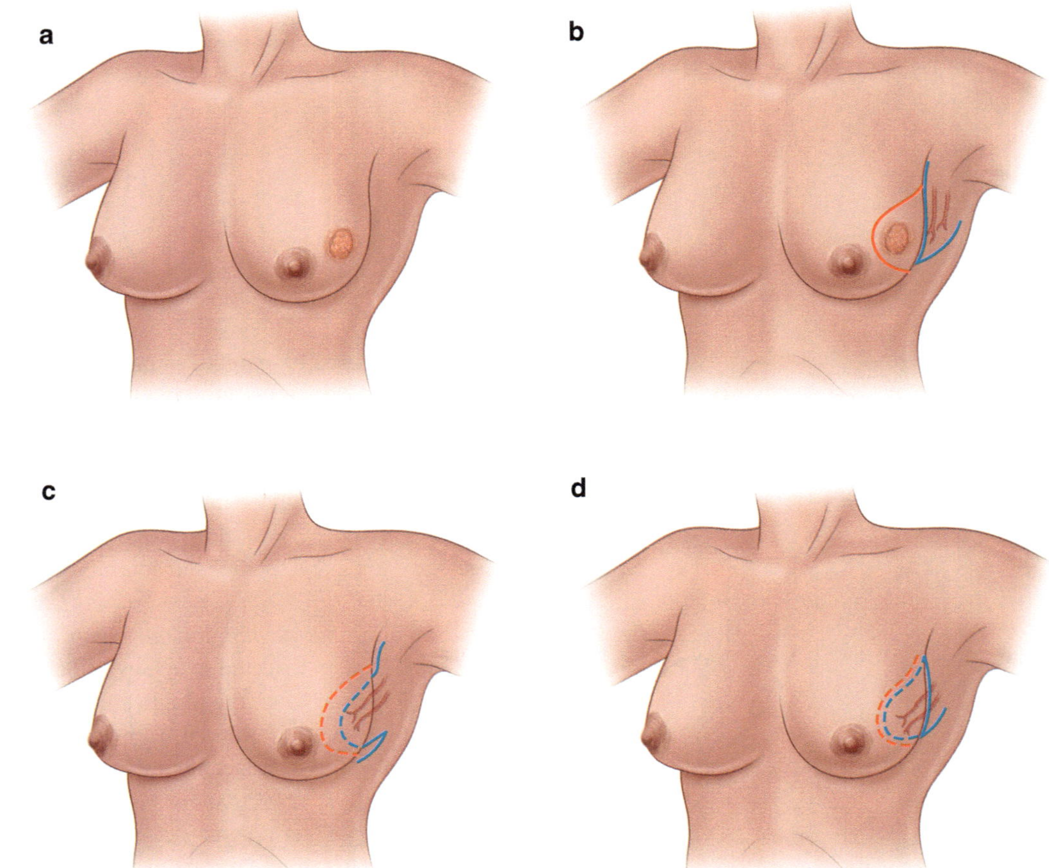

Fig. 13.11 The scheme of the lateral thoracic flap with upper base. (**a**) location of the tumor; (**b**) surgical markings of the flap (blue line) which medial border coincide the lateral contour of the breast—the location of surgical access; orange solid line poin at the area of skin and parenchyma mobilization around the tumor (**c**) tumor area is excised under the skin (red dotted line). The flap is mobilized with the preservation of feeding perforant vessels and is moved to the defect under the skin; (**d**) the deepidermized flap has filled the defect. The wound is closed along the lateral border of the breast (blue line)

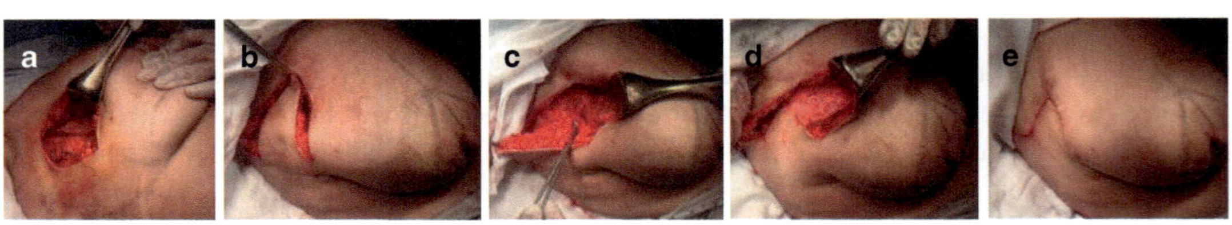

Fig. 13.12 Lateral thoracic flap with lower base, intraoperative photos. (**a**) contour access along the lateral border of the breast with tumor bed; (**b**) lateral thoracic flap is formed according to the presurgery markings; (**c**) flap is mobilized and set aside, instrument point to the intercostal perforant feeding flap; (**d**) flap is deepidermized according to the geometry of the wound and fixed in the tumor bed under the skin; (**e**) final view on the table

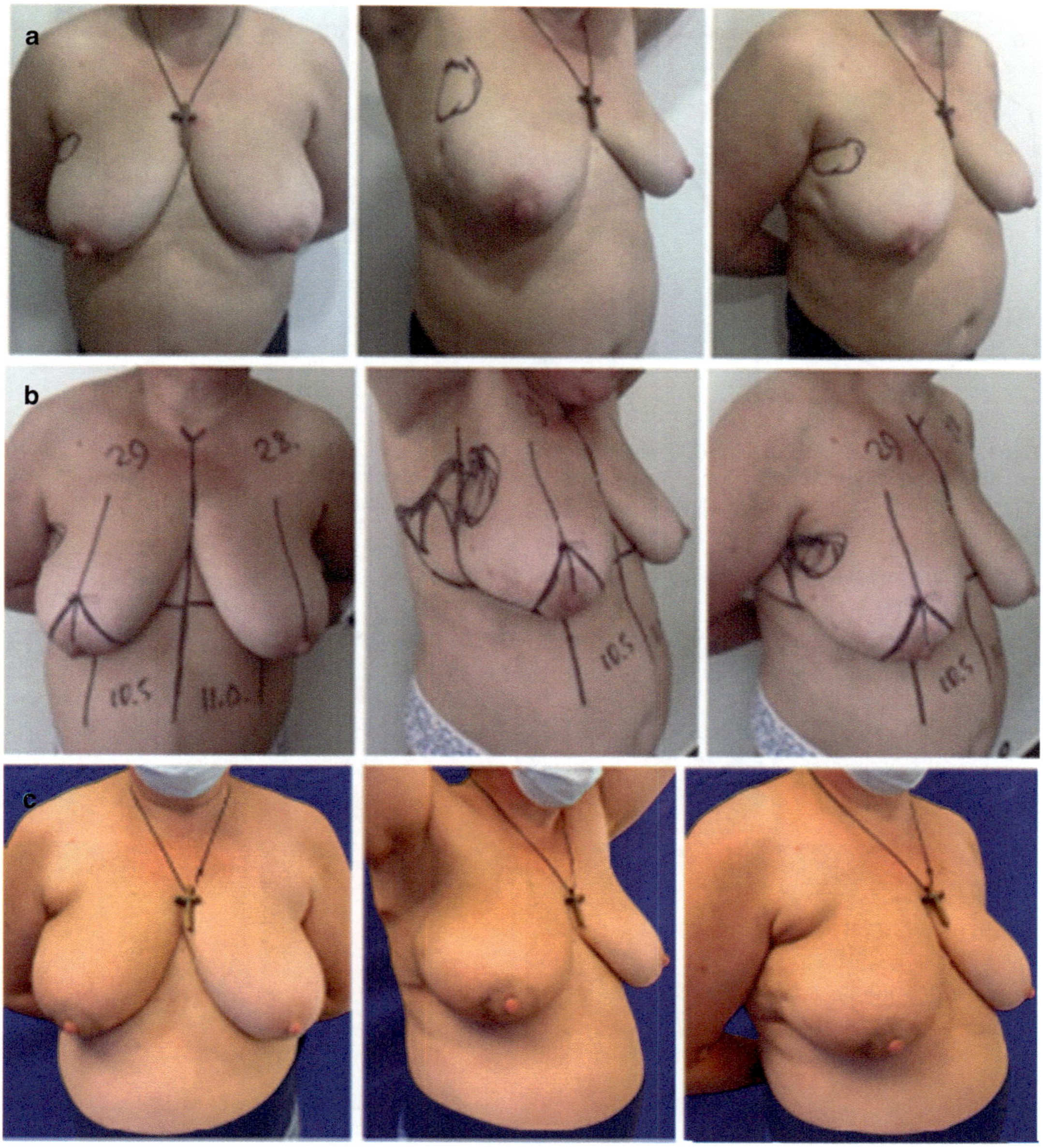

Fig. 13.13 Lateral thoracic flap with a lower base. (**a**) presurgery view with the position of the tumor; (**b**) presurgery markings with taking into account different scenarios (lateral thoracic flap, LTAP/LICAP flap, therapeutic mammoplasty); (**c**) postsurgery view after 14 months, after radiotherapy. The weight of the specimen was 58 g. The same patient as in Fig. 13.12

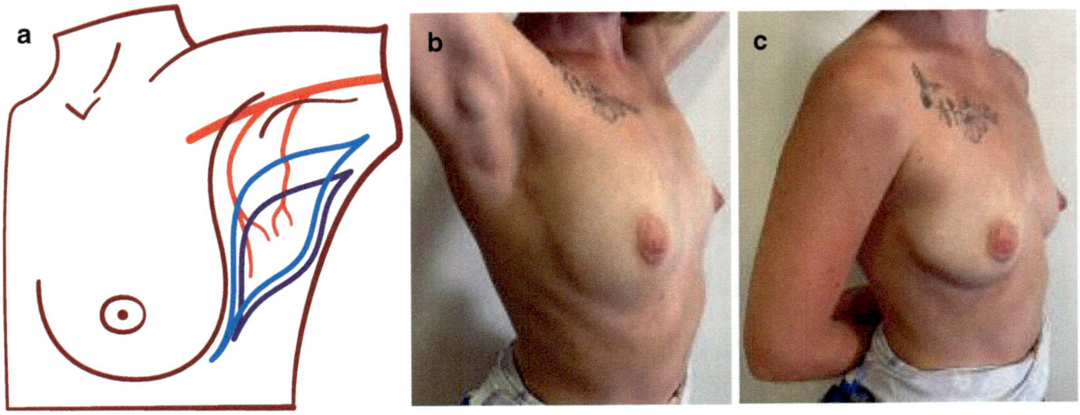

Fig. 13.14 Marking of the LTAP/LICAP flap with two curvilinear lines. (**a**) the scheme of marking with partial coincide the flap with breast contour along the lateral border of the breast. Different positions of the flaps; (**b**, **c**) patient with LICAP partial breast reconstruction. Tumor was located in upper-lateral quadrant. Postsurgery view after 17 months, after radiotherapy. The weight of the specimen was 14 g

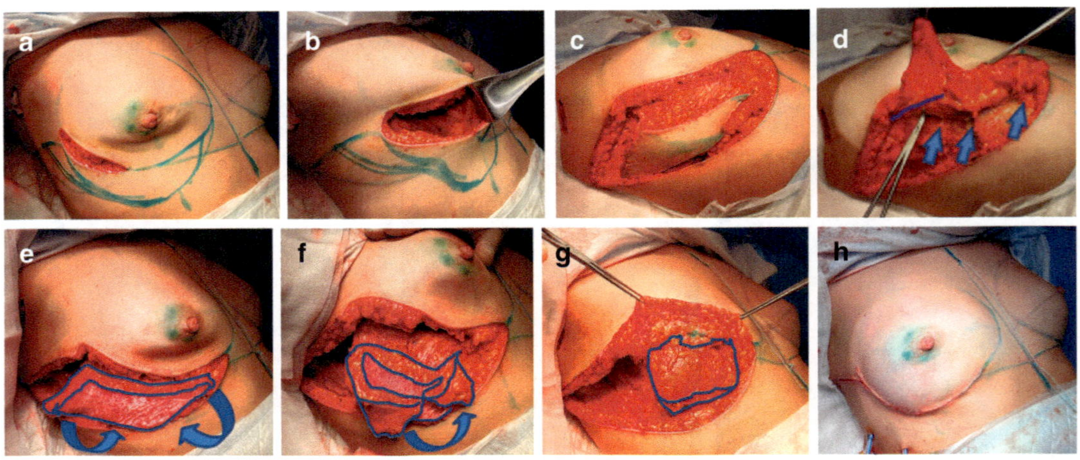

Fig. 13.15 Combined LTAP/LICAP/AICAP flap, intraoperative photos. (**a**) contour access along the lower-lateral border of the breast. The tumor is excised with almost all lower part of the breast parenchyma. Flap marking changed during the surgery according to the size and position of the defect; (**b**) tumor bed; (**c**) flap is mobilized according to the size of the final defect; (**d**) blood supply of the flap: instrument point to the branch of the lateral thoracic artery (marked by violet line), the lateral intercostal and two anterior perforants pointed by arrows; (**e**) flap is deepidermized; (**f**) flap is folded once from both corners; (**g**) flap is folded twice like a snail to get more volume according to the geometry of the defect; (**h**) final view on the table: flap is fixed in the tumor bed under the skin and submammary fold is restored

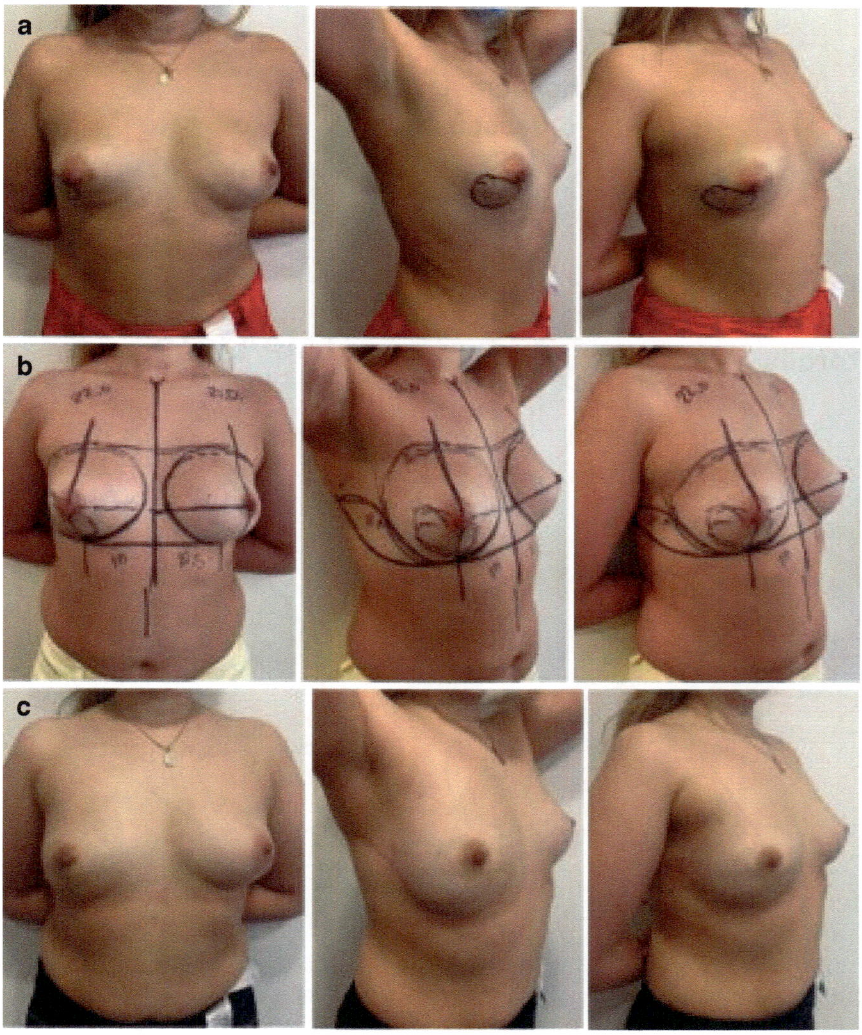

Fig. 13.16 Combined LTAP/LICAP/AICAP flap. (**a**) presurgery view with the position of the tumor; (**b**) presurgery markings with taking into account different scenarios (LTAP/LICAP flap, NAC-sparing mastectomy); (**c**) postsurgery view after 7 months, after radiotherapy. The weight of the specimen was 98 g. The same patient as in Fig. 13.15

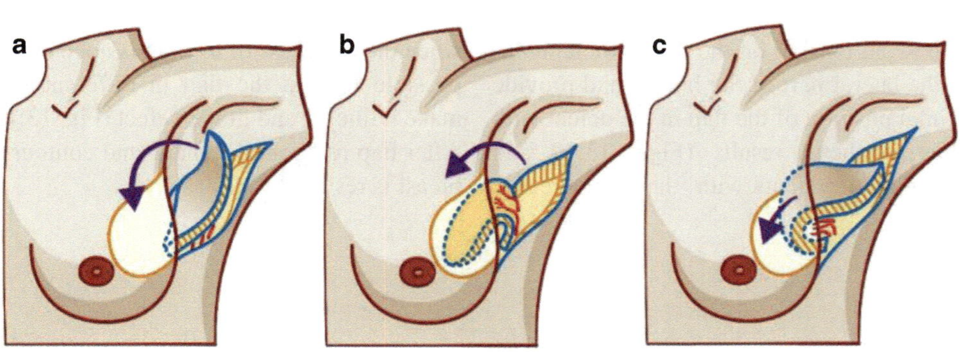

Fig. 13.17 The scheme of moving the LTAP/LICAP flap. (**a**) flap is moved like a propeller around the lateral intercostal perforant (point of rotation). Deepidermized skin of the flap stays anteriorly under the skin of the breast; (**b**) flap is flipped over like the book page. Deepidermized skin of the flap lies on the chest wall in the defect area. The fatty layer of the flap is under the skin; (**c**) flap is moved frontally and can be folded. Deepidermized skin of the flap stays anteriorly under the skin of the breast

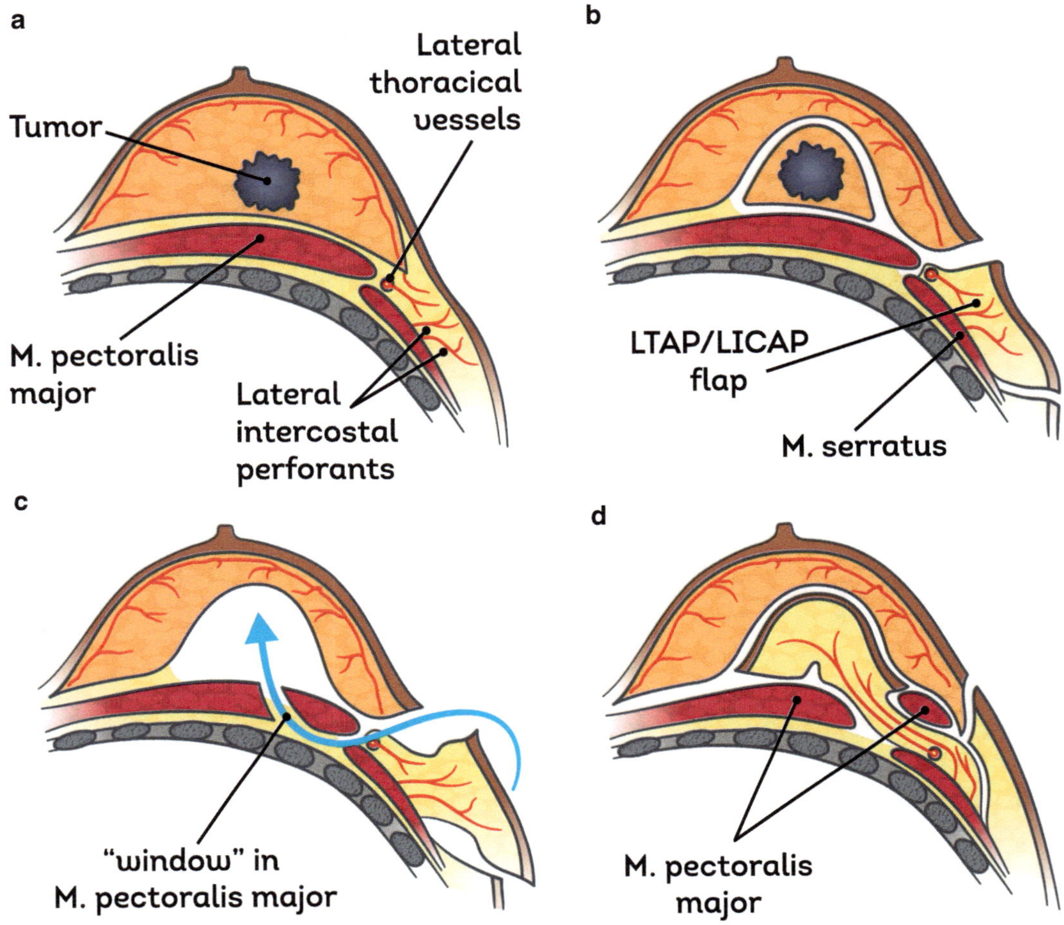

Fig. 13.18 The scheme of partial LTAP/LICAP flap reconstruction with moving the flap through the "window" in the m. pectoralis major. (**a**) the position of the tumor and vessels; (**b**) lateral contour access with the mobilization of the breast parenchyma along with the retromammary space, tumor excision, and mobilization of the flap; (**c**) flap is mobilized and "window" in the m. pectoralis major is prepared along the fibers of the muscle; (**d**) the flap is moved frontally through the "window" in the muscle to the tumor bed; the flap is in a new position. The wound is closed

helps to avoid tension on the flap pedicle, bulking in the lateral part of the breast, and provide an optimal position of the flap in the defect with excellent aesthetic results (Figs. 13.19 and 13.20). In slim patients with glandular breasts, when the thickness of the flap is not enough, it is possible to fold the flap in different ways to make it thicker and fit the defect (Fig. 13.15f, g). After flap rotation, the shape and contour of the breast is restored.

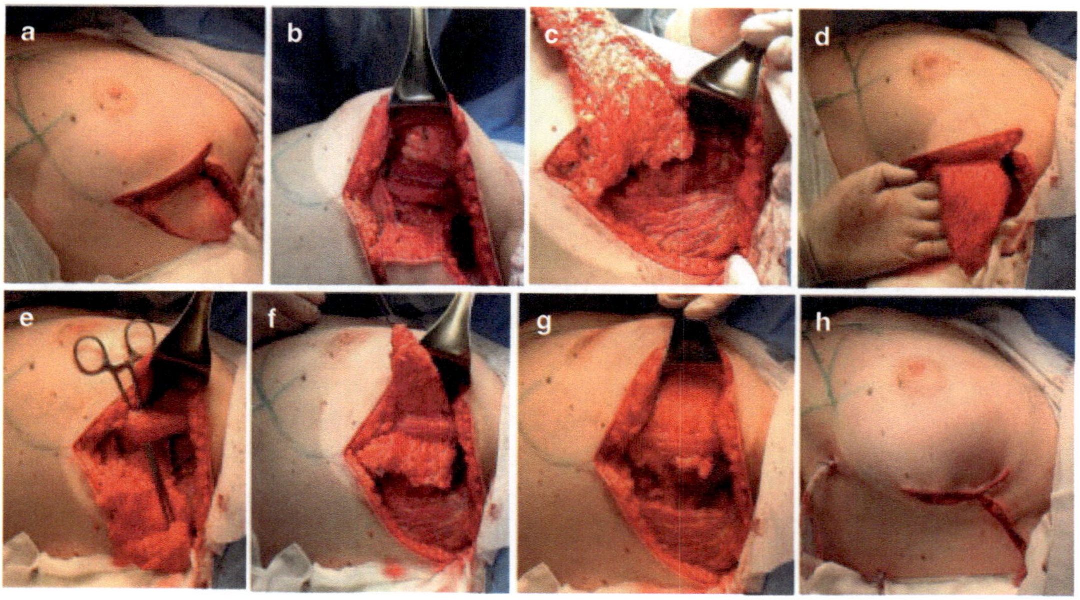

Fig. 13.19 Combined LTAP/LICAP flap transposed through the "window" in the m. pectoralis major, intraoperative photos. (**a**) contour access along the lateral border of the breast. The flap is prepared according to the size and position of the defect; (**b**) tumor bed; (**c**) flap is mobilized and set aside anteriorly to show feeding vessels; (**d**) flap is mobilized and deepidermized; (**e**) the "window" in the m. pectoralis muscle is prepared. The clamp is passed through the hole in the muscle; (**f**) flap is moving through the "window"; (**g**) flap is in the final position. It is fixed to the parenchyma medially; (**h**) final view on the table. No bulking in the lateral part of the breast without making the tunnel in the parenchyma

We use the additional mobilization of the parenchyma in the retromammary space, the fasciotomy on the posterior surface of the breast, and even nondeep incisions of the parenchyma (like in the "from inside" technique (Fig. 13.3c, d)). This maneuver helps to release and redistribute the tissue of the parenchyma and to prepare the tumor bed for better positioning of the flap. The flap is usually fixed to the parenchyma in the defect area to provide it stable position. It is especially important when folding is needed. When the wound is closed, the contour of the breast is restored by partial fixation of the wound margins to the chest wall along the lateral contour with LICAP/LTAP flaps, or along the submammary fold, with its reconstruction with the AICAP or MICAP or SEAP flap.

Wound margins should be mobilized widely before closure to avoid tension in the wound, but with preservation of feeding perforants coming to the skin in the axillary and epigastric area. We always put drains in the wound through the contraperture. If the drain tube is close to the vessel pedicle, we use nonsuction drainage to avoid the damage to the vessels. During wound closure, the lateral border of the breast should be restored. For this, the lower-lateral wound margin is mobilized widely, pulls up and fixed along the lateral border of the breast to the chest wall (m. serratus) together with the upper-medial wound margin from the breast side. Usually, three layers of sutures are used—fascial (with partial fixation to the chest wall along the breast border), dermal, and subcuticular. Wound closure

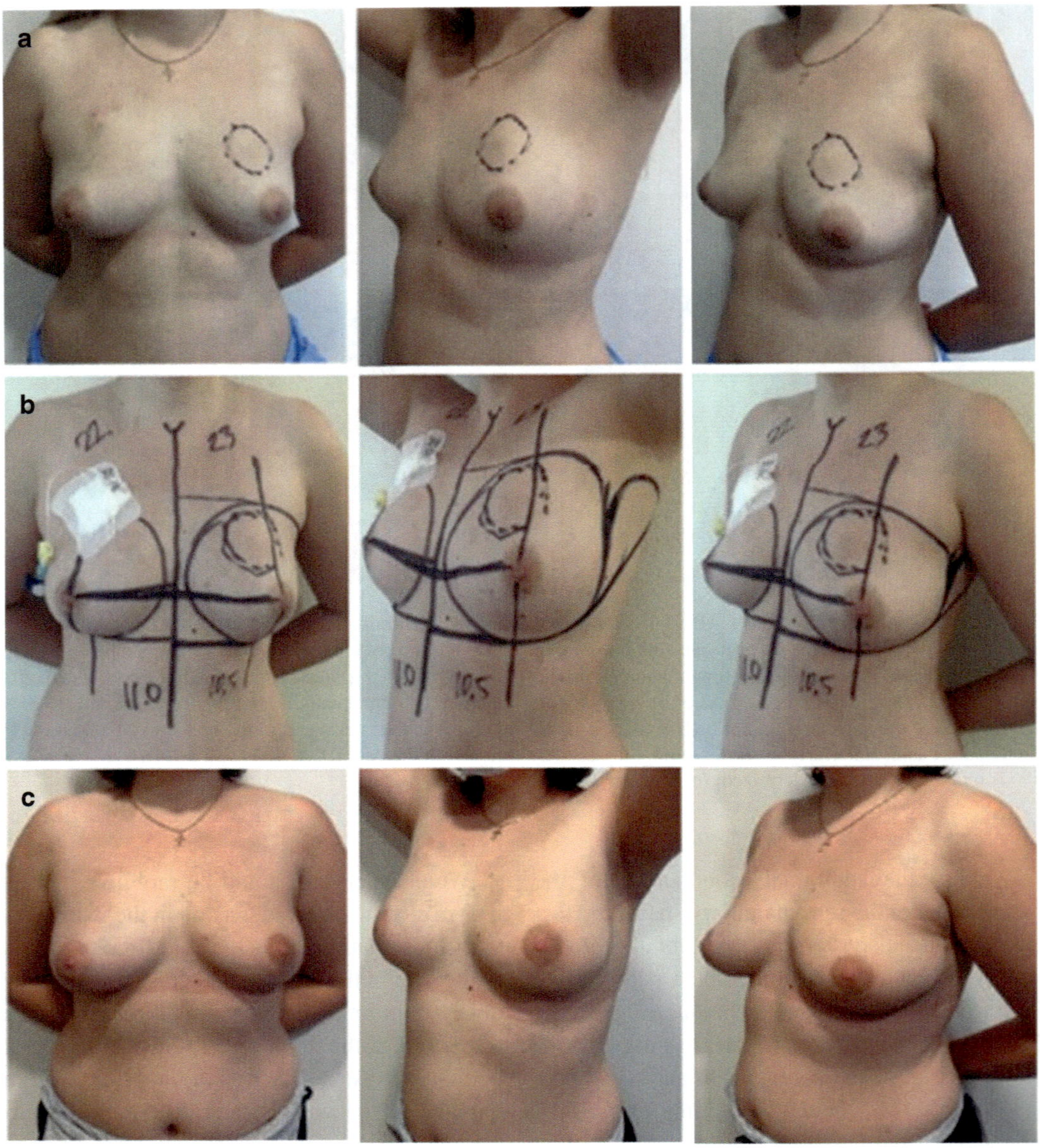

Fig. 13.20 Combined LTAP/LICAP flap. (**a**) presurgery view with the position of the tumor; (**b**) presurgery markings with taking into account different scenarios (LTAP/LICAP flap, NAC-sparing mastectomy); (**c**) postsurgery view after 15 months, after radiotherapy. The weight of the specimen was 108 g. The same patient as in Fig. 13.19

should be done in the sitting position of the patient to avoid distortions and deformations of the tissue. It also helps to find the optimal shape of the wound and to avoid the dog ears in the distal part of the scar. In cases with a lower position of the tumor when the surgeon needs to damage and then restore the submammary fold, non-absorbable sutures are used.

Tips

- Careful planning of the surgery taking into account the best aesthetic result and possible changes of the scenario during the procedure due to the final size and shape of the defect. All possible scenarios should be discussed with the patient. The equipment and devices for all scenarios shall be prepared.
- Marking the vessels for the flap with Doppler ultrasound before the surgery taking into account potential sources of blood supply.
- Intraoperative Doppler ultrasound is useful for the evaluation of the vessels coming to the flap.
- Avoiding incisions on the breast skin, using just contour incisions along the border of the breast and on surrounding areas—axillary and epigastric zones. All incisions have to be adapted to the real anatomical borders of the breast.
- Lumpectomy and all parenchyma and skin mobilization should be performed from the base of the glad—"from inside."
- Wide mobilization of the skin and parenchyma around the tumor and defect area but with careful preservation of the blood supply. If it is possible, maximal preservation of the lateral part of breast parenchyma to provide the best shape of the restored breast and minimize the shrinkage of the skin.
- Close cooperation with the pathologist and radiologist. The final decision about the shape and size of the flap has to be done after the final confirmation of the free margins of the specimen. The color marking of the margins of the specimen by a surgeon with an intraoperative evaluation of the specimen by a pathologist with the frozen section of the margins is strongly recommended.
- It is better to do de-epidermization of the flap just after the final mobilization of the flap pedicle. It helps to evaluate the blood supply of the flap by adequate oozing of the de-epidermized area.
- To get better redistribution and position of the breast tissue and the flap, the wide mobilization of breast parenchyma with incisions of the posterior fascia has to be done.
- The flap has to be mobilized enough and lie freely in the tumor bed without any tension in the sitting position of the patient.
- If the tumor is located centrally or medially, or in the case of a short pedicle, the flap can be moved to the defect area through the "window" in the m. pectoralis major.
- The flap can be folded in different ways to get better shape according to the shape and size of the defect.
- For better restoration of the lateral contour of the breast, the fascia of wound margins has to be fixed to the chest wall.
- In the case of AICAP or MICAP flaps, the submammary fold has to be fixed by nonabsorbable sutures.
- To avoid deformity and distortion of the breast, all final fixations of the flap or breast borders have to be done in the sitting position of the patient.
- Due to the large wound area, we always put the drains. We do it through the contraperture and use a suction drain if the tube is located far from the vessels and nonsuction if it is close to the pedicle.

Pitfalls

- For skinny patients with pronounced glandular breasts, the flap should be planned with a bigger size. Then it folds and can adequately close the defect.
- Inadequate mobilization of the flap can cause the deformation and "lateralization" of the breast—"stuck breast." Restoration of the lower ("hanging") parts of the breast needs a "freely hanging" flap.
- Twisting or compressing of the flap pedicle can cause acute or chronic ischemia with necrosis or fat fibrosis which intensifies after adjuvant radiotherapy.
- Some patients experience chronic pain in the area of the surgery. Most probably due to the damage of the intercostal nerves during the flap mobilization.
- Tension during wound closure can lead to the delayed healing and even dehiscence.
- Aggressive mobilization of the skin leads to scarring and depression. It can be effectively managed by delayed lipografting.
- In the case of the big size of the flap, the suboptimal planning of the flap shape could lead to the dog ear deformity.
- The AICAP and MICAP flap partial breast reconstruction needs careful fixation of the submammary fold.

After-Care

Usually, patients do not need special care and have to follow general recommendations. In our practice, the wound is always drained due to the large wound area. Drain is removed when the amount of daily discharge is less than 20–30 mL. Day after surgery the patient is advised to wear special compression garments and begin exercises according to the individual program. The program is selected by a physiotherapist according to the type of operation on the breast and axillary region. The scar is closed by hypo allergic tapes for a few weeks. Usually, patients discharge from the hospital after 2–3 days. We ask them to come to the visit after 10 days, 1 month (before the next stage of treatment), 3, 6, 12, and 24 months after the surgery for the clinical and radiological evaluation, clinical photos, and interviews about the quality of life. The examination includes an ultrasound to evaluate the blood supply and status of the flap and seroma formation. All patients are recommended to take painkillers for 2–3 weeks after the surgery as planned.

13.5 Conclusions

Modern oncoplastic breast surgery has many techniques and methods allowing for complete restoration and even improving breast appearance after oncological operation. Regional flaps, especially island pedicled flaps, are the useful tool for partial breast reconstruction which helps to make the signs of the surgery almost invisible. Together with some other techniques, they constitute the concept of "invisible surgery." Aiming for the best possible aesthetic result, these techniques are combined into "scenario strategy" when one procedure can swiftly move into another depending on the final size of the defect after tumor removal. This concept requires surgeons who truly strive to achieve the best aesthetic result of the oncological surgery, and who have "plastic surgeon's way of thinking." It also needs more time for the surgery and close teamwork with the radiologist and pathologist in the perioperative period. However, it gives the patient the most personalized approach in oncoplastic breast surgery.

Further Reading

Almahariq MF, Quinn TJ, Siddiqui Z, Jawad MS, Chen PY, Gustafson GS, Dilworth JT. Breast conserving therapy is associated with improved overall survival compared to mastectomy in early-stage, lymph node-negative breast cancer. Radiother Oncol. 2020;142:186–94. https://doi.org/10.1016/j.radonc.2019.09.018. PMID: 31615634.

Carmichael AR, Mokbel K. Evolving trends in breast surgery: oncoplastic to onco-aesthetic surgery. Arch Plast Surg. 2016;43:222–3. https://doi.org/10.5999/aps.2016.43.2.222.

Clough KB, Kaufman GJ, Nos C, Buccimazza I, Sarfati IM. Improving breast cancer surgery: a classification and quadrant per quadrant atlas for oncoplastic surgery. Ann Surg Oncol. 2010;17:1375–91. https://doi.org/10.1245/s10434-009-0792-y.

Corduff N, Taylor GI. Subglandular breast reduction: the evolution of a minimal scar approach to breast reduction. Plast Reconstr Surg. 2004;113(1):175–84.

Corradini S, Reitz D, Pazos M, Schönecker S, Braun M, Harbeck N, Matuschek C, Bölke E, Ganswindt U, Alongi F, Niyazi M, Belka C. Mastectomy or breast-conserving therapy for early breast cancer in real-life clinical practice: outcome comparison of 7565 cases. Cancers. 2019;11(2):160. https://doi.org/10.3390/cancers11020160. PMID: 30709048; PMCID: PMC6406394.

Hamdi M, Spano A, Van Landuyt K, D'Herde K, Blondeel P, Monstrey S. The lateral intercostal artery perforators: anatomical study and clinical application in breast surgery. Plast Reconstr Surg. 2008;121:389.

Hamdi M, Van Landuyt K, de Frene B, Roche N, Blondeel P, Monstrey S. The versatility of the intercostal artery perforator (ICAP) flaps. J Plast Reconstr Aesthet Surg. 2006;59:644–52.

Kim K, Park HJ, Shin KH, Kim JH, Choi DH, Park W, Ahn SD, Kim SS, Kim DY, Kim TH, Kim JH, Kim J. Breast conservation therapy versus mastectomy in patients with T1-2N1 triple-negative breast cancer: pooled analysis of KROG 14-18 and 14-23. Cancer Res Treat. 2018;50(4):1316–23. https://doi.org/10.4143/crt.2017.575. PMID: 29334604; PMCID: PMC6192926.

Mátrai Z, Újhelyi M, Kovács T, Kelemen P, Sávolt A, Kovács E, Éles K, Mészáros N, Kenessey I, Stamatiou A, Pukancsik D. Evaluation of a retroglandular oncoplastic technique as a standard level I oncoplastic breast-conserving surgery: a retrospective clinicopathologic study of 102 patients with breast cancer. Clin Breast Cancer. 2019;19(3):e459–67.

McCulley SJ, Schaverien MV, Tan VKM, Macmillan RD. Lateral thoracic artery perforator (LTAP) flap in partial breast reconstruction. J Plast Reconstr Aesthet Surg. 2015;68:686–91.

Munhoz AM, Montag E, Gemperli R. Oncoplastic breast surgery: indications, techniques and perspectives. Gland Surg. 2013;2(3):143–57. https://doi.org/10.3978/j.issn.2227-684X.2013.08.02.

Nebril BA, Ramírez SB, Novoa AG, Lamas CV. Rotational flaps in oncologic breast surgery. Anatomical and technical considerations. Cir Esp. 2016;94(7):372–8.

Ng ET, Ang RZ, Tran BX, Ho CS, Zhang Z, Tan W, Bai Y, Zhang M, Tam WW, Ho RC. Comparing quality of life in breast cancer patients who underwent mastectomy versus breast-conserving surgery: a meta-analysis. Int J Environ Res Public Health. 2019;16(24):4970. https://doi.org/10.3390/ijerph16244970.

Ogawa T, Hanamura N, Yamashita M, Kimura H, Ito M, Nakamura T, Kashikura Y, Nohara Y, Noro A. Oncoplastic technique combining an adipofascial flap with an extended glandular flap for the breast-conserving reconstruction of small dense breasts. J Breast Cancer. 2012 December;15(4):468–73. https://doi.org/10.4048/jbc.2012.15.4.468.

Sun Y, Kim S-W, Heo CY, Kim D, Hwang Y, Yom CK, Kang E. Comparison of quality of life based on surgical technique in patients with breast cancer. Jpn J Clin Oncol. 2014;44(1):22–7. https://doi.org/10.1093/jjco/hyt176.

Wan Q, Su L, Ouyang T, Li J, Wang T, Fan Z, Fan T, Lin B, Xie Y. Comparison of survival after breast-conserving therapy vs mastectomy among patients with or without the BRCA1/2 variant in a large series of unselected Chinese patients with breast cancer. JAMA Netw Open. 2021;4(4):e216259. https://doi.org/10.1001/jamanetworkopen.2021.6259. PMID: 33890992; PMCID: PMC8065382.

Zhu L, Li S, Tan L, Zhang X, Wu J, Su F, Chen K, Song E. In pursuit of a flawless Aphrodite: paving the way to scarless oncoplastic breast surgery. Cancer Commun. 2019;39:82. https://doi.org/10.1186/s40880-019-0422-4.

Zhygulin A, Fedosov A, Palytsia V. Invisible Surgery Concept and Scenario Strategy: How to Get the Best Aesthetic Results in Oncoplastic Breast-Conserving Surgery. Plast Reconstr Surg. 2021;148(6):1209–13. https://doi.org/10.1097/PRS.0000000000008518. PMID: 34847109.

Chest Wall Perforator Flaps in Breast-Conserving Surgery: Nottingham Approach

14

Stephen McCulley

Contents

Oncoplastic techniques can broadly be divided into parenchymal redistribution (most classically in the form of an Oncoplastic Mammaplasty/Therapeutic Mammaplasty) [1–5] or parenchymal volume replacement techniques [4–9]. Both techniques can also replace skin when required.

S. McCulley (✉)
Nottingham City Hospital, Nottingham University Hospitals, Nottingham, UK
e-mail: stephen.mcculley@nuh.nhs.uk

M. Hamdi et al. (eds.), *Pedicled Flaps in Partial Breast Reconstruction*,
https://doi.org/10.1007/978-3-031-08483-6_14

The complexity of oncoplastic techniques will vary from relatively simple excisions such as small batwing excision to more complex mammaplasty work and then onto chest wall perforator flaps (CWPF) requiring the dissection and delivery of flaps based on perforators around the breast. These procedures require more experience in raising such flaps, and they have been slower to adopt until more recently.

The need to use more complex oncoplastic techniques to optimise cosmetic outcomes may be in up to 25% of breast-conserving cases depending upon approach and philosophy of use [10]. However, regardless of how often they are genuinely required, there is consensus that oncoplastic techniques extend the role of BCS, reduce re-excision rates [11], and allow a higher rate of BCS with the safety of oncological outcomes [12, 13]. The addition of CWPF further adds to those aims.

The approach described in this chapter is based on the evolving oncoplastic techniques developed in Nottingham since 2000 (Fig. 14.1). The leading developers of this described approach are the author Stephen McCulley and his Oncoplastic surgery colleague Douglas Macmillan. CWPF were introduced for primary breast cancer in Nottingham in 2007 and used in approximately 50 cases per year. The Nottingham service has around 1000 new cancers annually. It is vital to state and understand that our default oncoplastic option in appropriate patients would be a mammaplasty technique. Most patients with sufficient volume or ptosis will have a mammaplasty option [14]. This is generally simpler and confines all scars to the breast in a standard cosmetic position. However, patients not suitable for mammaplasty techniques that may be candidates for CWPF procedures are those with non-ptotic breasts, breasts of minimal volume, and insufficient volume related to tumour size to perform a mammaplasty still, also, for those insisting on maintaining breast volume or refusing contralateral surgery. Ideally, CWPF are performed in patients with no or minimal ptosis.

Worldwide one of the most described pedicled perforator flaps in partial breast reconstruction is

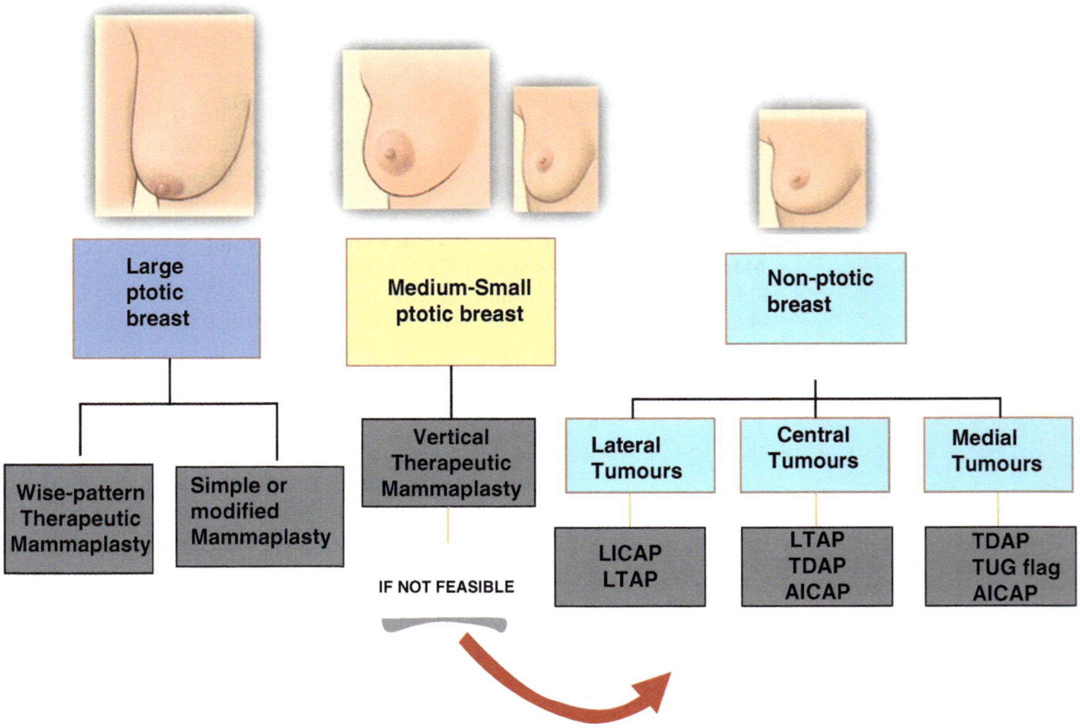

Fig. 14.1 Nottingham algorithm of oncoplastic surgery 2000–2020. (Courtesy of Prof. McCulley, all rights reserved)

the Thoracodorsal Artery Perforator (TDAP) flap [15]. This flap remains a remarkably versatile flap in terms of pedicle length, and hence flap reaches into the breast and volume of the available flap. However, the TDAP uses the main thoracodorsal pedicle preventing the use of Latissimus Dorsi flap (LD) or future TDAP reconstruction. It is also a more lengthy and complex dissection compared to the supplies options we would recommend for the majority of cases, namely, Lateral Intercostal Artery Perforator (LICAP) flap [16], the Lateral Thoracic Artery Perforator (LTAP) flap [6], Combined LICAP/LTAP flaps [6] or Anterior Intercostal Artery Perforator (AICAP) flap.

The CWPF aim to replace, or if appropriate, overcorrect the lost volume and skin from cancer excision. Therefore, the flap needs to have a good blood supply to avoid fat necrosis and be robust for adjuvant radiotherapy. In addition, the flap should be delivered as much as possible into the breast without disrupting the natural breast boundary. Indeed, try and avoid changing lateral or inferior breast boundary as best possible. In order to achieve these goals, the surgeon must understand the principles of each type of flap in terms of pedicle options, flap delivery options, and flap reach into the breast. Once understood, the best options can be planned.

14.1 Lateral Intercostal Artery Perforator (LICAP) Flap

This flap is based on the lateral intercostal perforators. Hamdi has described these perforators for the LICAP flap. This description suggests these perforators tend to lie 3–4 cm in front of the latissimus dorsi muscle border [16]. The commonly described perforators lie in the third to sixth intercostal spaces. Our investigations and experience of these flaps are similar but show that the fourth to sixth is the most used and numerous. We have also found that the triangle created by the lateral breast border, the inframammary fold and the anterior axillary line houses many exceptionally reliable intercostal perforators, and I sometimes refer to this "Triangle of plenty". Similarly, most usable perforators are within 10–20 mm from the lateral breast crease. The lateral breast crease or fold is defined to different extents in different patients, particularly in higher BMI patients. In such cases, the edge of the breast needs to be judged clinically. These clinical based observations on perforator positions do vary to literature descriptions.

As the blood supply is based on the intercostal perforators, the pivot points of these flaps will be based on these perforators, and any surrounding tissue left undissected lateral to them. This is a vital point to understand the reach of the LICAP flap. Indeed, the more lateral tissue that is left attached, the more it will limit the flap reach and create lateral fullness. Similarly, it is crucial to understand that the LICAP flap cannot be transposed into the centre of the breast without removing or tunnelling the lateral breast tissue if the tumour defect is more medial. Therefore, a limitation of the LICAP flap is the need to remove normal lateral breast tissue to reach some more central tumour defects. Hence LICAP flaps are ideal for lateral breast tumour defects and less ideal for central and upper breast defects.

The base of the LICAP flap will always remain slightly to the outside of the breast. When starting to use these flaps, it is a common mistake to try and leave too many intercoastal perforators that lie more than 3 cm away from the lateral breast border. This will result in lateralising the breast's crease.

The LICAP flap remains the workhorse of immediate chest wall perforator flaps despite the limitations mentioned above. The LICAP perforators, to a varying degree, are available in all patients. However, the surgeon must decide and delineate the best perforator in terms of size and signal on a handheld Doppler and then plan which would be potentially the most useful in delivering a flap to fill the defect.

14.2 LICAP Steps

14.2.1 Assessing Available Perforators

The perforators can be mapped using an 8 MHz handheld Doppler. It is helpful to draw the lateral breast fold, the inframammary fold and the anterior border of the latissimus dorsi muscle as this gives a framework in which to predict the most likely place for the perforators (Fig. 14.2). Each intercostal space can be assessed and the signals marked. When looking for the LICAP perforators, you will commonly encounter the main trunk and potential perforators of the lateral thoracic vessels. These should always be marked, and if one has a linear signal suggesting the path of the lateral thoracic artery, this can be noted and added to the potential planning.

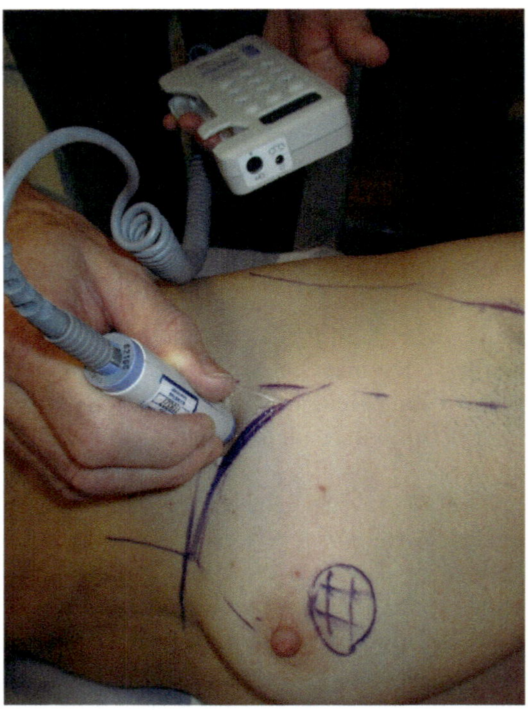

Fig. 14.2 Assessing perforators with a probe

14.2.2 Flap Markings and Planning

The LICAP flaps can be delivered either as a traditional propeller type flap or as a turnover flap (Fig. 14.3a–d). The propeller type delivery would usually be based on a single or a small local collection of perforators. If there is a good perforator with any visible pulsation, then a single perforator will be reliable for the vascularity of the entire flap. These flaps have the potential of being up to 25 cm long with a diameter of 10 cm. The vascularity of these larger flaps should be assessed on the table. However, they are frequently much smaller for the use of partial breast reconstruction, and it is vital that the vascularity of a flap is assessed, and any doubtful areas can be removed regardless of flap size. This can easily be assessed within the skin of the flap. The average flap will likely be 5–8 cm wide with a length of approximately 12–18 cm.

The turnover flap can be based on a linear line of LICAP perforators, or as is recommended, be performed as a combination of LICAP and lateral thoracic perforators and vessels. Turnover flaps will leave the dermis face down, although they can be folded at the tip, creating some skin if the skin needs replacing.

The propeller flap more easily keeps the dermis or skin side in its standard orientation and therefore is easier to be used for skin replacement.

The markings of the flap will be based on the principles of the volume needed to fill the cancer defect. The design will be dictated by the position of the perforators that are planned to be used. It is helpful to slightly curve the anterior part of the flap to fractionally narrow the tightest point of closure which is from the edge of the breast crease to the lower border of the flap (Fig. 14.4a, b). Narrowing this area does run the risk of reducing vascularity to the flap however does reduce the lateralisation of the breast crease by reducing skin closure tension. Another consideration for the markings is to allow any

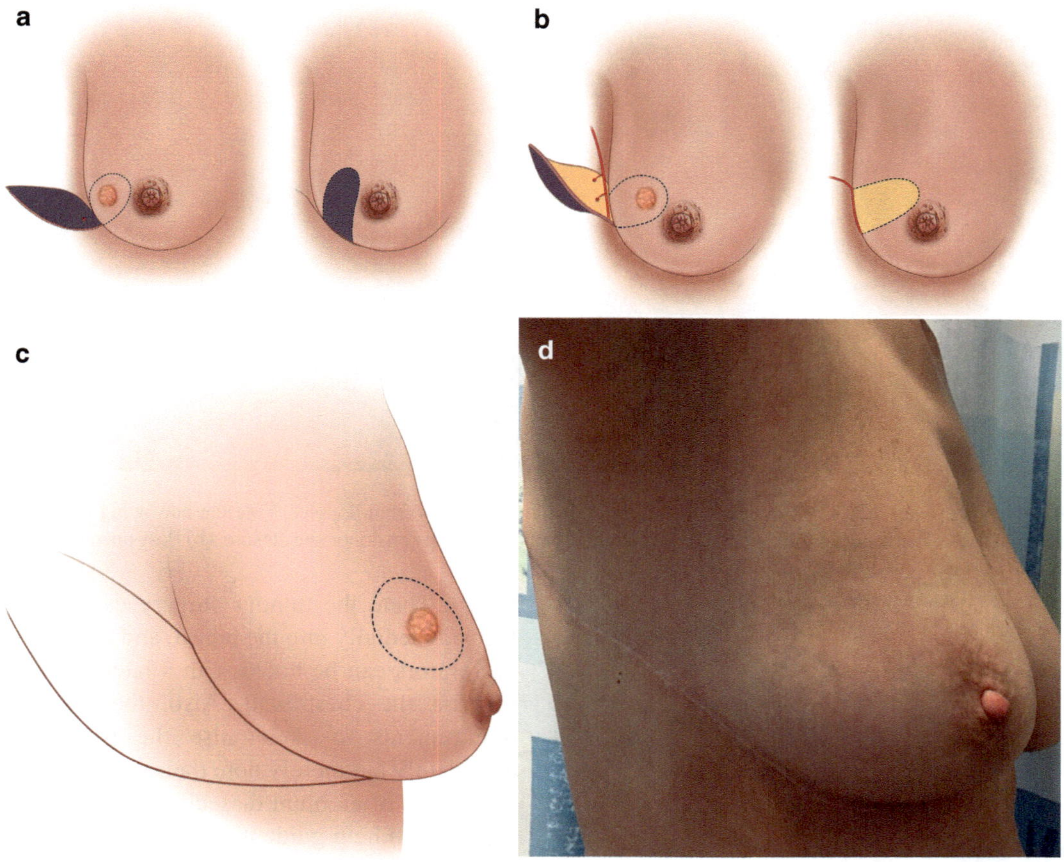

Fig. 14.3 (**a**) Propeller or turnover flap delivery. (**b**) LICAP/LTAP flap as a turnover flap into defect based. (**c**) Flap with sixth LICAP perforator. (**d**) Post-operative LICAP flap propellered into defect based

axillary surgery, as it is helpful to access the required nodal surgery from the upper aspect of the flap. Therefore, this can also be considered in deciding the exact position of the flap. It is, of course, possible to do a separate small incision, especially for a sentinel node, if this is more helpful.

14.2.3 Patient Positioning

For many patients, there is no requirement to be in a true lateral position as these flaps do not encroach too far into the back due to their size (Fig. 14.5). This also makes patient positioning easier and oncology surgery more straightforward and familiar. The patient is usually put in a half lateral position with a 3-L inflatable bag or large sandbag under the scapular. This lifts the chest walls slightly away from the operating table, allowing the posterior aspect of the flap to be efficiently closed. The arm can be placed on a bar either across the patient or externally rotated up and out away from the patient.

14.2.4 Dissection

The flap will have been drawn and planned on the above factors, but there is no requirement to commit to the exact dimensions of the flap during surgery (Fig. 14.6a, b). Usually, the tumour excision is done from the upper medial border of the flap, and this incision can be made initially. This will be an 8–10 cm curvilinear incision around the lateral border of the

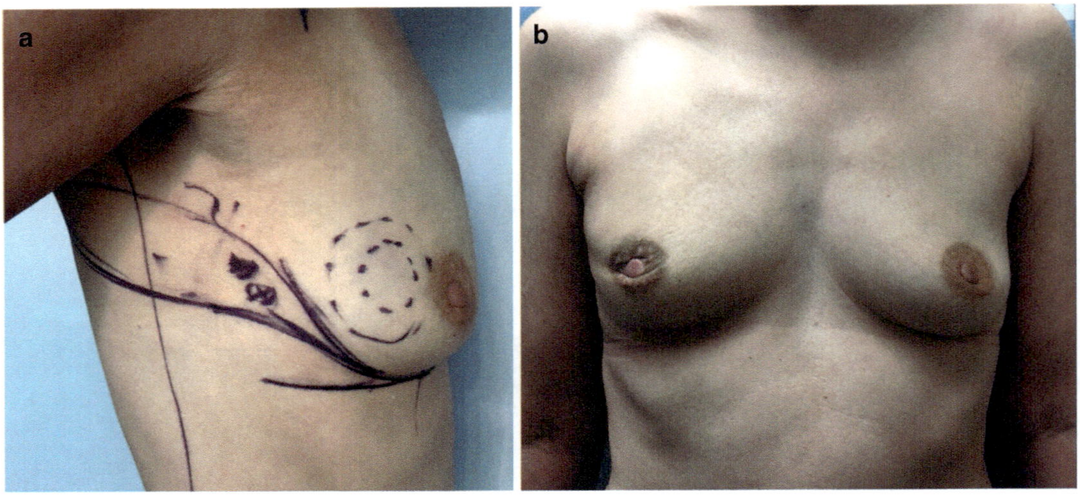

Fig. 14.4 (**a**) Flap design—The flap is based on available perforators from doppler. Note the narrowing of the flap adjacent to the lateral breast fold so as to limit lateral pulling of the breast on donor site closure. (**b**) Post-operative result

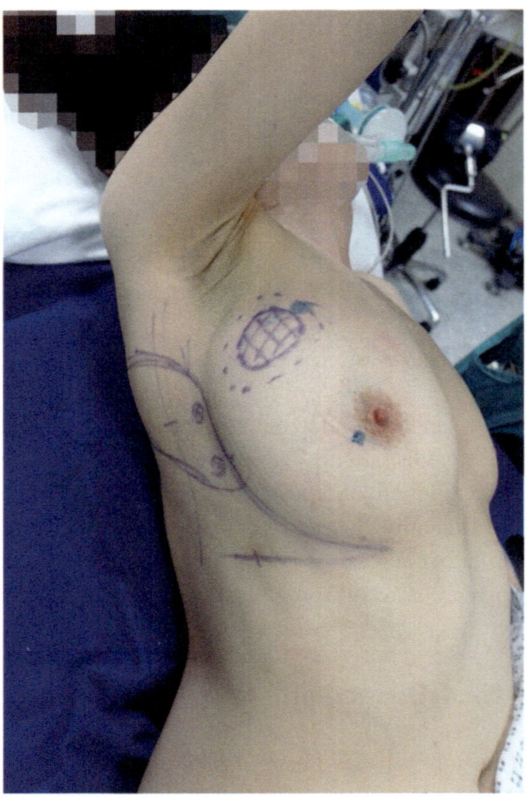

Fig. 14.5 Patient positioning

breast. Then, the tumour surgery can be performed medially into the breast, and the LICAP perforators can be noted with a lateral dissection on the chest wall. Also, there are no requirements to skeletonise the perforators completely but merely note their presence with gentle and often blunt dissection. The Doppler signals will help guide to the most likely position to observe the perforators. The superior dissection can then take place for any nodal surgery. Once the oncological surgery has been completed, the flap dimensions can then be rechecked with relation to the likely pivot point and the volume required, and the final flap is then raised from the chest wall. One can choose to de-epithelialise the flap before raising the flap from the chest wall (which make de-epithelialisation easier but does create some more bleeding), or the de-epithelialisation can be done at the end of the procedure. If one is planning larger flaps, I would always recommend leaving some skin on the tip of the flap to assess vascularity at the end of the operation and before the flap inset. If the skin looks healthy, it can then be removed at inset.

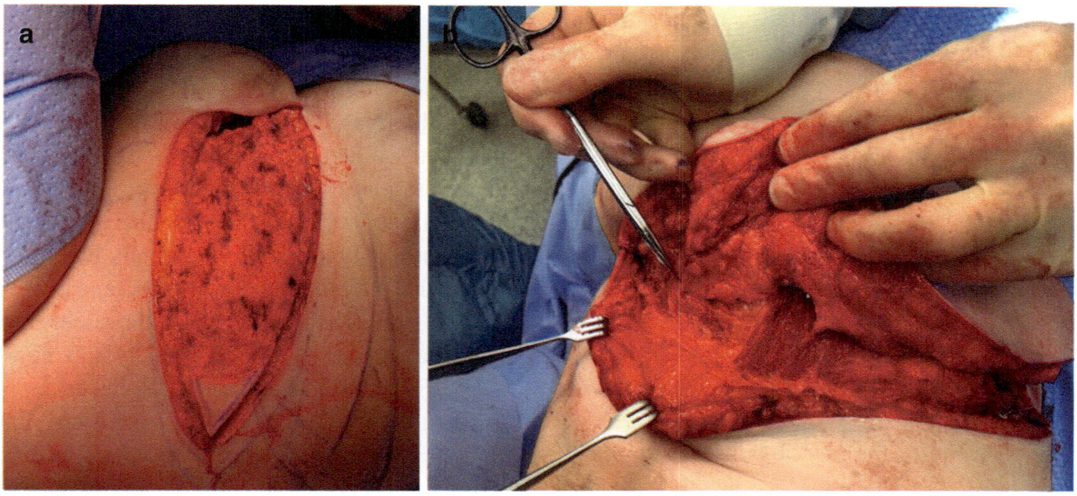

Fig. 14.6 (a) Dissection starts at the medial and upper border to complete oncology surgery and to identify perforators as needed. The flap can then be dissected and resized as required. (b) Scissors pointing to the position of LICAP vessels. Note the LD muscle and TDAP perforators that are freed

14.2.5 Flap Inset and Skin Closure

The flap will be delivered either by propeller or turnover and can be shortened to fit neatly into the cavity or folded if more bulk is required. The flap does not always require suturing into the cavity itself, but it is helpful to do some dermal sutures near the lateral border of the breast to encourage the flat to stay in position and literally "not fall out laterally". Occasionally in very firm breast tissue, where any visible or palpable edge can be felt to the breast tissue, one can put some gentle sutures to hold the flap position. However, it is preferred to stop the flap from falling out of the cavity and find its way within the defect. This prevents some tethering which can occur with true suturing of the flap. If one does suture the flap due to palpable parenchymal edges, then suture to the breast tissue and not to the chest wall. The flap donor site can then be closed in layers from the fascia, dermis and skin. A drain can be inserted for 24 h if required, although the patient can usually have this surgery as a day case. Smaller cases do not require a drain.

14.3 LTAP Flap

The LTAP flap [13] is based on perforators from the lateral thoracic artery and vein and, as such, have very different properties to the LICAP flap. It has a true vascular pedicle that can be dissected all the way back to the axillary vessels if required. Therefore, the pedicle can be a few centimetres up to 10–12 cm, depending on the level of dissection. In practice, a very long pedicle is rarely required. However, the pedicle does allow for a proper transposition of the flap into the centre of the breast. This makes the flap a very versatile and elegant solution for central and upper central two more defects. It also allows the lateral breast tissue uninvolved in the tumour excision to be left intact (unlike with the LICAP flap) with easy tunnelling of this flap or simple splitting of the lateral breast tissue to allow the pedicle to access central defects. Therefore, it is in principle and functionality more like the TDAP flap but only sacrifices the lateral thoracic vessels as its pedicle.

The lateral thoracic artery can have a variable course, and in approximately 5–10% of patients, it does not appear to consistently run down the lateral border of the breast as is required for this flap. In these cases, the artery seemed to enter the breast at a higher level, preventing an LTAP from being raised. However, the lateral thoracic vessels can be found just below Scarpa's fascia 1–2 cm lateral to the lateral breast crease in the remaining patients.

14.4 LTAP Steps

14.4.1 Markings

The principle of the markings is very similar to the LICAP flap. Using the Doppler, the linear signal of the lateral thoracic vessels should attempt to be confirmed and its likely position. However, even without a confirmed doppler signal of the lateral thoracic artery, this vessel should always be looked for at surgery as either an option for an LTAP flap or an augment to the LICAP flap options. Again, the positioning of the markings for the flap will be dictated by the likely present vasculature. Ideally, one would be looking for an intensity of a perforator(s) that lies along the linear signal of the lateral thoracic vessels.

It can be challenging to interpret if perforators are genuinely from the lateral thoracic or intercostal vessels, and the surgeon should remain open-minded to the final blood supply and hence delivery of the flap. However, if an ideal linear signal of the Lateral thoracic vessels is identified or pulsatile lateral thoracic vessels are seen entering the flap near the perforator signal, this flap is very safe and robust to raise.

14.4.2 Dissection of the LTAP Flap

As with the LICAP flap, the upper border of the flap can be incised and the lateral thoracic vessels identified just below Scarpa's fascia. These will need to be followed superiorly to perform any nodal surgery. This does require great care as the sentinel lymph node classically lies adjacent to the lateral thoracic vessels, and therefore care is needed to ensure that the vessels are not damaged during the sentinel lymph node biopsy. For this reason, one would never commit to an LTAP flap until all the oncology surgery is performed. If an axillary clearance is required, preserving the lateral thoracic vessels is feasible, although this makes the clearance more challenging. Again, if it was not feasible to preserve the lateral thoracic vessels or they were injured, then one can revert to a LICAP based flap.

Once the oncology surgery is performed and the suitable nature of the vessels has been identified, the flap can be raised, and any other preserved LICAP perforators can be dissected free, and the entire flap is lifted on the lateral thoracic vessels (Fig. 14.7a–e). The vessels can be left with a small collar of fat around them to make dissection easier. The proximal dissection is then just continued as required to allow tension-free transposition of the flap into the breast. The flap is de-epithelialised and can be either shaped, folded, or placed directly into the cavity depending on the dimensions and requirements. The donor site is closed in the same manner as a LICAP flap.

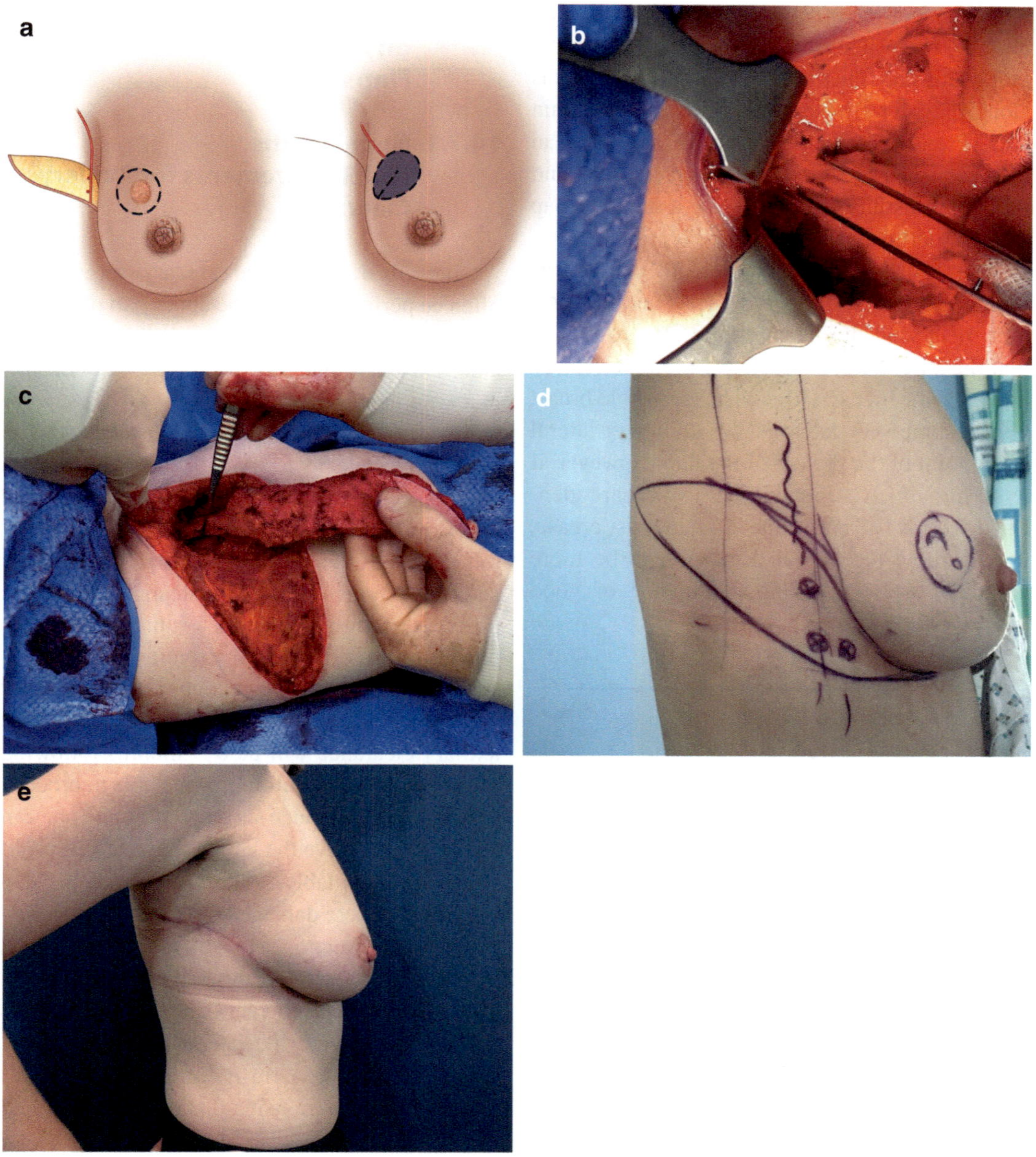

Fig. 14.7 (**a**) LTAP flap. (**b**) LTAP vessels just under Scarpa's fascia on superior aspect flap. (**c**) Flap raised on LTAP pedicle. (**d**) Pre-op LTAP. (**e**) Post-op LTAP

14.5 Combined LTAP/LICAP Flaps

The use of both lateral intercostal perforators and the lateral thoracic artery perforators has already been described above in the LICAP flaps. However, it is essential to discuss this combined flap approach in detail as it is a very reliable and relatively simple way of delivering the chest wall perforated flaps. In addition, it is helpful for those early on in their learning curve with these flaps as it allows the surgeon to keep a greater number of vessels, increasing the vasculature of the flap and reducing decision making, which is always more difficult early in the learning curve. In simple terms, this flap relies on a "mesentery" of vessels along the lateral breast border that may contain LICAP and LTAP based vessels. The flap can then be turned over based on this mesentery, and therefore this flap will always be a turnover flap with the dermis face down in the breast.

It is still helpful to doppler out the area as with all CWPF to identify vessels and perforators. It is vital during the dissection to ensure that the surgeon does not leave too much tissue lateral to the breast. Otherwise, the whole breast will become very lateralised with a very lateral pivot point of the breasts of the flap. However, if a mixture of LICAP and LTAP vessels are identified within 1–2 cm of the lateral breast crease, it will allow the lateral dissection to be more complete while allowing confidence of good vascularity.

14.6 Choosing Between the LICAP, LTAP, and Combined Flap?

These procedures are based on a series of principles and surgical techniques, including the identification of perforators, understanding of flap dimensions and pivot points to enable flap delivery, understanding the basic but distinct differences between the pedicle options of these differing flaps, and working out the requirements of the defect to be filled. Although the surgeon will make a clear plan prior to surgery, all options must remain possible, and the surgeon will be free to change the plan as the procedure evolves. This will be based on the findings of the relative perforators or vessels to supply these flaps and any untoward changes to the oncology surgery in terms of resection margins and, therefore, the size of the defect to be filled. Similarly, the surgeon must be adaptive in choosing the flap to achieve the overwhelming goal of suitably filling the defect with well-vascularised tissue.

14.7 Decisions that Impact on Chest Wall Perforated Flaps

14.7.1 Nodal Status and Requirements for Axillary Clearance

As described above, the axillary surgery can often be performed from the upper part of the flap or through a separate incision it felt more suitable. The LTAP flap requires more care in the primary surgery to complete the nodal surgery without damaging the pedicle. However, this is very achievable in nearly all cases. Even with axillary clearance, it is feasible to preserve the lateral thoracic vessels in most cases. If a patient returns a positive axillary sentinel lymph node and then requires an axillary clearance, there are different potential scenarios for this. Usually, the patient returning a positive sentinel node result will be receiving adjuvant chemotherapy in most cases. In this situation, the requirements for the axillary clearance will be 6–9 months following the surgery, and therefore it is feasible to proceed with axillary clearance surgery. Although one can attempt to preserve the lateral thoracic vessels, it would be acceptable to the viability of the flap even if they were damaged.

If, in the situation, the axillary surgery needs to occur a few weeks following the initial surgery, then evidently, great care does need to be taken in preserving the lateral thoracic vessels. Therefore, this scenario is infrequent and not a practical problem in using this flap.

14.7.2 Single-Stage or Two-Stage Surgery?

As with any breast-conserving surgery, a certain percentage of patients will have incomplete margins, usually from DCIS. Occasionally the involved margins will also be positive for invasive tumours. Fortunately, oncoplastic techniques such as CWPF do reduce positive margins.

However, 5–7% in our experience do have positive margins. There can be different philosophies to the approach of single versus two-stage surgery to delineate the margins. In the vast majority, it is our practice to do the chest will perforator flaps as a single stage and immediate partial breast reconstruction to fill the wide local excision defect. Advantages are that this allows a single procedure for the patient, and the perforators and flaps are much easier to dissect and be identified in the primary surgery. Similarly, the cancer defect does not have time to retract or create scarring, which can become problematic within a few weeks of surgery. However, this approach will result in some flaps being discarded for widespread incomplete margins. That can be reduced by meticulous attention to preoperative assessment and with the use of intraoperative radiology to assess margins and, if available, the use of frozen sections intraoperatively. The frozen section is very helpful for an invasive disease but can be more problematic in identifying DCIS, which is the main issue in the majority of incomplete margins.

If a two-stage approach is to be adopted [17], then the tumour can be excised through the preplanned upper margin of the flap and then the cavity filled with water and not saline. Water maintains itself far better in the body, and water can be re-injected into the cavity in the outpatients clinic every 7–10 days until margin analysis has been completed. This approach is more commonly planned if there is significant uncertainty about the margins of the tumour or if the patient has very few other full-back options away from the back in terms of breast reconstruction. Therefore, be more cautious about margins if the CWPF would prevent using the TDAP or LD flap, and these are the main total reconstruction options.

When incomplete margins are found, it is feasible to re-explore these flaps, and indeed the cavities are quite well delineated within the first few weeks; therefore, further margin excisions can easily be performed and the flaps replaced. If surgery follows chemotherapy, clips shall be placed within the tumour cavity, which should be routine practice. If there are multiple positive margins, then one must discuss the likelihood of achieving a complete margin, and in some cases, mastectomy may be decided upon. If patients go on to have mastectomy and reconstruction performed, the surgeon can choose whether to keep the CWPF as part of the reconstruction or discard it depending on the reconstruction type and the usefulness of the CWPF remaining.

14.8 Anterior Intercostal Artery Perforator (AICAP) Flaps and Internal Mammary Artery Perforator (IMAP) Flaps

The central and medial lower parts of the breast can be volume replaced from flaps based just below the inframammary fold (IMF), based upon the anterior perforators of the sixth intercostal vessels, the internal mammary perforators. However, the lateral lower breast is still better managed with LICAP flaps. These flaps can be raised as a linear transposition flap with the closure of the inframammary fold or as a crescent-shaped flap (Fig. 14.8). These flaps can be raised randomly if small, but it is always preferable to ensure the flap base is planned on an identified perforator.

The IMAP flap can be based on the fifth or sixth perforators and can at times create a slight bulge medially which can be corrected later if required.

Patients for these flaps need to have available tissue just below or at the IMF and some upper abdominal laxity to allow advancement

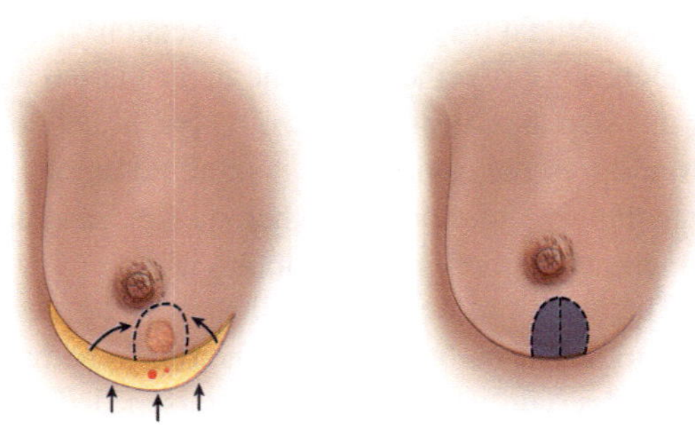

Fig. 14.8 AICAP Flap

of the lower border of these flaps to prevent inferior migration of the IMF or to, at least, minimize this.

14.8.1 Planning and Dissection

The doppler can identify perforators at or just below the IMF or at the medial end of the IMF for the IMAP flap. Once identified, the decision to use a linear or crescent-shaped flap will depend on where the available tissue is related to the tumour defect. As these flaps tend to be narrow, a central perforator within a crescent design is likely better vascularised but has less reach.

The patient can be positioned as usual, and the superior aspect of the flap is used for access to the tumour. A separate axillary incision is used for any nodal surgery. The flap is raised and de-epithelialised. Separating the inferior dermis is vital to allow movement of the flap as best possible.

The upper abdominal tissue can be undermined as required and advanced to allow a tension-free closure as possible.

14.8.2 Complications of Chest Wall Perforator Flaps

Overall, these flaps are well perfused and tolerate radiotherapy well. Total or sub-total flap failure is rare. However, some of the flaps can undergo fat necrosis if the flaps have poor vascularity supplying them or the flap's dimensions are too large. This process can be managed in line with fat necrosis in other scenarios, such as observation, liposuction, fat transfer or formal excision.

Deformity or tethering of the flap can be seen if the flap has been incorrectly positioned or sutured into the cavity. This is more common in very thin or ptotic breasts, where these flaps can sometimes be more problematic to use.

The scars on the chest wall tend to be very well tolerated but can be thickened or hypertrophic in certain patients. This is worsened if the flaps are made too wide, creating tension on the closure. For this reason, the flap should be planned for what is required but not overly large to minimise any donor site problems. Similarly, there can be potentially slight altered sensation or discomfort on the lateral chest wall, although this has been uncommon and considerably less common compared to major back flap procedures such as the latissimus dorsi flap.

Most flaps will heal with no clinically apparent fat necrosis and feel soft. As with most oncoplastic procedures, the use of mammograms remains adequate, with benign changes easily distinguishable from recurrence [18].

14.9 Conclusion

CWPF offer an alternative to mastectomy for many patients, especially those with small volume breasts who would get unsatisfactory outcomes from simple breast-conserving techniques and are not suitable for a mammaplasty repair of the defect. This complex patient group can achieve good cosmetic outcomes and patient-reported scores with CWPF techniques and is certainly comparable to mastectomy and total reconstruction with considerably simpler surgery and quicker recovery [19].

There is undoubtedly a learning curve to their use, but different levels of flap harvest can be attempted depending upon the experience available.

References

1. Macmillan RD, James R, Gale KL, McCulley SJ. Therapeutic mammaplasty. J Surg Oncol. 2014;110(1):90–5. https://doi.org/10.1002/jso.23659.
2. McCulley SJ, Macmillan RD. Planning and use of therapeutic mammoplasty--Nottingham approach. Br J Plast Surg. 2005;58(7):889–901. https://doi.org/10.1016/j.bjps.2005.03.008.
3. Clough KB, Lewis JS, Couturaud B, Fitoussi A, Nos C, Falcou MC. Oncoplastic techniques allow extensive resections for breast-conserving therapy of breast carcinomas. Ann Surg. 2003;237(1):26–34. https://doi.org/10.1097/00000658-200301000-00005.

4. Munhoz AM, Montag E, Gemperli R. Oncoplastic breast surgery: indications, techniques and perspectives. Gland Surg. 2013;2(3):143–57. https://doi.org/10.3978/j.issn.2227-684X.2013.08.02.
5. Hamdi M. Oncoplastic and reconstructive surgery of the breast. Breast. 2013;22(Suppl 2):S100–5. https://doi.org/10.1016/j.breast.2013.07.019.
6. McCulley SJ, Schaverien MV, Tan VK, Macmillan RD. Lateral thoracic artery perforator (LTAP) flap in partial breast reconstruction. J Plast Reconstr Aesthet Surg. 2015;68(5):686–91. https://doi.org/10.1016/j.bjps.2015.01.008.
7. Hamdi M, Van Landuyt K, de Frene B, Roche N, Blondeel P, Monstrey S. The versatility of the intercostal artery perforator (ICAP) flaps. J Plast Reconstr Aesthet Surg. 2006;59(6):644–52. https://doi.org/10.1016/j.bjps.2006.01.006.
8. Veber M, Ho Quoc C, Fakiha M, Toussoun G, Delay E. Reconstruction par lambeau perforant de l'artère intercostale latérale (LICAP) d'une séquelle sévère de traitement conservateur du cancer du sein [Lateral Intercostal Artery Perforator (LICAP) flap for lateral breast defect reconstruction]. Ann Chir Plast Esthet. 2011;56(6):568–73. https://doi.org/10.1016/j.anplas.2011.07.004.
9. Macmillan RD, Carstensen L, Tan V, McCulley SJ. Local perforator flaps in oncoplastic breast conserving surgery: Nottingham's experience. In: Losken A, Hamdi M, editors. Partial breast reconstruction: techniques in oncoplastic surgery. 2nd ed. St. Louis, MO: Quality Medical Publishing; 2017.
10. Clough KB, Acosta-Marín V, Nos C, et al. Rates of neoadjuvant chemotherapy and oncoplastic surgery for breast cancer surgery: a French national survey. Ann Surg Oncol. 2015;22:3504–11. https://doi.org/10.1245/s10434-015-4378-6.
11. Heeg E, Jensen MB, Hölmich LR, Bodilsen A, Tollenaar R, Laenkholm AV, Offersen BV, Ejlertsen B, Mureau M, Christiansen PM. Rates of re-excision and conversion to mastectomy after breast-conserving surgery with or without oncoplastic surgery: a nationwide population-based study. Br J Surg. 2020;107(13):1762–72. https://doi.org/10.1002/bjs.11838.
12. Losken A, Hart AM, Chatterjee A. Updated evidence on the oncoplastic approach to breast conservation therapy. Plast Reconstr Surg. 2017;140(5 S):14S–22S. https://doi.org/10.1097/PRS.0000000000003951.
13. Mele S, Wright D, Paramanathan N, Laws S, Peiris L, Rainsbury R. Long-term effect of oncoplastic breast-conserving surgery using latissimus dorsi miniflaps on mammographic surveillance and the detection of local recurrence. J Plast Reconstr Aesthet Surg. 2017;70(9):1203–9. https://doi.org/10.1016/j.bjps.2017.06.030.
14. Macmillan RD, McCulley SJ. Oncoplastic breast surgery: what, when and for whom? Curr Breast Cancer Rep. 2016;8:112–7. https://doi.org/10.1007/s12609-016-0212-9.
15. Soumian S, Parmeshwar R, Chandarana M, Marla S, Narayanan S, Shetty G. Chest wall perforator flaps for partial breast reconstruction: surgical outcomes from a multicenter study. Arch Plast Surg. 2020;47(2):153–9. https://doi.org/10.5999/aps.2019.01186.
16. Hamdi M, Spano A, Landuyt KV, D'Herde K, Blondeel P, Monstrey S. The lateral intercostal artery perforators: anatomical study and clinical application in breast surgery. Plast Reconstr Surg. 2008;121(2):389–96. https://doi.org/10.1097/01.prs.0000298317.65296.cf.
17. Roy PG, Tenovici AA. Staged approach to partial breast reconstruction to avoid mastectomy in women with breast cancer. Gland Surg. 2017;6(4):336–42. https://doi.org/10.21037/gs.2017.03.08.
18. Tan VK, Cornford EJ, McCulley SJ, Macmillan RD. Qualitative mammographic findings and outcomes of surveillance mammography after partial breast reconstruction with an autologous flap. J Surg Oncol. 2015;111(4):377–81. https://doi.org/10.1002/jso.23838.
19. Kelsall JE, McCulley SJ, Brock L, Akerlund M, Macmillan RD. Comparing oncoplastic breast conserving surgery with mastectomy and immediate breast reconstruction: case-matched patient reported outcomes. J Plast Reconstr Aesthet Surg. 2017;70(10):1377–85. https://doi.org/10.1016/j.bjps.2017.05.009.

Complications with Breast Volume Replacement Local Perforator Flaps: Avoidance, Recognition and Treatment

15

John Murphy, Francisco Moura, and Edel Marie Quinn

Contents

Abbreviations

AICAP	Anterior intercostal artery perforator
BCS	Breast conserving surgery
BMI	Body mass index
CT	Computed tomography
CWPF	Local chest wall perforator flaps
ICAP	Intercostal artery perforator
IMF	Inframammary fold
LD	Latissimus dorsi
LICAP	Lateral intercostal artery perforator
LTAP	Lateral thoracic artery perforator
MICAP	Medial intercostal artery perforator
MRI	Magnetic resonance imaging
NAC	Nipple-areolar complex
NPWT	Negative pressure wound therapy
RT	Radiotherapy
SSI	Surgical site infection
TAP	Thoracodorsal artery perforator

J. Murphy (✉) · F. Moura · E. M. Quinn
Nightingale Breast Unit, Wythenshawe Hospital, Manchester University NHS Foundation Trust, Manchester, UK
e-mail: john.murphy@mft.nhs.uk; Francisco.serraemoura@mft.nhs.uk; Edel.quinn@mft.nhs.uk

M. Hamdi et al. (eds.), *Pedicled Flaps in Partial Breast Reconstruction*,
https://doi.org/10.1007/978-3-031-08483-6_15

15.1 Introduction

Local perforator volume replacement flaps provide surgeons with further options to increase breast conservation rates for breast cancer patients, bringing with it associated improvements in patient satisfaction, re-excision rates and similar overall survival compared to Breast Conserving Surgery (BCS) [1–4]. BCS has been shown to be oncologically and surgically safe, with a long-term survival comparable to that of total mastectomy; indeed long-term data from several National Cancer registries suggests improved overall survival associated with BCS [5–7]. They are also utilised to avoid poor outcomes in volume sensitive parts of the breast during BCS (Fig. 15.1). Local flaps also aid maintenance of cosmesis when tumour volume resection would otherwise lead to poor outcomes without such techniques (Fig. 15.2). In addition, they are very useful in the delayed setting to address difficult to correct defects affecting the breast from previous BCS (Fig. 15.3). When the correct flap is performed on the right patient, local

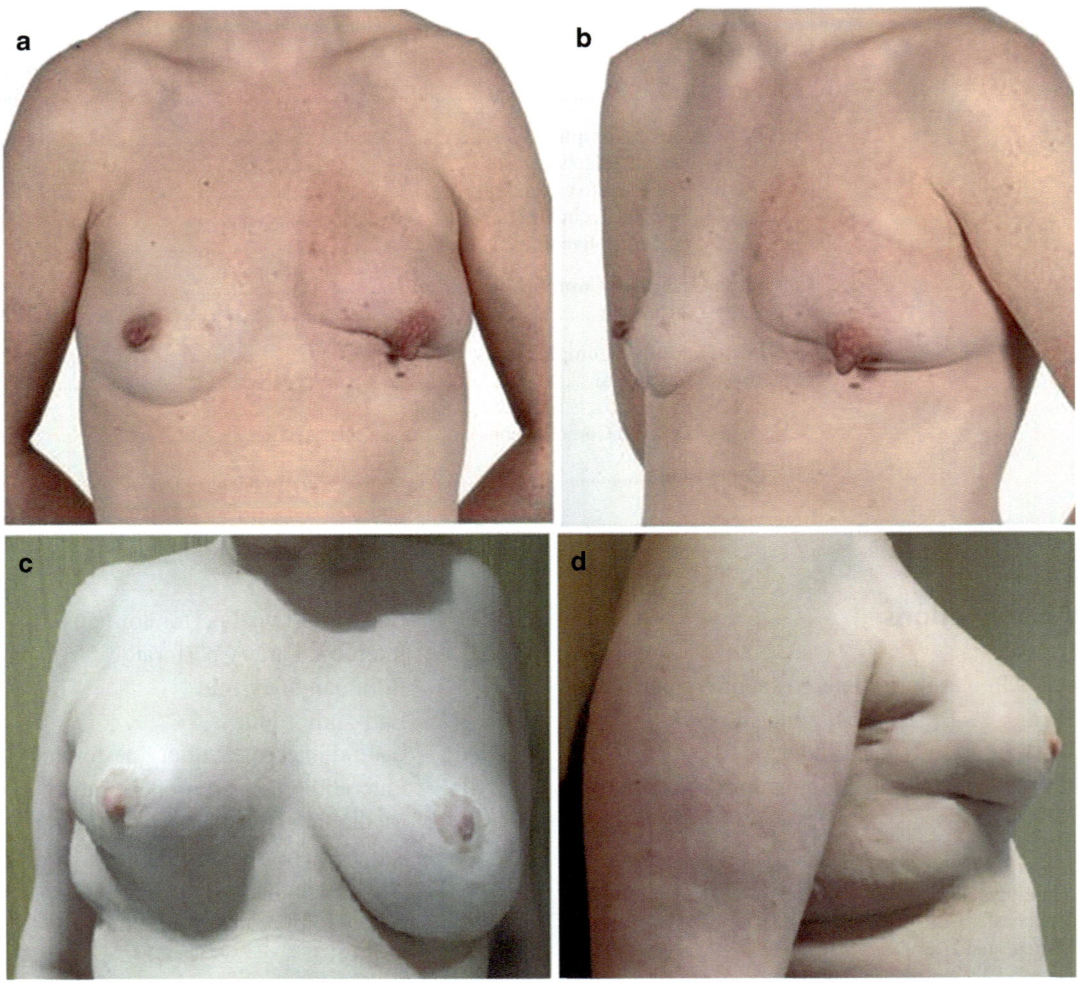

Fig. 15.1 Example of a poor aesthetic outcome in BCS without partial breast reconstruction. Partial breast reconstruction using local perforator flaps enables avoidance of poorer aesthetic outcomes which can be very difficult to correct. Demonstrated here (Upper panel—**a**, **b**) is a classical birds beak deformity secondary to BCS. Defects in the lateral quadrant (lower panel—**c**, **d**) also cause nipple areolar complex deviations alongside the volume deficit associated with suboptimal aesthetic outcomes. In this situation the patient had undergone breast reduction surgery 15 years prior to BCS

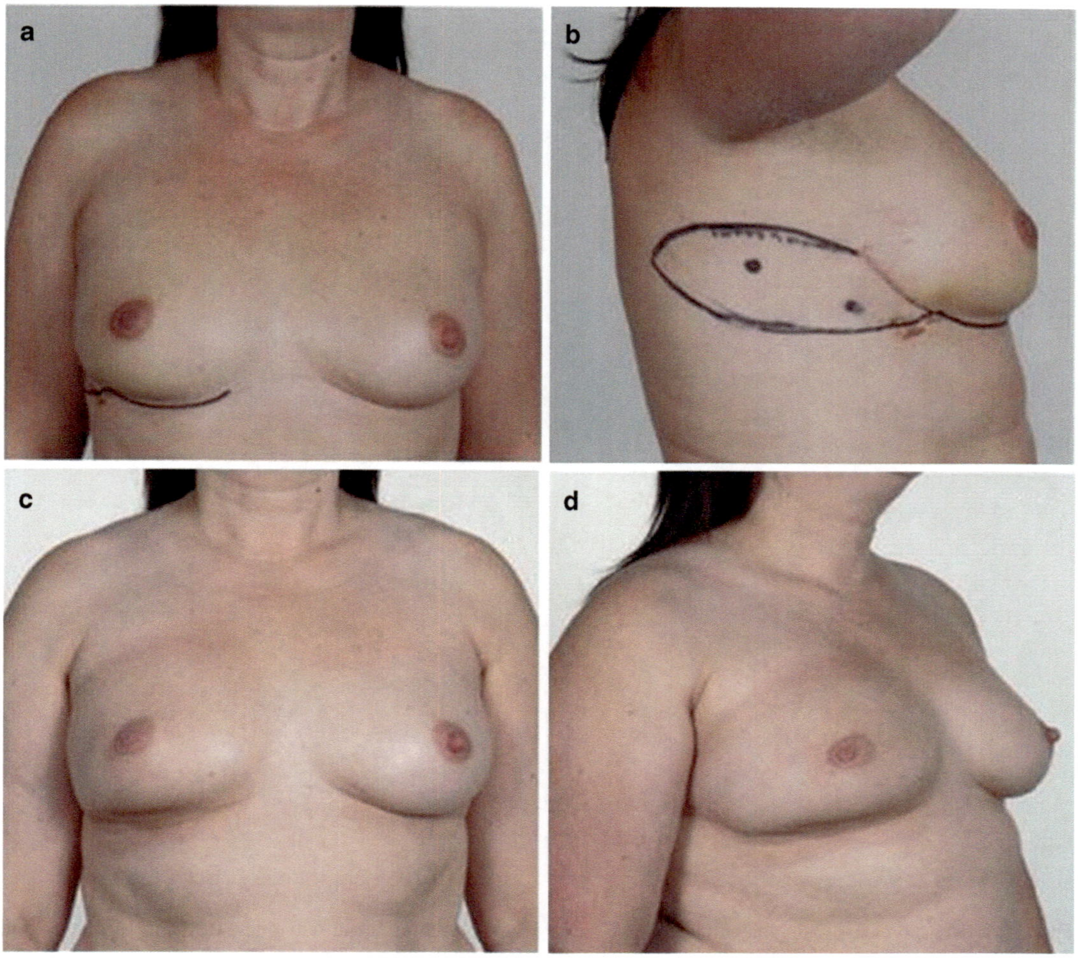

Fig. 15.2 Outcome following partial breast reconstruction using a lateral CWPF with adjuvant radiotherapy. Pre-operative marking demonstrated in (**a**) and (**b**). The procure was performed as a two-stage procedure in which a fully excised 49 mm Grade 2 Invasive Ductal Carcinoma and Sentinel node biopsy was performed at the first stage with the defect cavity held open with water (H_2O). The second surgery was performed within 2 weeks with a lateral CWPF providing the patient with a natural looking contour of the breast with good cosmetic outcome. (**c**) and (**d**) show post-operative results at 24 months following radiotherapy

flaps deliver excellent results. However, as with all surgical procedures, complications can occur. Therefore, knowledge of prevention, recognition and management of complications is as important as learning how to perform the procedure.

The prevention of complications is particularly important in breast reconstruction because not only do complications threaten the cosmetically sensitive breast area, they add to the patient's psychological burden and most importantly, can cause delay in adjuvant postoperative cancer treatments. Fortunately, most complications from oncoplastic breast reconstruction do not increase length of hospital stay nor interfere with adjuvant treatment [8]. In addition to becoming familiar with potential complications, surgeons must anticipate these undesirable events and take appropriate measures to help prevent their occurrence. This chapter will focus on the prevention, recognition and management of complications of local flaps used in volume replacement BCS.

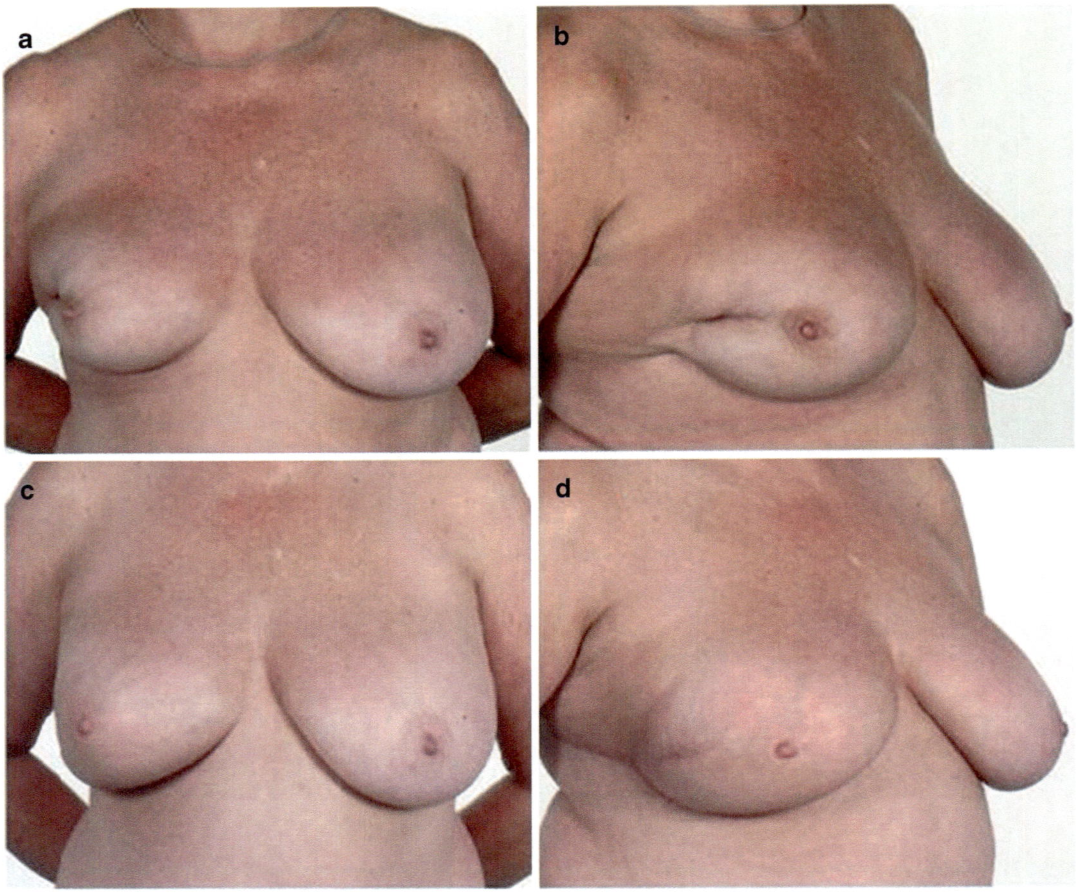

Fig. 15.3 Revision case using lateral CWPF. Female patient with poor outcome of BCS affecting the lateral aspect of the right breast (upper panel). Defects in the lateral quadrant (**a**, **b**) also cause nipple areolar complex deviations alongside the volume deficit associated with suboptimal aesthetic outcomes. Revision surgery with a lateral CWPF provided the patient with a natural looking contour of the breast with good cosmetic outcome (lower panel) (**c**, **d**)

15.2 Prevention of Complications

Avoidance of complications begins in the preoperative period with a comprehensive history and physical examination, along with Oncoplastic Multi-Disciplinary Team discussion examining the oncological considerations of the particular case. Careful patient selection, surgical planning, technical execution and peri-operative care are essential to the success of the surgical treatment.

15.2.1 Patient Selection

Appropriate patient selection will reduce complications and improve cosmetic outcomes. Moreover, pragmatic pre-operative counselling of the patient will reduce the likelihood of complications. Informed consent should include an open discussion of potential problems that can occur.

Besides the surgeon's experience, the incidence of complications is related to the patient's co-morbidities, with the most relevant factors being a high (>30) body mass index (BMI), smoking history, overall skin quality (breast and potential donor sites), evidence of prior radiation and the need for simultaneous procedures such as mastopexy and axillary dissection [9, 10]. Other factors such as hypertension, diabetes, liver failure, immunosuppression, renal failure, inherited blood disorders, inflammatory skin conditions and a history of complicated scarring can all negatively affect the surgical result [11]. Working closely together with different specialities, where necessary, is crucial to optimise patients with multiple risk factors for surgery.

Tobacco use has a well-documented detrimental effect on tissue perfusion resulting in more severe skin sloughing and possible flap necrosis [12]. This effect places the donor site at risk of delayed wound healing in patients undergoing partial breast reconstruction. Heavy alcohol use should be avoided as this affects the hepatic system, which in turn affects both the clotting cascade and drug metabolism, which can contribute to haematoma formation [13].

Patients with a history of irradiation usually have subcutaneous and deep scar tissue which contributes to decreased vascularity of the skin and poorer outcomes [14]. Using reconstructive local flaps from adjacent non-irradiated tissue is especially relevant in those patients undergoing delayed reconstruction, following previous BCS, in which the non-irradiated tissue can regenerate the damaged area caused by scar tissue with radiotherapy.

Adipose tissue has a poor vascular supply which decreases the blood supply to the wound site and prevents cellular oxygenation and nutrients necessary for wound healing [15]. A high BMI is likely to result in increased post-operative complications due to the increased operative time as there is increased dissection of tissues and a subsequent increased risk of bleeding [16]. In addition, it is likely that obese patients have other co-morbidities that further increase their risk of complications [17].

Volume displacement techniques are a useful alternative in those patients with large ptotic breasts who gain benefit from a therapeutic mammoplasty [18]. However, Panhofer et al. [10] identified an increased risk of post-operative wound infection and partial flap necrosis in those undergoing reduction oncoplastic breast surgery (doughnut or other techniques) in 39 patients compared to 318 undergoing BCS alone. This is due to the increased mobilization of the breast parenchyma [19].

15.2.2 Peri-operative Planning

Establishing a consistent perioperative routine is the first step in preventing complications. The reconstructive options available are primarily determined by location and by the tumour to breast volume ratio. The selection of the site and size of the flap should be based on the site and volume of breast defect, site of perforators, aesthetics and assessment of skin and subcutaneous tissue determined by a pinch test. Hand-held unidirectional Doppler can be used with the patient lying supine with the shoulder abducted mimicking the operative position prior to surgery to confirm the presence of suitable perforators (Fig. 15.4). Planning a flap in reverse and with an extra margin will avoid tension on closing. As the flap's blood supply is inversely proportional to the distance from the base of the flap, it is important that undue tension is prevented, especially along the distal aspect of the flap. Additional imaging such as computed tomography (CT) angiography is not usually required to assess calibre of perforators, as the diameter of vessels is usually very small and such imaging modalities offers little extra knowledge to that which is gained from the use of Doppler assessment. Occasionally, when assessing the Thoracodorsal vessels for a TDAP flap, it may be appropriate to formally assess the Thoracodorsal pedicle with duplex scanning or CT angiography if there is a clinical concern about the absence of such vessels if an axillary procedure has been performed previously in which the pedicle may have been damaged as part of the oncological treatment. The authors also recommend assessing for suitable perforators well in advance in the delayed setting as perforators situated around the periphery of the breast are fre-

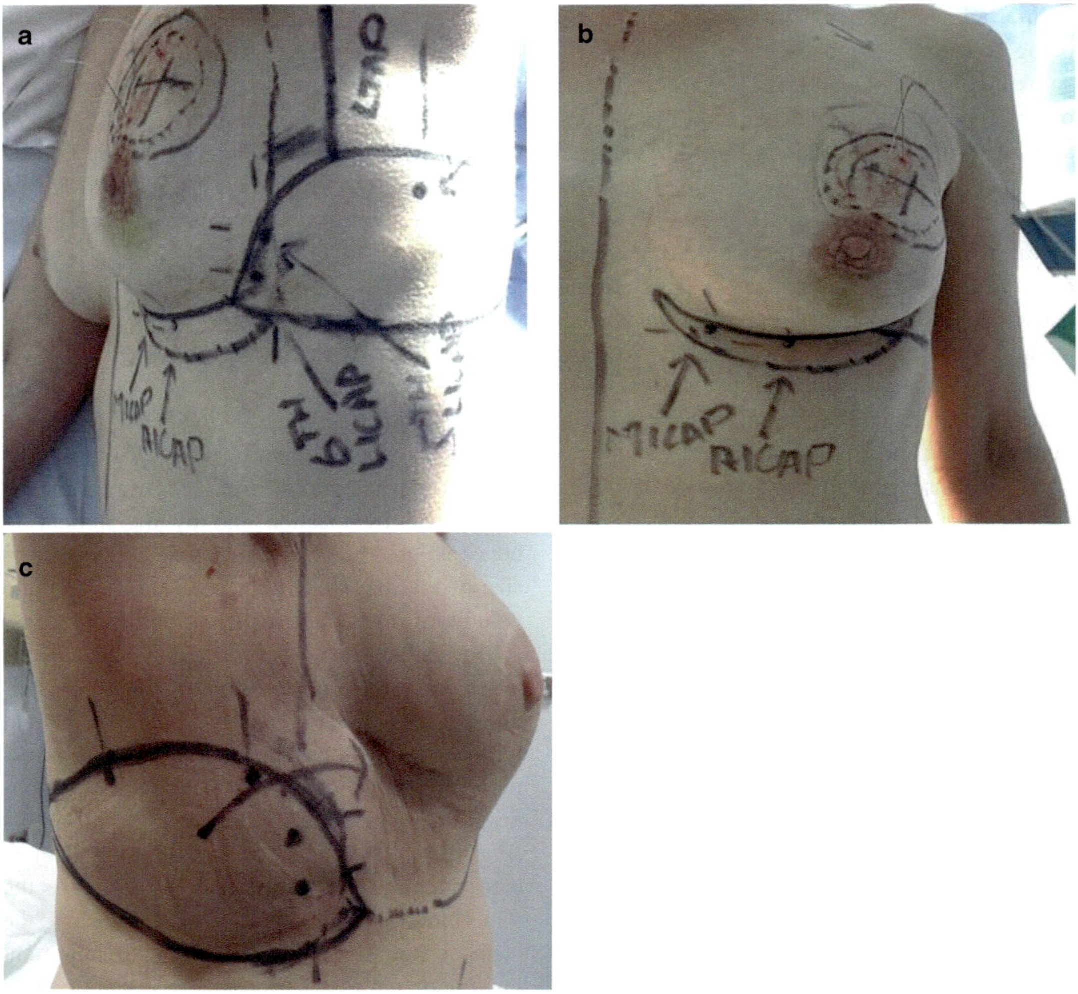

Fig. 15.4 Pre-operative markings demonstrating the location of anterior and lateral CWPF. The anterior chest wall perforators are located in the inframammary crease whereas the lateral perforators are present around the anterior axillary line. This patient had a tumour affecting the supero-lateral area of her left breast and, therefore, a lateral chest wall perforator flap would be suitable (upper panel—**a**, **b**). In the delayed setting, marking the flap to be used follows the same principles ensuring that the perforators are present and haven't been damaged during the previous procedures (lower panel—**c**)

quently damaged during the original oncological surgical episode. In this situation, the use of other perforator flaps may well be indicated, such as the TDAP flap, for which appropriate theatre time, patient positioning, assessment of vessels needs to be considered to ensure complications are kept to a minimum (Fig. 15.4).

The incidence of complications can be related to the surgeon's learning curve. Progression along the learning curve will allow the surgeon to carry out a greater variation in the types of perforator flaps performed, excision of increasing size of cancerous lesions deemed suitable for BCS, increase the proportion of day case surgery and reduce operative time. Local perforator volume replacement flaps can be performed immediately (ie. at the same timing of tumour excision), early (once negative margins have been confirmed) and delayed (once adjuvant therapy has been completed). If a surgeon has limited experience, it may be worth considering carrying out the procedure in a two-stage early fashion to ensure tumour margin clearance and axillary nodal assessment is completed before partial breast reconstruction. This can be of upmost importance in those patients in whom the LTAP flap is planned, as preservation of the LTAP vessels during an axillary dissection is particularly challenging. Indeed, a safer option maybe utilizing an alternative perforator-based flap to correct the defect in such cases. If, however, the LTAP has been utilised as the flap of choice during a one stage procedure and axillary sentinel lymph node biopsy has returned a positive result alternate choice exists, rather than proceeding directly to axillary dissection. We have found that in many such cases, adjuvant chemotherapy will be indicated. We would advocate the patient undergoing chemotherapy first and by the time completion axillary dissection is performed around 8 months later, the flap is also neovascularised from the surrounding tissue and dependence on the LTAP vessels less relevant. In this situation, inadvertent damage to the LTAP during dissection does not lead to flap loss. The other safe option is to include the axilla in the radiation field following BCS and utilise RT as the definite treatment for the node positive axilla.

Several local flaps have been described in oncoplastic breast surgery [20–25]. These flaps may be positioned into the defect by different movements including 'turnover', propeller, advancement or pedicled techniques. Each of these flaps (Table 15.1) and their movements have associated limitations that should be accounted for when planning an oncoplastic operation. For instance, the 180° rotation of a propeller flap can be associated with a risk of fat necrosis due to venous congestion compared to other methods. Venous congestion can be prevented by avoiding excessive skeletonization of the perforator, dissection of the perforator

Table 15.1 Advantages and Limitations of different perforator flaps used in oncoplastic breast surgery

Flap (source vessel)	Reach (quadrants)	Advantages	Limitations	References
TDAP (Thoracodorsal artery)	All quadrants	Covers large defects	Difficulty in locating the perforator	Jeong [26], Hamdi et al. [23], Santanelli et al. [27], Kim et al. [28]
		Preserves LD muscle	Unpredictable course, diameter and vein calibre	
		Reduces donor site complications and hospital stay compared to LD (e.g. seromas)	Dissection of perforators can be challenging	
		Similar colour and texture to breast	Requires intra-operative change in position	
LTAP (Lateral Thoracic Artery)	Lateral	Preserves TDAP/MS-TD/LD for future use	Anatomy of LTA has been shown to be variable and absent in up to 25% cases	Taylor and Daniel [29], Rowsell et al. [30], Bhattacharya et al. [31], McCulley et al. [32], Martellani et al. [24]
		Use of sandbag may prevent need for intra-operative movement	Technically challenging dissection during axillary clearance procedure	
		Scar hidden in brassiere strap		
		Similar colour and texture to breast		
		Can be used with LICAP to increase perfusion of flap		
		Greater reach than LICAP flap when pedicle fully mobilised		

(continued)

Table 15.1 (continued)

Flap (source vessel)	Reach (quadrants)	Advantages	Limitations	References
LICAP (Lateral Intercostal Artery)	Lateral	Preserves TDAP/MS-TD/LD for future use	Perforator are short in length	Hamdi et al. [21], Munhoz et al. [25], Kim et al. [28], Martellani et al. [24]
		Use of sandbag may prevent need for intra-operative movement	Variable position	
		Scar hidden in brassiere strap	92% have dominant pedicle	
		Similar colour and texture to breast	Higher risk of developing fat necrosis and flap necrosis at farthest from the perforators	
		Easier identification of vessels and quicker dissection		
		Further anterior position of perforators compared to TAP		
		Sensate flap can be harvested		
AICAP (Anterior Intercostal Artery)	Inferior	No intra-operative movement	Relatively small amount of tissue that can be used	Hamdi and De Frene [33], Hamdi et al. [34], Munhoz et al. [25]
		Scar along IMF	Effects of radiotherapy in delayed reconstruction may affect vascular supply of this tissue	
		Could be used as transposition island flap V-Y advancement flap for lateral defects	Increased tension of donor site closure may cause lowering of IMF	
MICAP (Medial Intercostal Artery)	Medial	No intra-operative movement	As per AICAP	Hamdi et al. [34, 35]
		Scar along IMF		
Thoraco-epigastric (Superior Epigastric Artery)	Inferior	Scar along IMF	As per AICAP	Hamdi et al. [34], Uemura [36], Lee et al. [37]
	Central	Arc of rotation allows reach to upper inner quadrant		
	Supero-medial	Longer pedicle than AICAP		

together with the adjacent fascia, and moving the flap by a turnover method.

15.2.3 Surgical Technique

Attention to detail and adherence to safe surgical principles minimizes the risk of unfavourable outcomes. A sterile field reduces likelihood of infection [38]. In addition to flap design, delicate technique is the cornerstone to a successful surgical result. The technical aspects include tissue handling, adequate undermining and suture placement. Raising the flap in the correct plane and achieving haemostasis without causing excess trauma reduces the risk of excess bleeding and subsequent haematoma formation. Following this, care should be taken when mobilising the flap into the defect to avoid kinking and compression at the pedicle. The use of toothed forceps and skin hooks can cause damage to the flap margins, leading to ischaemic compromise. Adequate undermining is essential to create a tension-free closure. Dermal sutures, where appropriate, play a vital role to accomplish this too. Closing the wound without tension is fundamental to prevent skin necrosis and dehiscence. The authors no longer routinely use drains unless a specific indication is identified and advocate the routine use of negative pressure wound therapy (NPWT) on closed incisions at risk of dehiscence and surgical site infection (SSI). These are applied at the time of wound closure as shown in Fig. 15.5. NPWT dressings remain in place for 7 days and are associated with a reduction in dehiscence, SSI, tissue oedema and reduction in seroma formation [39, 40].

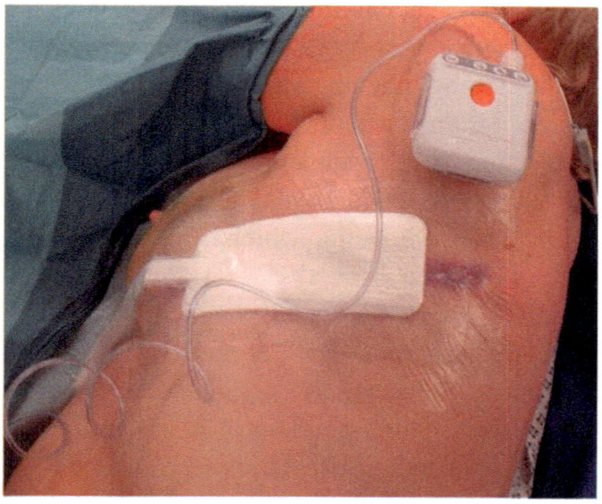

Fig. 15.5 Application of NWPT dressing (PICO™) over the donor site. This patient underwent a lateral CWPF for partial breast reconstruction of a defect to the inferolateral quadrant of the left breast. The application of NWPT is routinely used to reduce the risk of post-operative wound dehiscence, seroma formation and surgical site infection

15.2.4 Post-operative Care

Post-operative review prior to discharge (most patients can be treated as a day case procedure) and outpatient review of the patient at week 1, 2 and 4 will facilitate early recognition and treatment of complications. Some complications are reversible, and expeditious treatment may prevent a reversible complication from becoming an irreversible one. In general, most patients should develop long-term disease-free and excellent cosmetic outcomes (Fig. 15.6).

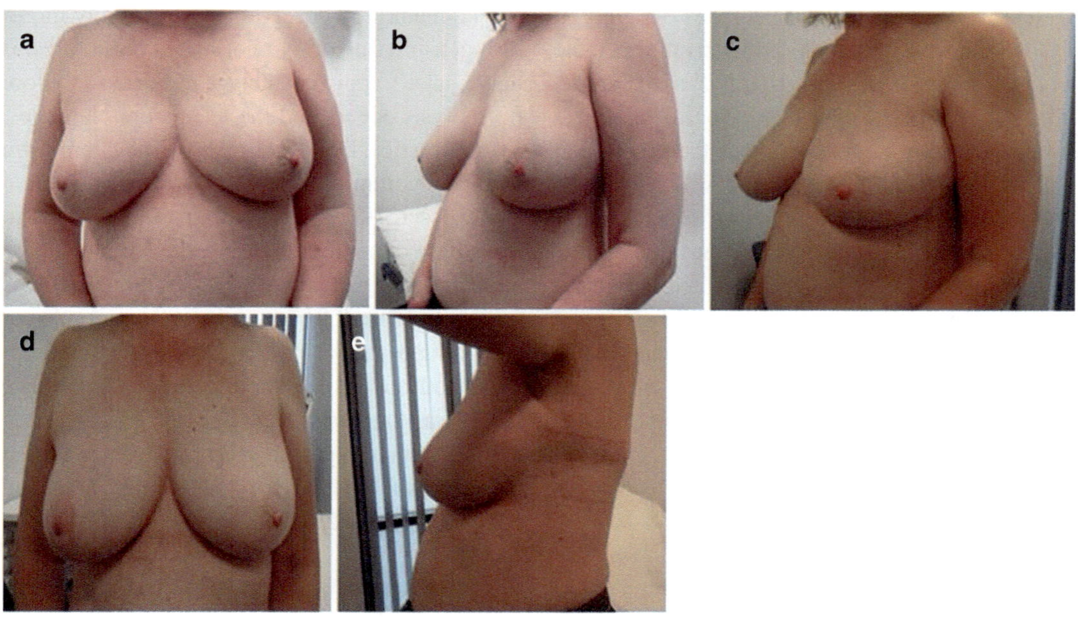

Fig. 15.6 Long-term 5-year post-operative outcome following lateral CWPF for partial breast reconstruction after resection of a large breast tumour. The tumour was located in the upper outer quadrant of the left breast (**a**, **b**—Pre-operative images); initially a 48 mm Grade 2 invasive lobular carcinoma was resected alongside axillary dissection for node positive disease. The patient underwent adjuvant chemotherapy, whole breast radiotherapy as well as endocrine therapy. Represented here are the results 5 years post initial resection and partial breast reconstruction (**c**–**e**)

15.3 Intra-Operative Complications

15.3.1 Ischaemia

A pale flap with slow capillary refill heralds impending ischaemia and this is always disquieting for the operating surgeon. Thankfully given the local nature of flaps, the size of the flap relative to vessel(s) diameter ensures this is an unusual occurrence. Intra-operative clinical assessment and judicious use of doppler are indicated to ensure no flap compromise. When using local chest wall perforator flaps (CWPFs), it may be that the use of more than one perforator for the flap (e.g. combination of LICAP and LTAP) is entirely suitable and further ameliorates any concerns regarding flap perfusion. A tension-free flap inset should be performed to avoid rupture of the perforator. When insetting the flap and signs of ischaemia are recognised, additional undermining to relieve tension or modifying the skin suture type may improve the perfusion of skin edges. Consideration of post-operative oedema is critical when placing sutures as this may result in strangulation of parts of the flap.

It is also important to consider the possibility of flap ischaemia secondary to avulsion of the pedicle from its origin, as the vessels are of small calibre. If at all possible, we would advocate leaving a small mesentery of tissue around the vessels (so long as the flap placement allows), which gives the flap more protection from the risk of avulsion in the intra- and immediate post-operative period.

Venous congestion may also lead to ischaemia. This presents within the first post-operative hours to days with oedema and blueish discolouration (if a skin paddle is present). If no intervention is carried out, flap epidermolysis to full-thickness necrosis can occur.

15.4 Post-Operative Complications

15.4.1 Immediate

15.4.1.1 Haematoma

A haematoma typically presents in the intra-operative or the immediate post-operative setting. Flaps that are tense and demonstrate a change in colour often indicate hematoma formation. Drug-associated coagulopathy and inadequate haemostasis are the most common causes of haematoma. The risk is related to the extent of flap harvesting [41]. Haematomas may compromise the viability of the flap by inducing vasospasm or separating the flap from the wound bed. The free radical production in a haematoma can lead to flap necrosis. A haematoma may also predispose the surgical site to infection which leads onto inflammatory oedema.

Intra-operatively, haemorrhage is averted with meticulous haemostasis. Careful ligation or cauterization of secondary segmental pedicles is essential to achieve good haemostasis, as well as careful inspection of the breast parenchyma which can often be an unsuspecting cause of haematoma formation. Closure of dead space can also be useful to prevent haematoma occurrence. Drains are rarely used in our practice. The exception to this rule is when there is significant dead space and the wound bed or flap are excessively oozy.

If the haematoma is small and not tense, this can be managed conservatively by merely monitoring, aspirating or by releasing some sutures. It may take approximately 2 weeks before fibrinolysis occurs and the haematoma liquefies. In our practice, however, if there is any doubt, we would recommend exploration under general anaesthesia. If the haematoma is significant in size, tense or painful, then expedient treatment by returning the patient to the operating theatre is critical to prevent flap vascularity compromise or sloughing of the wound. This is treated by evacuation and controlling the bleeding vessels. The risk of haematoma in local flap oncoplastic breast reconstruction requiring evacuation is reported at 1.7–5% [42–45] and 0.9–4.4% when managed conservatively [42, 45].

15.4.2 Early

15.4.2.1 Wound Dehiscence

Wound dehiscence occurs as a result of skin necrosis or infection. Excessive tension can give rise to ischaemia which in turn causes skin necrosis. Dehiscence can be characterised according to its severity: superficial (limited to the dermis or above) or full thickness (deeper to the dermis). The rate of wound dehiscence is reported at 0.9–24% [25, 45–48]. However, in comparison, the rates are higher at 19–25% in those undergoing volume displacement reduction mammoplasty [49, 50].

The tensile strength of a wound is almost negligible until Day 5 post-operatively at which point there is a rapid gain in strength lasting approximately 6 weeks [51]. This highlights the importance of deeper subcutaneous and dermal stitching in providing stability to the wound in the early phase of healing. In addition, we advocate the use of NWPT dressing for at least 7 days, with the preference being 14 days if the patient is tolerating the dressing with no obvious skin excoriation.

The management of these patients depends on the time since operation, cause and severity of the dehiscence. Causative factors such as infections and modifiable patient-specific factors such as nutrition and smoking should be addressed. In most cases, the dehiscence is left to heal by secondary intention. There may be a role for NPWT in larger and deeper dehiscence in order to accelerate granulation. Skin grafting may be required to accelerate the wound healing process so that the patient may proceed with adjuvant therapies if required. Poor scarring from any resultant wound dehiscence can be addressed later on.

15.4.2.2 Seroma

A seroma results from the accumulation of serous fluid in dead space. An important advantage of local flaps is that any underlying muscle is preserved which improves donor site morbidity but does not eradicate it. Seromas are more commonly seen following large local or pedicled flaps. Thus, they are widely reported after Latissimus Dorsi (LD) flap reconstruction [52, 53]. The incidence in thoracodorsal flaps has been reported as high as 5.5–14.7% [47, 54]. However, a recent systematic review of Oncoplastic BCS reports a seroma rate of 1% [55]. Furthermore, Hamdi et al. reported no seroma occurrence in BCS perforator flaps other than in thoracordorsal flaps [47]. Seromas are generally minor complications that can most times be managed conservatively. Occasionally seromas require aspiration for symptomatic purposes or antibiotics due to infection. Operative strategies that may reduce the incidence of seroma include the use of quilting if there is a large dead space. In our institution, NPWT dressing is usually applied to wound for which some evidence exists to reduce seroma formation. In addition, a seroma capsulectomy is sometimes performed when the second part of a two-stage procedure is delayed for more than 2 weeks. This maintains a natural soft texture to the breast at the site of the defect reconstruction. The authors do not routinely use drains, tissue adhesives or steroid injections to prevent the formation of seroma.

15.4.2.3 Infection

Infections usually manifest as erythema, pain and swelling generally around Day 5–7 postoperatively. It can also present several weeks post-operatively. Infections are either limited to the superficial skin, deeper layers (in the form of an abscess) or both. The incidence of Oncoplastic BCS-associated infection is reported to be as low as 2% [47, 48, 55]. There is a lack of detail in the available literature relative to partial breast reconstruction with regards to the varying severities (Superficial or abscess) of infection and its subsequent management. To prevent its occurrence, stringent sterility in the operating theatre should be employed. Ensuring that the flap is well perfused throughout and using minimal suturing material to oppose the skin edges will reduce the likelihood of infection. Tissue oxygenation is crucial to prevent wound bacterial colonisation [56]. Drains should be limited or not used where possible. Pre-operative antibiotic prophylaxis reduces the risk of SSIs for patients undergoing breast cancer surgery [57]; however, a systematic review could not find a consensus on the necessary duration of antibiotic prophylaxis following all forms of breast reconstruction, but did not find any benefit for patients who received them for longer than 24 h [58]. In our institution, prophylactic antibiotics are not routinely given post-operatively.

Depending on the severity of infection, most of these cases are managed by performing gram stain and culture of any discharge from the wound or on an aspirate of any associated collection, followed by appropriate broad-spectrum antibiotic until culture sensitivities are available.

15.4.2.4 Flap Necrosis

Flap necrosis is one of the most significant complications and can present as either partial or complete loss. Partial flap necrosis can be specific to the overlying skin or to the underlying fat. The necrosis tends to affect the most distal aspect of the flap as this is not usually an axial flap. The rate of flap necrosis is difficult to assess as it depends upon the defect and the type of local flap. Literature indicates a 2.5–14% partial flap loss in LTAP/ICAP/TDAP flaps [20–23, 28, 35, 59]. McCulley et al. [32] report no flap loss in their report on LTAP with or without conjunction with LICAP.

To reduce the risk of necrosis, optimisation of patient factors, flap planning and surgical technique as described earlier is critical. Venous congestion, post-operative oedema and infection are the most common causes of flap necrosis. When a large flap is necessary, a convex flap design allows for a larger amount of skin and makes the base narrower which in turn circumvents wound tension closure [60].

The objective in managing flap necrosis is to speed up the healing process for the patient to resume breast cancer treatment. Management is generally conservative. Time should be given for the tissue to declare its viability. If the flap is clearly necrotic, as manifested by dark and dry tissue, or if the patient is systemically unwell as a result, then debridement should be performed to remove necrotic tissue and allow more prompt healing by secondary intention. This can be complimented by NPWT, skin grafting and basic wound care. Further reconstruction can be considered once oncological treatment is fully complete. Uncomplicated fat necrosis does not usually require any acute intervention.

15.4.2.5 Injury to Adjacent Structures

Injury to important adjacent structures is a rare occurrence in oncoplastic breast surgery. Local flaps, predominantly those based on tissue on the lateral aspect of the chest wall, do carry the risk of damaging the thoracodorsal and intercostal nerves. The TDAP perforator, for instance, is dissected free and isolated from the thoracodorsal nerve. Injury to this nerve may result in complications related to LD function including difficulties in adduction and internal rotation of the shoulder. Hamdi et al. [20] reported that shoulder function (LD strength) was maintained when comparing the operated to the unoperated side in 22 patients that underwent TDAP flap volume replacement. Theoretically, damage to the lateral intercostal nerve branches may result in sensory damage to parts of the breast and nipple-areolar complex (NAC).

15.4.2.6 Fat Necrosis

Fat necrosis is a relatively common complication in many different types of autologous reconstructive breast surgery that results from poor tissue perfusion. Isolated fat necrosis can lead to a feeling of lumpiness, pain and asymmetry. Naturally, this can be quite distressing for the patient and may cause concern in relation to cancer recurrence. The rate of fat necrosis in local flap oncoplastic volume replacement which is reported as managed conservatively ranges from 0.9% to 7.7% [25, 42, 45]. The rate of fat necrosis which requires surgical management ranges from 2.5% to 5% [47, 59].

If the sequelae of adjuvant therapy have subsided and the lump persists, further tissue sampling is often necessary to rule out tumour recurrence, as surgical scarring and fat necrosis may appear very similar to a breast cancer recurrence both clinically and on imaging (see Fig. 15.7). If fat necrosis is confirmed, surgical correction may be considered. Excision of fat necrosis is sometimes warranted if this is a large area and to address the patients' anxiety. Besides excision, surgical corrections may include NAC reposition or fat grafting. If a large defect requires

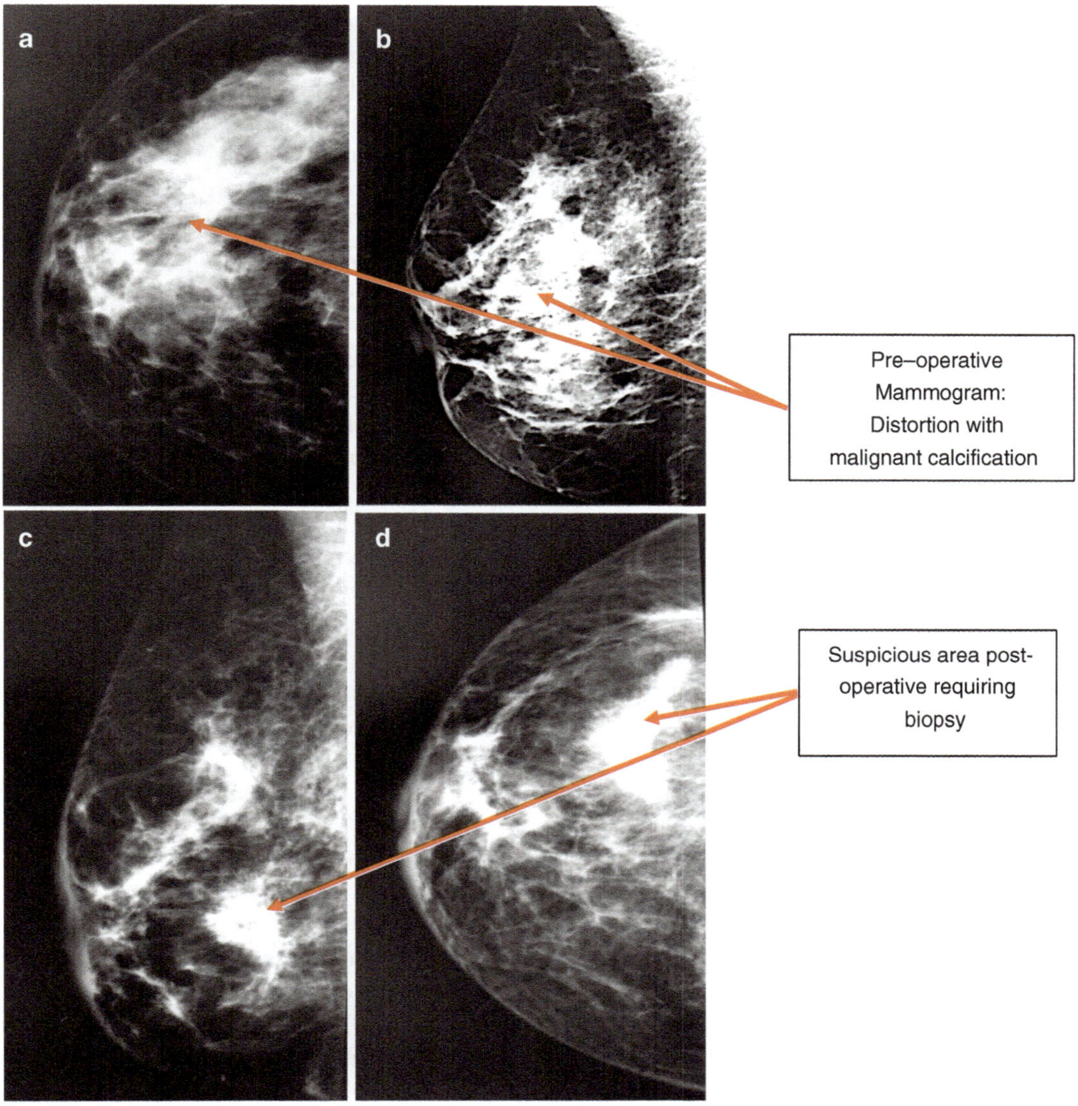

Fig. 15.7 (**a**, **b**) Pre-operative mammograms demonstrating a spiculate mass with microcalcification indicative of the breast carcinoma (upper panel). (**c**, **d**) Following partial breast reconstruction, post-operation scarring can appear suspicious mandating biopsy as shown (lower panel). The biopsies demonstrated post-operative benign change only

reconstruction, then using another pedicled flap from an uncompromised and non-irradiated region may be an option for volume replacement. Symmetrisation surgery to the contralateral breast may also be performed.

15.4.2.7 Oncological Considerations

Positive Margins

Oncoplastic techniques allow wider oncological resections compared with standard BCS. As a result, this reduces the positive margin rate and results in less re-excisions [3]. There is no international consensus on what constitutes a positive margin. The Association of Breast Surgery in the UK [61] considers a 1 mm minimum clear radial margin for both DCIS and invasive breast cancer whilst other international societies [62] differ by recommending a 2 mm excision margin for DCIS.

In standard BCS, positive margins occur in 20–40% of all standard BCS and one in five patients undergoing BCS require re-operation [63, 64]. A systematic review evaluated over 5000 patients treated with Oncoplastic BCS (including local flaps and reduction mammoplasty) in 49 studies reporting a weighted average positive margin rate of 10.8%, re-excision rate of 6.0% and conversion to mastectomy rate of 6.2% [55]. Our re-excision rate for positive margins is 9% with a conversion to mastectomy rate of fewer than 3%. However, Hamdi [47] report an even lower a re-operation rate of 2.5% for positive margins. Despite the lack of high-quality evidence, the available comparative observational studies and systematic review to date report that, at the very least, there are no poorer outcomes compared with standard BCS [65].

Surgical experience plays a key role in managing surgical margins. To avoid positive margins, a delayed strategy should be employed if there is concern about ability to achieve clear margins in one-stage alone. This is particularly true to those at the start of the learning curve. Additional techniques to reduce positive margins that have been reported include the use of bed biopsies with frozen section at the time of surgery and carrying out full cavity re-excision until the new margins are confirmed clear [66].

Should a surgeon be faced with positive margins, a decision should be made to proceed with completion mastectomy or further re-excision of margins. This is largely dependent on remaining breast volume, cancer type and the patient's wishes. Importantly, re-excision of margins can be performed successfully after local flap reconstruction, even if it has been performed as a single-stage procedure [43, 45]. This should be done so promptly to prevent delay to adjuvant therapy. However, one should appreciate that re-excision is associated with the increased risks of further surgical intervention, including delay to adjuvant therapy, stress to patients and their families, compromise of cosmetic outcomes and increased healthcare costs.

Local Recurrence

A meta-analysis carried out by Losken et al. [3] compared 3165 patients that had oncoplastic procedures (both reduction and oncoplastic flaps) and 5494 patients that had BCS alone. Local recurrence was reported in 4% in the oncoplastic group compared to 7% in the BCS group with an average 37-month and 64-month follow-up, respectively. This is a similar result to the systematic review reported by De La Cruz et al. [55] assessing oncologic outcomes after oncoplastic BCS for T1-T2 breast cancer which reported 3.2% local recurrence rate. A separate retrospective cohort study reviewed 1800 consecutive patients in a single centre comparing BCS alone with oncoplastic surgery revealing that there was no statistical difference in local recurrence-free survival between the conventional and oncoplastic BCS groups with a 75-month median follow-up time [67]. Currently our group have a 0% local recurrence rate with a median follow-up of 38 months in over 100 patients. Post-operative mammographic and, when needed, magnetic resonance imaging surveillance, in addition to self and clinical examination, is important to identify, preferably early, any suspicion of recurrence (Fig. 15.8).

15.4.3 Delayed Complications

15.4.3.1 Scarring

Scarring is a consequence of surgical incisions. These can be complicated by hypertrophic and keloid scarring. The healing process can result in painful scars, unsightly appearance and contracture causing distortion of the breast. Skin contracture may affect the curvature of the breast or distort and malposition the NAC. Identifying patients at increased risk of complications such as those with dark skin or a prior history of abnormal scarring is important to apply preventative strategies. Similarly, well planned oncoplastic incisions can be hidden in less visible areas (preferably in natural skin creases) and not extending over the breast skin. It is preferable to design the donor site of a lateral chest wall based oncoplastic flap in a transverse plane. This allows the scar to be hidden under the brassiere.

Several methods can be applied to address scarring complications. Intra-operatively, care should be taken to evert the skin edges and

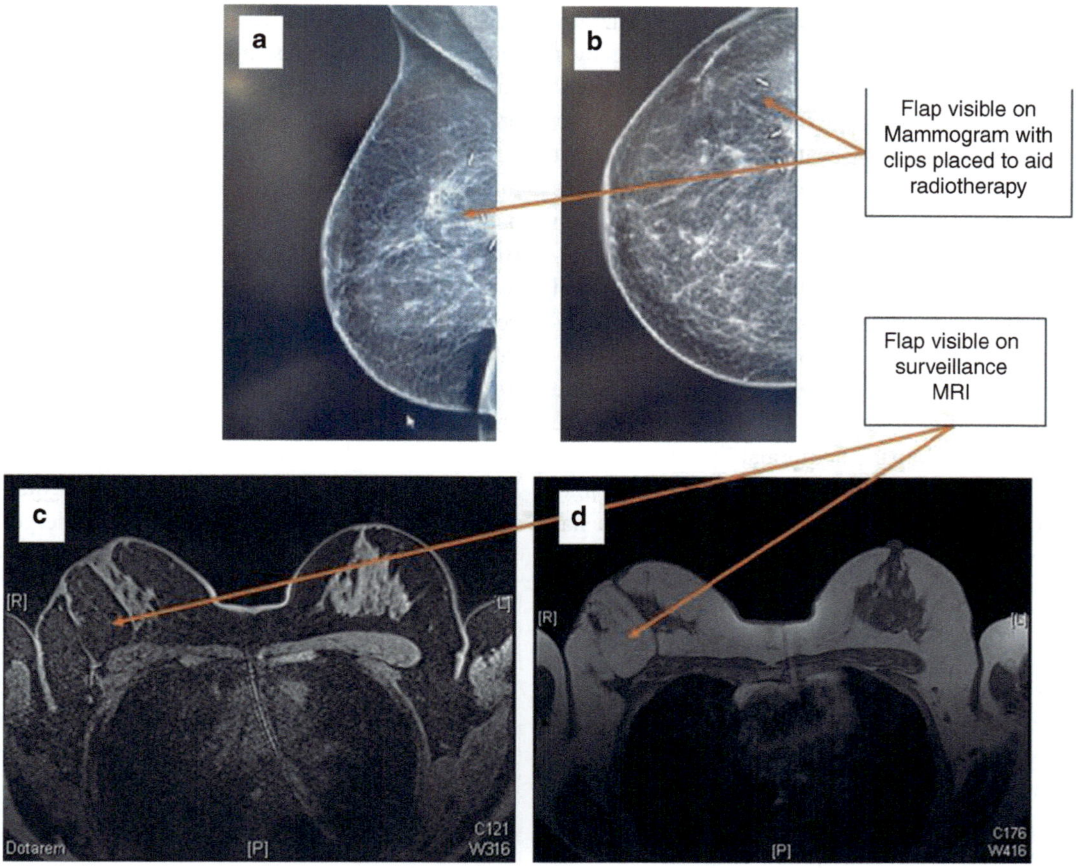

Fig. 15.8 Post-operative mammographic (MLO and CC views) (**a**, **b**) and MRI surveillance (**c**, **d**) in patients who have undergone BCS with local flap volume replacement. The mammogram demonstrating the surgical margin clips in situ. MRI surveillance may also be indicated in certain circumstances which can give excellent views of the flap used in partial breast reconstruction (lower panel). *CC* cranio-caudal, *MLO* medio-lateral oblique

reduce tension at the closure site. Post-operative methods include advising the patient to massage the scar site on a daily basis once it has healed. With regard to general management of scars, the use of silicone sheets or pressure compression garments are popular conservative approaches [68]. A short course of corticosteroid injections can be useful particularly in keloid scarring as it leads to hypotrophy. However, it can lead to depigmentation, telangiectasia and systemic effects. Other techniques include surgical scar revision or excision, radiotherapy, laser abrasion, use of 5-fluorouracil injection and other medications [69, 70]. However, there is a lack of evidence in the literature specific to local flap breast reconstruction.

15.4.3.2 Cosmetic Complications

"Trap-Door" Deformity

Incisions that take a U- or C-shaped closure can result in "trap-door" effect. The flap may become depressed and the tissue circumscribing it tends to bulge. This can result due to scar contracture, redundant subcutaneous tissue, bevelled wound edges or lymphatic obstruction [71]. Undermining of the peripheral recipient site can prevent this deformity.

Loss of Breast Volume and Contour Abnormalities

Patients undergoing BCS with oncoplastic volume replacement typically undergo radiotherapy post-operatively. The effect of radiotherapy together with the effect of tissue healing over time can result in loss of breast volume and subsequent asymmetry to the contralateral breast. Fujimoto et al. [72] evaluated the longevity of flap volume using CT and magnetic resonance imaging volumetry comparing BCS alone with CWPFs. This study reported that CWPFs maintain their volume over at least 5 years and that they have improved cosmetic outcomes compared to BCS alone. Various options exist for volume asymmetry correction but lipofilling is the commonest intervention. The reported incidence of patients requiring additional lipofilling ranges from 1.7% to 27% [43, 73]. NAC reposition may also be a valuable option if the loss of volume has affected NAC position and its symmetry compared to the contralateral side.

15.4.3.3 Pain

Early excessive pain at the wound site may be a sign of haematoma or infection. However, pain may be present for several weeks after therapy is completed. Theoretically, local oncoplastic flaps are likely to result in less chronic pain compared to other options that require dissection of muscle as is the case of a LD flap. The pain can be related to the extent of the size of the flap, but also the patient's physical and psychological state. It is therefore important to provide patients with early physiotherapy to achieve complete and prompt shoulder rehabilitation.

15.5 Conclusion

The overall goal of oncoplastic BCS is control of disease and maintenance of natural breast shape and symmetry. The key to minimizing complications lies with appropriate perioperative planning. Complication rates can be decreased by proper patient selection, understanding predictors of complications, choice of flap and familiarity with surgical technique. In addition, this procedure has a learning curve and specific training is required to achieve positive results. Despite the relatively recent development of oncoplastic breast surgery, comparative observational studies and systematic reviews report no poorer oncological outcomes compared with standard BCS [55, 74]. In addition, oncoplastic breast surgery has demonstrated better health-related quality of life and no increased physical discomfort for breast cancer patients as compared to patients treated with BCS [4]. Prospective larger studies with longer follow-up will significantly contribute to the generation of stronger evidence and more accurate prediction in the outcomes and complications of oncoplastic BCS. Most complications encountered after local flap volume replacement surgery can be managed non-operatively. Prevention and early detection are key to reducing the morbidity burden for patients undergoing these surgeries.

Key Points

- Prevention, recognition and managing complications is as important as learning how to perform the procedure.
- Cosmetic outcomes can be improved whilst complication rates can be decreased by appropriate patient selection, understanding the underlying causes of complications, choice of flap and familiarity with surgical technique.
- The selection of the site and size of the flap should be based on the site and volume of breast defect, site and quality of perforators, aesthetics and assessment of skin and subcutaneous tissue.
- Delicate surgical technique is the cornerstone to a successful surgical result.
- Regular post-operative reviews are essential to identify potentially reversible complications.
- Flap necrosis is an unusual complication of local oncoplastic volume replacement flaps.
- Most complications after local flap surgery can be managed on an outpatient basis, with a low return to theatre rate.

- CWPFs maintain their volume over at least 5 years and they have improved cosmetic outcomes compared to BCS alone.
- Evidence of decreased positive margins, lower recurrence rates and increased overall survival after oncoplastic breast surgery compared to BCS alone or mastectomy, shows oncoplastic breast surgery to be, at least, equivocal to traditional surgery in terms of oncological safety and carries with it improved cosmetic outcomes.
- Local perforator flaps are excellent options to correct volume and contour deformities following BCS associated with poor aesthetic outcomes.

References

1. Chakravorty A, et al. How safe is oncoplastic breast conservation? Comparative analysis with standard breast conserving surgery. Eur J Surg Oncol. 2012;38(5):395–8. https://doi.org/10.1016/j.ejso.2012.02.186.
2. Chen JY, et al. Comparison of oncoplastic breast-conserving surgery and breast-conserving surgery alone: a meta-analysis. J Breast Cancer. 2018;21(3):321–9. https://doi.org/10.4048/jbc.2018.21.e36.
3. Losken A, et al. A meta-analysis comparing breast conservation therapy alone to the oncoplastic technique. Ann Plast Surg. 2014;72(2):145–9. https://doi.org/10.1097/SAP.0b013e3182605598.
4. Rose M, et al. Patient-reported outcome after oncoplastic breast surgery compared with conventional breast-conserving surgery in breast cancer. Breast Cancer Res Treat. 2020;180(1):247–56. https://doi.org/10.1007/s10549-020-05544-2.
5. Almahariq MF, et al. Breast conserving therapy is associated with improved overall survival compared to mastectomy in early-stage, lymph node-negative breast cancer. Radiother Oncol. 2020;142:186–94. https://doi.org/10.1016/j.radonc.2019.09.018.
6. Fisher B, et al. Twenty-year follow-up of a randomized trial comparing total mastectomy, lumpectomy, and lumpectomy plus irradiation for the treatment of invasive breast cancer. N Engl J Med. 2002;347(16):1233–41. https://doi.org/10.1056/NEJMoa022152.
7. Veronesi U, et al. Twenty-year follow-up of a randomized study comparing breast-conserving surgery with radical mastectomy for early breast cancer. N Engl J Med. 2002;347(16):1227–32. https://doi.org/10.1056/NEJMoa020989.
8. Munhoz A, Gemperli R. The role of local flaps as volume replacement. In: Losken A, Hamdi M, editors. Partial breast reconstruction. 2nd ed. New York, NY: Thieme Medical Publishers; 2017. p. 321.
9. Chen CL, et al. The impact of obesity on breast surgery complications. Plast Reconstr Surg. 2011;128(5):395e–402e. https://doi.org/10.1097/PRS.0b013e3182284c05.
10. Panhofer P, et al. Standardization of morbidity assessment in breast cancer surgery using the Clavien Dindo Classification. Int J Surg. 2014;12(4):334–9. https://doi.org/10.1016/j.ijsu.2014.01.012.
11. Salasche SJ, Grabski WJ. Complications of flaps. J Dermatol Surg Oncol. 1991;17(2):132–40. https://doi.org/10.1111/j.1524-4725.1991.tb01606.x.
12. Kinsella JB, et al. Smoking increases facial skin flap complications. Ann Otol Rhinol Laryngol. 1999;108(2 I):139–42. https://doi.org/10.1177/000348949910800206.
13. Salem RO, Laposata M. Effects of alcohol on hemostasis. Am J Clin Pathol. 2005;123:S96. https://doi.org/10.1309/113n8eufxyueccna.
14. Patterson TJS, Berry RJ, Wiernik G. The effect of x-radiation on the survival of skin flaps in the pig 1. Br J Plast Surg. 1972;25:17.
15. Guo S, DiPietro LA. Critical review in oral biology & medicine: factors affecting wound healing. J Dent Res. 2010;89(3):219–29. https://doi.org/10.1177/0022034509359125.
16. Lee K, et al. The impact of obesity on breast cancer diagnosis and treatment. Curr Oncol Rep. 2019;21:41. https://doi.org/10.1007/s11912-019-0787-1.
17. Jarolimova J, Tagoni J, Stern TA. Obesity: its epidemiology, comorbidities, and management. Prim Care Compan J Clin Psychiatry. 2013;15(5):PCC.12f01475. https://doi.org/10.4088/PCC.12f01475.
18. Losken A, Urquia LN. Partial breast reconstruction. In: Breast reconstruction. Cham: Springer; 2020. p. 7–23. https://doi.org/10.1007/978-3-030-34603-4_2.
19. Spear SL, et al. Experience with reduction mammaplasty combined with breast conservation therapy in the treatment of breast cancer. Plast Reconstr Surg. 2003;111(3):1102–9. https://doi.org/10.1097/01.PRS.0000046491.87997.40.
20. Hamdi M, Decorte T, et al. Shoulder function after harvesting a thoracodorsal artery perforator flap. Plast Reconstr Surg. 2008a;122(4):1111–7. https://doi.org/10.1097/PRS.0b013e31818459b4.
21. Hamdi M, Spano A, et al. The lateral intercostal artery perforators: anatomical study and clinical application in breast surgery. Plast Reconstr Surg. 2008b;121(2):389–96. https://doi.org/10.1097/01.prs.0000298317.65296.cf.
22. Hamdi M, et al. The role of oncoplastic surgery in breast cancer. Acta Chir Belg. 2008c;108(6):666–72. https://doi.org/10.1080/00015458.2008.11680313.

23. Hamdi M, Salgarello M, et al. Use of the Thoracodorsal Artery Perforator (TDAP) flap with implant in breast reconstruction. Ann Plast Surg. 2008d;61(2):143–6. https://doi.org/10.1097/SAP.0b013e318158fd7b.
24. Martellani L, et al. Use of licap and ltap flaps for breast reconstruction. Acta Chir Plast. 2019;60(1):4–8. http://www.ncbi.nlm.nih.gov/pubmed/30939877. Accessed 23 Jun 2020
25. Munhoz AM, et al. Immediate conservative breast surgery reconstruction with perforator flaps: new challenges in the era of partial mastectomy reconstruction? Breast. 2011;20(3):233–40. https://doi.org/10.1016/j.breast.2011.01.001.
26. Jeong TK. Two options for perforator flaps in the flank donor site: latissimus dorsi and thoracodorsal perforator flaps. Plast Reconstr Surg. 2005;115(3):755–63. https://doi.org/10.1097/01.PRS.0000152427.09893.80.
27. Santanelli F, et al. Total breast reconstruction using the thoracodorsal artery perforator flap without implant. Plast Reconstr Surg. 2014;133(2):251–4. https://doi.org/10.1097/01.prs.0000436843.15494.ad.
28. Kim JB, et al. The usefulness of pedicled perforator flap in partial breast reconstruction after breast conserving surgery in Korean women. Arch Plast Surg. 2018;45(1):29–36. https://doi.org/10.5999/aps.2017.01200.
29. Taylor GI, Daniel RK. The anatomy of several free flap donor sites. Plast Reconstr Surg. 1975;56(3):243–53. https://doi.org/10.1097/00006534-197509000-00001.
30. Rowsell AR, et al. The anatomy of the subscapular-thoracodorsal arterial system: study of 100 cadaver dissections. Br J Plast Surg. 1984;37(4):574–6. https://doi.org/10.1016/0007-1226(84)90152-8.
31. Bhattacharya S, et al. The lateral thoracic region flap. Br J Plast Surg. 1990;43(2):162–8. https://doi.org/10.1016/0007-1226(90)90156-T.
32. McCulley SJ, et al. Lateral thoracic artery perforator (LTAP) flap in partial breast reconstruction. J Plast Reconstr Aesthet Surg. 2015;68(5):686–91. https://doi.org/10.1016/j.bjps.2015.01.008.
33. Hamdi M, De Frene B. Pedicled perforator flaps in breast reconstruction. Semin Plast Surg. 2006;20(2):73–8. https://doi.org/10.1055/s-2006-941713.
34. Hamdi M, et al. The versatility of the inter-costal artery perforator (ICAP) flaps. J Plast Reconstr Aesthet Surg. 2006;59(6):644–52. https://doi.org/10.1016/j.bjps.2006.01.006.
35. Hamdi M, et al. Pedicled perforator flaps in breast reconstruction: a new concept. Br J Plast Surg. 2004;57(6):531–9. https://doi.org/10.1016/j.bjps.2004.04.015.
36. Uemura T. Superior epigastric artery perforator flap: preliminary report. Plast Reconstr Surg. 2007;120(1):1e. https://doi.org/10.1097/01.prs.0000263538.71343.b7.
37. Lee JW, et al. Oncoplastic volume replacement techniques according to the excised volume and tumor location in small- to moderate-sized breasts. Gland Surg. 2014;3(1):14–21. https://doi.org/10.3978/j.issn.2227-684X.2014.02.02.
38. Chauveaux D. Preventing surgical-site infections: measures other than antibiotics. Orthop Traumatol Surg Res. 2015;101:S77–83. https://doi.org/10.1016/j.otsr.2014.07.028.
39. Irwin GW, et al. Negative pressure wound therapy reduces wound breakdown and implant loss in prepectoral breast reconstruction. Plast Reconstr Surg. 2020;8(2):e2667. https://doi.org/10.1097/GOX.0000000000002667.
40. Strugala V, Martin R. Meta-analysis of comparative trials evaluating a prophylactic single-use negative pressure wound therapy system for the prevention of surgical site complications. Surg Infect. 2017;18(7):810–9. https://doi.org/10.1089/sur.2017.156.
41. Delay E, Ganz OM, Quoc CH. Autologous latissimus dorsi breast reconstruction. In: Oncoplastic and reconstructive breast surgery. Cham: Springer; 2019. p. 541–51. https://doi.org/10.1007/978-3-319-62927-8_41.
42. Hillberg NS, et al. Delay of adjuvant radiotherapy due to postoperative complications after oncoplastic breast conserving surgery. Breast. 2018;39:110–6. https://doi.org/10.1016/j.breast.2018.04.005.
43. Quinn E, Highton L, Murphy J. Five-year experience of oncoplastic volume replacement using local perforator flaps. 2020 Annual Meeting Official Proceedings, Volume XXI. Ann Surg Oncol. 2020;27:223. https://doi.org/10.1245/s10434-020-08630-3.
44. Roy PG, Tenovici AA. Staged approach to partial breast reconstruction to avoid mastectomy in women with breast cancer. Gland Surg. 2017;6(4):336–42. https://doi.org/10.21037/gs.2017.03.08.
45. Soumian S, et al. Chest wall perforator flaps for partial breast reconstruction: surgical outcomes from a multicenter study. Arch Plast Surg. 2020;47(2):153–9. https://doi.org/10.5999/aps.2019.01186.
46. Kim J, et al. Electroactive-paper actuator made with cellulose/NaOH/urea and sodium alginate. Cellulose. 2007;14:217. https://doi.org/10.1007/s10570-007-9111-6.
47. Hamdi M. Oncoplastic and reconstructive surgery of the breast. Breast. 2013;22(S2):S100–5. https://doi.org/10.1016/j.breast.2013.07.019.
48. Jonczyk MM, et al. Trending towards safer breast cancer surgeries? Examining acute complication rates from a 13-year nsqip analysis. Cancers. 2019;11(2):253. https://doi.org/10.3390/cancers11020253.
49. Clough KB, et al. Oncoplastic techniques allow extensive resections for breast-conserving therapy of breast carcinomas. Ann Surg. 2003;237(1):26–34. https://doi.org/10.1097/00000658-200301000-00005.

50. Losken A, et al. The role of reduction mammaplasty in reconstructing partial mastectomy defects. Plast Reconstr Surg. 2002;109(3):968–75. https://doi.org/10.1097/00006534-200203000-00025.
51. Ireton JE, Unger JG, Rohrich RJ. The role of wound healing and its everyday application in plastic surgery: a practical perspective and systematic review. Plast Reconstr Surg. 2013;1:e10. https://doi.org/10.1097/GOX.0b013e31828ff9f4.
52. Randolph LC, et al. Prediction of postoperative seroma after latissimus dorsi breast reconstruction. Plast Reconstr Surg. 2005;116:1287–90. https://doi.org/10.1097/01.prs.0000181517.20122.36.
53. Titley G, Spyrou GE, Fatah MF. Preventing seroma in the latissimus dorsi flap donor site. Br J Plast Surg. 1997;50:106.
54. Munhoz AM, et al. The role of the lateral thoracodorsal fasciocutaneous flap in immediate conservative breast surgery reconstruction. Plast Reconstr Surg. 2006;117(6):1699–710. https://doi.org/10.1097/01.prs.0000209943.13682.42.
55. De La Cruz L, et al. Outcomes after oncoplastic breast-conserving surgery in breast cancer patients: a systematic literature review. Ann Surg Oncol. 2016;23(10):3247–58. https://doi.org/10.1245/s10434-016-5313-1.
56. Schaffer K, Taylor CT. The impact of hypoxia on bacterial infection. FEBS J. 2015;282(12):2260–6. https://doi.org/10.1111/febs.13270.
57. Gallagher M, Jones DJ, Bell-Syer SV. Prophylactic antibiotics to prevent surgical site infection after breast cancer surgery. Cochrane Database Syst Rev. 2019;(2):CD005360. https://doi.org/10.1002/14651858.CD005360.pub5.
58. Phillips BT, et al. A systematic review of antibiotic use and infection in breast reconstruction: what is the evidence? Plast Reconstr Surg. 2013;131:1–13. https://doi.org/10.1097/PRS.0b013e3182729c39.
59. Roy PG. One-stage vs. two-stage approach for partial breast reconstruction with lateral chest wall perforator flaps. Cancer Treat Res Commun. 2016;9:56–61. https://doi.org/10.1016/j.ctarc.2016.06.003.
60. Holmström H, Lossing C. The lateral thoracodorsal flap in breast reconstruction. Plast Reconstr Surg. 1986;77(6):933–41. https://doi.org/10.1097/00006534-198606000-00010.
61. Association of Breast Surgery. ABS consensus margin width in breast conservation surgery. London: ABS; 2015. www.associationofbreastsurgery.org.uk. Accessed 14 Jun 2020.
62. Morrow M, et al. Society of Surgical Oncology-American Society for Radiation Oncology-American Society of Clinical Oncology consensus guideline on margins for breast-conserving surgery with whole-breast irradiation in ductal carcinoma in situ. J Clin Oncol. 2016;34(33):4040–6. https://doi.org/10.1200/JCO.2016.68.3573.
63. Haloua MH, et al. A systematic review of oncoplastic breast-conserving surgery: current weaknesses and future prospects. Ann Surg. 2013;257:609–20. https://doi.org/10.1097/SLA.0b013e3182888782.
64. Jeevan R, et al. Reoperation rates after breast conserving surgery for breast cancer among women in England: retrospective study of hospital episode statistics. BMJ. 2012;345(7869):e4505. https://doi.org/10.1136/bmj.e4505.
65. Campbell EJ, Romics L. Oncological safety and cosmetic outcomes in oncoplastic breast conservation surgery, a review of the best level of evidence literature. Breast Cancer Targets Ther. 2017;9:521–30. https://doi.org/10.2147/BCTT.S113742.
66. Rusby JE, et al. Immediate latissimus dorsi miniflap volume replacement for partial mastectomy: use of intra-operative frozen sections to confirm negative margins. Am J Surg. 2008;196(4):512–8. https://doi.org/10.1016/j.amjsurg.2008.06.026.
67. Niinikoski L, et al. Resection margins and local recurrences in breast cancer: comparison between conventional and oncoplastic breast conserving surgery. Eur J Surg Oncol. 2019;45(6):976–82. https://doi.org/10.1016/j.ejso.2019.02.010.
68. Monstrey S, et al. Updated scar management practical guidelines: non-invasive and invasive measures. J Plast Reconstr Aesthet Surg. 2014;67:1017–25. https://doi.org/10.1016/j.bjps.2014.04.011.
69. Gold MH, et al. Updated international clinical recommendations on scar management: Part 2 - Algorithms for scar prevention and treatment. Dermatol Surg. 2014;40(8):825–31. https://doi.org/10.1111/dsu.0000000000000050.
70. Ogawa R. The most current algorithms for the treatment and prevention of hypertrophic scars and keloids. Plast Reconstr Surg. 2010;125(2):557–68. https://doi.org/10.1097/PRS.0b013e3181c82dd5.
71. Koranda FC, Webster RC. Trapdoor effect in nasolabial flaps: causes and corrections. Arch Otolaryngol. 1985;111(7):421–4. https://doi.org/10.1001/archotol.1985.00800090035002.
72. Fujimoto H, et al. Oncoplastic breast-conserving surgery using chest wall perforator flaps: three-dimensional quantitative analysis of the percentage of breast volume excised and changes over time in flap volume. J Surg Oncol. 2020;121(2):216–23. https://doi.org/10.1002/jso.25809.
73. Youssif S, et al. Pedicled local flaps: a reliable reconstructive tool for partial breast defects. Gland Surg. 2019;8(5):527–36. https://doi.org/10.21037/gs.2019.09.06.
74. Cil TD, Cordeiro E. Complications of oncoplastic breast surgery involving soft tissue transfer versus breast-conserving surgery: an analysis of the NSQIP database. Ann Surg Oncol. 2016;23(10):3266–71. https://doi.org/10.1245/s10434-016-5477-8.

Radiotherapy and Local Chest Wall Perforator Flaps in Partial Breast Reconstruction

16

J. Murphy and E. M. Quinn

Contents

J. Murphy (✉) · E. M. Quinn
Nightingale Breast Unit, Wythenshawe Hospital, Manchester University NHS Foundation Trust, Manchester, UK
e-mail: John.murphy@mft.nhs.uk; Edel.quinn@mft.nhs.uk

16.1 Introduction

Local chest wall perforator flaps are most commonly performed as a means of oncoplastic partial breast reconstruction after breast conserving surgery (BCS) for invasive breast carcinoma or ductal

M. Hamdi et al. (eds.), *Pedicled Flaps in Partial Breast Reconstruction*,
https://doi.org/10.1007/978-3-031-08483-6_16

carcinoma in-situ (DCIS). The flaps are usually performed in the immediate setting but can also be used to correct deformities arising as a result of previous BCS. Most patients who undergo BCS will require adjuvant radiotherapy to complete their oncological treatment [1–3]. This means that flaps performed as immediate partial breast reconstruction will be exposed to radiotherapy in the adjuvant setting. For similar reasons, when chest wall perforator flaps are performed in the delayed setting to correct deformity arising from previous BCS, with the flaps are commonly placed into previously irradiated tissue. Therefore, it is important to understand the effects of radiotherapy in relation to the use of local chest wall flaps.

16.1.1 Indications for Radiotherapy After Breast Conserving Surgery

International guidelines from the UK, US and Europe make similar recommendations in relation to the role of radiotherapy in the management of invasive breast cancer treated by BCS. Randomised controlled trials have shown that whole breast radiotherapy produces clinically meaningful reductions in local recurrence rates and improved overall survival at 5–10 years for women with invasive breast cancer, treated with BCS with negative surgical margins [4]. UK, US and European guidelines all suggest that whole-breast radiotherapy should be offered to all women with invasive breast cancer who have had BCS with clear margins [2–4]. An additional boost of radiotherapy to the tumour bed (and, therefore, the site of the flap) is also recommended for women with higher risk of local recurrence—those under 50, with grade 3 tumours, lymphovascular invasion or close margins [3]. Whole breast radiotherapy should also be considered in women who have BCS for DCIS [1]. However, guidelines agree that it is appropriate to consider omission of radiotherapy in lower risk cases [1–3].

Radiotherapy can be omitted in some patients who undergo BCS for invasive cancer. Evidence of the benefit in terms of clinically meaningful reductions in local recurrence in women with invasive breast cancer aged 65 years and over is low and there is no evidence of overall survival benefit at 5- to 10-year follow-up for these women [4]. The benefits of radiotherapy to those with a very low absolute risk of recurrence are uncertain and radiotherapy may be omitted in women aged 65 and over with tumours that are T1N0, ER positive, HER2-negative and grade 1–2 [1]. However, this is a small proportion of those women who undergo BCS and usually relates to those with smaller tumours, who are less likely to need volume replacement following BCS. Therefore, the vast majority of women requiring chest wall perforator flap reconstruction following BCS will require adjuvant radiotherapy.

16.1.2 Postmastectomy Radiotherapy

Chest wall perforator flaps can also be used as a form of reconstruction after total mastectomy [5] or as revision surgery following previous mastectomy and reconstruction [6]. These patients may also have had previous radiotherapy. International guidelines recommend post-mastectomy radiotherapy (PMRT) be offered to patients with node-positive invasive breast cancer and should be considered in those with node-negative T3 or T4 invasive breast cancer [1–3]. Therefore, prior radiation exposure must also be taken into account when planning chest wall perforator flaps in such scenarios.

The relationship between radiotherapy and local flap reconstruction must be considered in relation to:

1. The effects of postoperative radiotherapy on the flap.
2. The effects of the flap on planning and delivery of radiotherapy.
3. Effects of prior radiotherapy on delayed flap-based reconstruction.

16.2 Consideration 1: Postoperative Radiotherapy After Local Perforator Flap Reconstruction

Data specifically relating to the effects of postoperative radiotherapy on chest wall perforator flaps is lacking. However, in published case series reporting the use of chest wall perforator flaps for immediate partial breast reconstruction, the majority of patients have had adjuvant radiotherapy. Reported significant complication rates from the combination of surgery and radiotherapy are low, suggesting perforator flaps handle radiotherapy well, which is indeed consistent with our experience [7–9]. One of the benefits of local perforator flaps is that the origin of the perforator vessel is usually not within the conventional whole breast radiotherapy field. This is likely beneficial in terms of reduction of complication rates. More detailed studies of the effects of radiotherapy on free flaps performed for reconstruction post total mastectomy have been performed and some of these results can be extrapolated to chest wall perforator flaps. Here, we will discuss effects of post-operative radiation in terms of complications, cosmetic outcomes and flap volumes.

16.2.1 Postoperative Radiotherapy and Complications

In studies of BCS with oncoplastic volume replacement using local flaps, most reported complications occur in the early postoperative phase, prior to radiotherapy. Few studies have looked specifically at the effect of radiotherapy on the complication rate. Potential complications which can occur following radiotherapy include fat necrosis (Fig. 16.1), infection, flap fibrosis and scar contracture.

In one study of 25 patients undergoing partial reconstruction with local perforator flaps, where all patients received adjuvant radiotherapy, one patient developed fat necrosis during radiotherapy requiring excision of the resultant hard mass [10]. A separate study has shown fibrosis of the flap and residual breast parenchyma, along with volume reduction to be noted after postoperative radiotherapy in thin patients or those flaps with little subcutaneous fat [11]. In a further study of

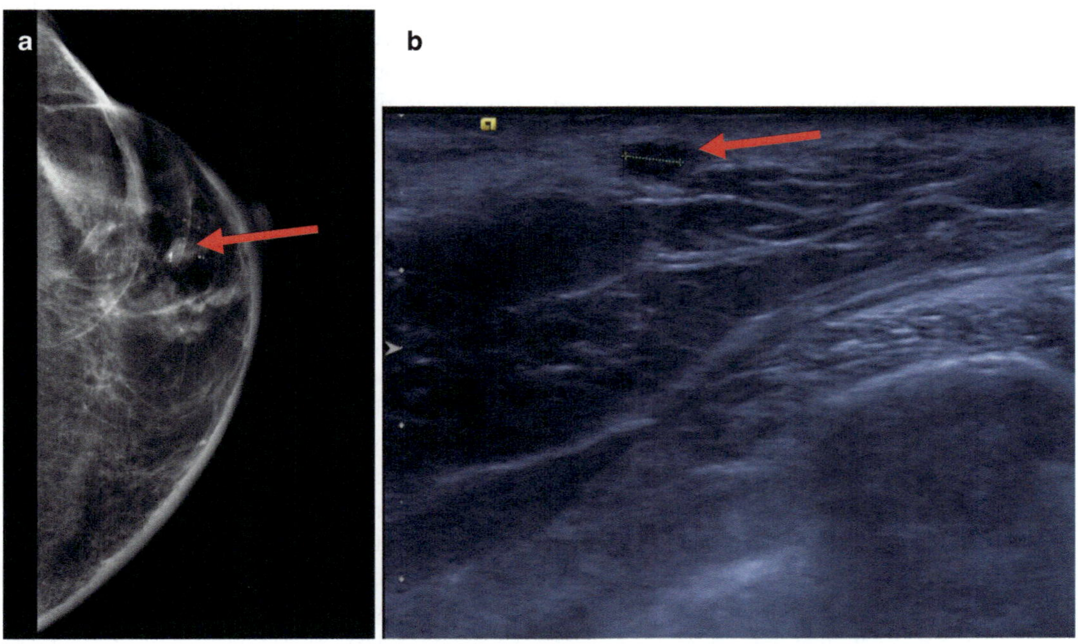

Fig. 16.1 (**a**) Mammographic and (**b**) Ultrasound Appearances of Fat Necrosis within Local Perforator Flaps

oncoplastic BCS, where just under half of the patients had undergone local flap reconstruction, 20.4% of complications occurred after adjuvant radiotherapy [9]. Reported complications in this study included fat necrosis, seroma, infection and wound problems. Three patients required surgical drainage of an abscess after radiotherapy [9]. In another study of 112 patients undergoing local flap reconstruction, no delayed complications were reported post radiotherapy [7].

Complications of radiotherapy have been more extensively studied in autologous flap-based breast reconstruction after mastectomy, particularly as comparator groups of non-irradiated patients are more commonly available. Pedicled flaps such as latissimus dorsi (LD) and transversus rectus abdominis (TRAM) have some similarities to local chest wall perforator flaps although the volume of tissue harvested is usually larger. Reported postoperative radiotherapy effects on TRAM flaps include mild and moderate skin erythema, desquamation and fat necrosis [12]. Radiotherapy was associated with a higher rate of late complications, occurring at a rate of 23.3%, in one series of irradiated patients compared to 13.6% in the non-irradiated group after TRAM flap reconstruction [13]. Fat necrosis resulting in larger masses was also seen more commonly in the radiotherapy group in this cohort. These patients had a higher rate of secondary surgery to remove fat necrosis, compared to those who had not received radiotherapy [13]. There was also a significant increase in flap contracture rates in the RT group [13].

Free flap reconstruction after mastectomy is most commonly performed using either a free TRAM or deep inferior epigastric perforator (DIEP) flap. Radiotherapy has been shown to result in fat necrosis, scar contracture and pigment changes in these free flaps. However, the association between radiotherapy and free flap fat necrosis is not shown uniformly across various studies. Some report higher rates of fat necrosis after radiotherapy compared to no radiotherapy [14] but others have shown no significant difference between irradiated and non-irradiated flaps [15–17]. Fat necrosis may be a complication of relative ischaemia of the flap itself, rather than directly related to postoperative radiotherapy.

Higher rates of skin contracture, hyperpigmentation and asymmetry have been reported in abdominal free flaps after postoperative radiotherapy compared to those performed without adjuvant radiotherapy [14]. Other studies have shown no effect of postoperative radiotherapy on major complications after autologous reconstruction [18]. Reoperation rates for complications after autologous free flap reconstruction and adjuvant radiotherapy have been reported at a high rate of 47% in one study [19]. Indications for reoperation in this series included fat necrosis, fibrosis and skin complications such as retraction and hypertrophic scarring [19]. However, there was no comparator group in this study so it is difficult to ascertain the true magnitude of the radiotherapy effect on these complications.

From the available literature, it is likely that radiotherapy after flap-based reconstruction may be associated with slightly increased rates of fat necrosis. However, it is clear that in the majority of cases this can be managed non-operatively. Effects can also be seen in relation to scar contracture and skin pigmentation, where skin paddles are maintained. In the majority of local flap-based reconstructions, however, the flap is buried without a visible skin paddle. The potential effects of such complications on cosmetic outcomes will now be examined in more detail.

16.2.2 Postoperative Radiotherapy and Cosmetic Appearance

Skin changes, contracture and fibrosis which can occur after radiotherapy may affect the cosmetic outcome of flap-based reconstruction. However, reports consistently show high patient and surgeon satisfaction levels with local flap-based reconstruction, even after radiotherapy.

Studies of patient reported outcomes after local flap reconstruction with adjuvant radiotherapy show high satisfaction rates, ranging from 84% to 90% [10, 20, 21]. In a small study of pre-

and post-surgery and radiotherapy BREAST-Q scores in women undergoing BCS, anterior intercostal artery perforator (AICAP) flap reconstruction and radiotherapy, there was no significant score differences observed post-treatment [22]. Within this study, it was noted that development of fibrosis within the flaps occurred after radiotherapy but the effect was no different to that of breast tissue treated with radiotherapy [22]. An example of pre-operative and post-radiotherapy cosmetic outcomes are shown in Fig. 16.2.

Assessment of cosmetic outcomes by physicians and computer software programmes is also generally favourable. In comparison to standard BCS, patients who underwent local chest wall perforator flap reconstructions after excision of >15% of breast volume, followed by radiotherapy, were found to have significantly more good or excellent outcomes 2 years post-treatment (96% versus 48%) when subjectively assessed by two independent physicians and when objectively assessed using software examination of frontal view photographs (91% versus 66%) [23]. Findings were similar in a small series of local flap reconstructions reviewed by two surgeons preoperatively and 12-months post-surgery and radiotherapy, where 90% were felt to have a good or excellent outcome [20]. The patients who had had less desirable outcomes in this study had developed postoperative complications, one a haematoma and one case of breast lymphoedema [20].

The pedicled LD flap has also been studied in the setting of partial breast reconstruction.

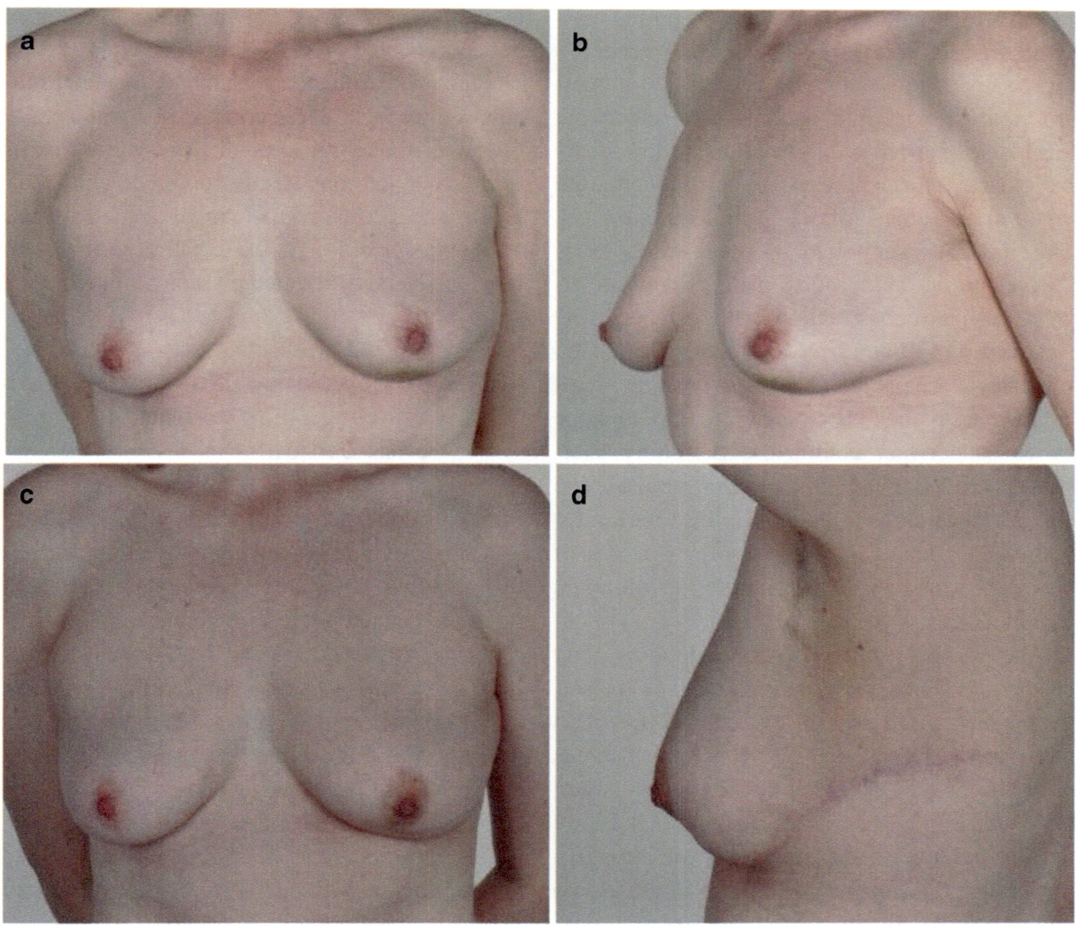

Fig. 16.2 (**a**, **b**) Preoperative appearance of a patient due to undergo left sided BCS with immediate local perforator flap reconstruction; (**c**, **d**) Post-treatment appearance 12 months after surgery and radiotherapy in the same patient

Again, high median psychosocial and physical well-being scores have been reported by patients' post-radiotherapy using the BREAST-Q instrument [24]. Independent subjective assessment of photographs by plastic surgeons and laypersons also showed high scores for symmetric volume, symmetric shape, overall symmetry, scar appearance and overall aesthetic result in this series [24]. However, the timing of assessment relative to radiotherapy treatment was not defined. The LD can be combined with other local flaps to fill large defects after BCS and a small series has again shown good patient reported outcomes in this setting after radiotherapy [25].

A surrogate marker of patient and surgeon satisfaction with cosmetic outcomes after local flap reconstruction is the need for revision or symmetrising surgery after radiotherapy. Reported revision surgery rates are low, suggesting generally high satisfaction rates. In one of the largest reported series of 112 patients who underwent local flap partial reconstruction followed by radiotherapy, no symmetrisation procedures were required at median follow-up of 15 months [7]. This has been supported by other small series [20]. A further study of 28 patients who underwent partial reconstruction with extended LD followed by radiotherapy reported two revision surgeries—one patient underwent bilateral breast augmentation due to personal preference and one patient underwent contracture deformity excision, scar release and implant insertion [26]. The authors' own case series of 116 local perforator flap reconstructions has shown a revision rate of 3% at median 36 months follow-up (unpublished).

There is also further evidence supporting good cosmetic outcomes after radiotherapy, in the setting of the more extensively studied free flap reconstruction. Free flap reconstruction studies offer the benefit of a comparator group, when assessing effects of radiotherapy, which is not usually possible in the assessment of local flap reconstruction. Cosmetic outcomes in those who undergo autologous free flap reconstruction with adjuvant radiotherapy compared to no radiotherapy have been shown to be comparable [15, 16]. In a series of 164 patients undergoing immediate abdominally-based free flap reconstruction, satisfaction scores were similar between the group who received radiotherapy (86% rated good or excellent) and the group who did not (87% rated good or excellent) [17]. There were lower physical well-being scores assessed by the BREAST-Q tool in the radiotherapy group but no difference in satisfaction with breast or psychosocial well-being scores in this study [17]. However, these findings are not uniform across all studies. Myung et al. have shown that radiotherapy does result in a drop in cosmetic outcome scores assessed by computer software after free flap reconstruction, when assessed at 1 year postoperatively and compared to patients who did not receive radiotherapy [14]. However, whilst scores dropped from baseline, the majority of patients in this cohort maintained scores of good or excellent.

Published evidence relating to cosmetic outcomes after local flap reconstruction is generally of low methodological quality but high satisfaction levels are consistently reported. This combined with a low revision surgery rate, suggests cosmetic outcomes of local flap reconstruction are not adversely affected by radiotherapy.

16.2.3 Postoperative Radiotherapy Effects on Flap Volume and Position

Fibrosis induced by radiotherapy can result in loss of flap volume over time. This could affect overall breast volume and symmetry, although there are limited studies looking at this in terms of local perforator flaps. One MRI-based study of local chest wall perforator flap volume over time after radiotherapy has shown that mean flap volume relative to baseline decreases to 89.7% at 1 year and decreases further to 77.7% at year 5. However, whilst 5-year flap volume was less than 60% of baseline in 15% of patients, it remained greater than 80% in 62% [23]. An illustration of maintenance of volume 5 years post treatment is shown in Fig. 16.3. As the origin of the feeding perforator vessel for local flaps does not usually lie within the radiotherapy field, it is not subject to radiotherapy effect and thus maintains good volume blood flow. This may contribute to the good volume preservation usually seen in local perforator flaps.

A study of the use of the extended LD flap in partial breast reconstruction showed an average volume decrease in the flap of 69% at 18 months post radiotherapy [26]. In this study, all patients also had routine resection of the motor nerve to LD. Previous studies have shown that the LD atrophies by as much as 54% even in those who do not undergo postoperative radiotherapy [27]. It has been suggested atrophy is a greater problem if there is more muscle in the flap as muscle atrophies more than fat [26]. Therefore, this may be less of a problem in the fasciocutaneous local chest wall perforator flaps.

Again, comparative studies are available when looking at the effects of radiotherapy in free flap reconstructions. A small study of abdominal free flap total breast reconstruction has shown that mean flap volume as measured by CT at 12–18 months post-radiotherapy had decreased by 12.3% compared to a 2.6% volume loss seen in flaps not exposed to radiotherapy [14]. However, it is more important to consider if this degree of volume loss is clinically significant. A further study of free flap reconstruction showed some flap shrinkage in 30% of those who received radiotherapy but only 10% experienced enough distortion to require revision surgery [15]. Chatterjee et al. have shown a mean volume difference in immediate DIEP reconstructions of 65 mL 1-year post-radiotherapy compared to non-irradiated DIEP flaps [28].

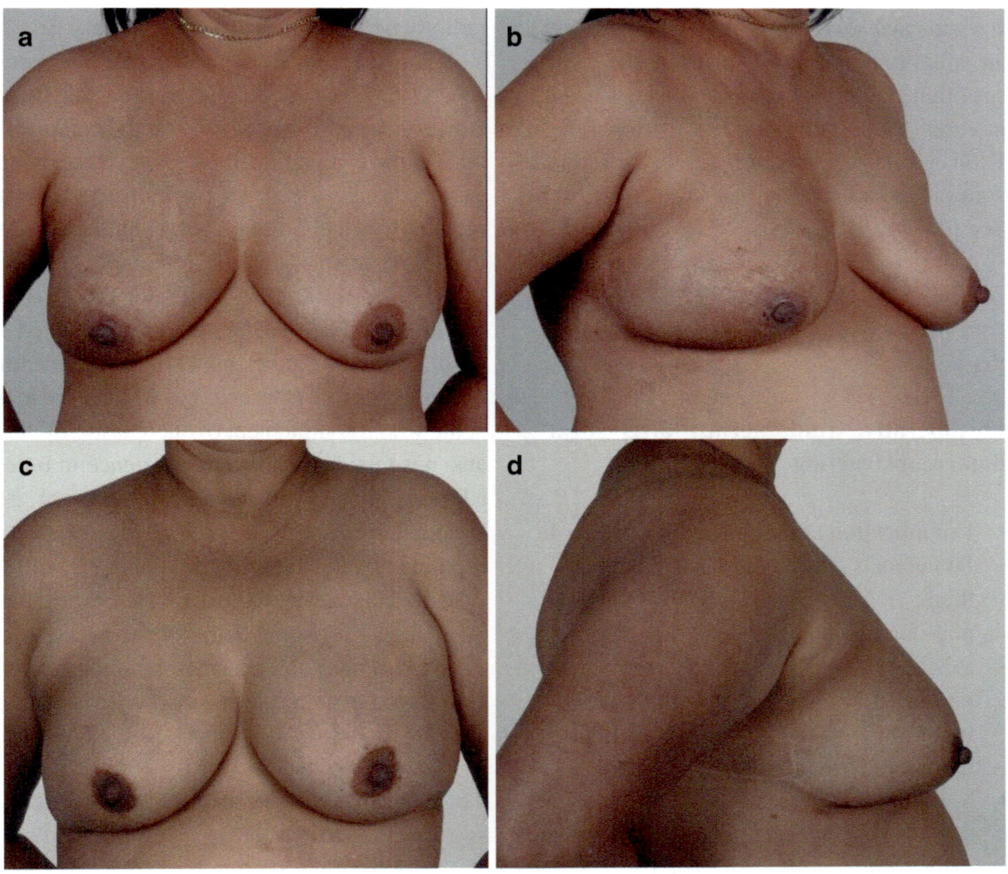

Fig. 16.3 (**a**, **b**) Immediate post-operative example of right sided local perforator flap reconstruction; (**c**, **d**) The same patient 4 years later showing maintenance of flap volume

They also looked at the volume difference between the reconstructed breast and the native contralateral breast, showing a mean volume difference of 75 mL for non-irradiated women and 100 mL for those who received radiotherapy, which was non-significant. Most importantly, those in the radiotherapy group were no more likely to have undergone volume adjustment surgery or volume symmetrising surgery than those in the no radiotherapy group [28]. A further study of patients who had undergone bilateral mastectomy with immediate DIEP flap reconstructions with unilateral radiotherapy used 3D photograph analysis to show there was no statistical difference in breast volume or projection between both sides when compared at least 6 months after radiotherapy [29]. However, the irradiated flaps were all found to sit significantly higher on the chest wall compared to the non-irradiated flaps [29].

It seems that some flap volume loss is likely to occur after radiotherapy. However, the volume loss is often small and not clinically significant in most cases. This is supported by the low rates of revision and symmetrisation surgery after local perforator flap reconstruction, as previously discussed [7, 20, 26].

Key Points

Postoperative radiotherapy after local flap reconstruction

- Complication rates are low, with rates of fat necrosis possibly increased by radiotherapy. Most cases can be managed non-operatively.
- Whilst quality of available evidence is low, high patient and surgeon satisfaction rates with cosmesis are consistently reported.
- Some flap volume loss may occur after radiotherapy but this is usually not clinically significant and does not translate to a requirement for revision surgery.

16.3 Consideration 2: The Effect of Flaps on Adjuvant Radiotherapy

16.3.1 Local Flaps and Timing of Adjuvant Radiotherapy

Most patients who undergo immediate reconstruction with local perforator flaps will require adjuvant radiotherapy, as a key component of their cancer treatment. It is important that restoration of cosmesis does not adversely affect timing, and potentially effectiveness, of oncological treatment. In a single study of 150 oncoplastic BCS procedures (46% local flaps), 8% of patients had a delay to commencement of adjuvant radiotherapy due to complications [9]. However, radiotherapy was still delivered at a median of 49 days postoperatively (range 35–81 days) in these patients and 55% of them commenced radiotherapy within 8 weeks of surgery [9].

Most reports of local flap reconstruction do not specifically address timing of adjuvant therapy. However, larger series show that the complication rate following this surgery is low and most complications usually occur in the early postoperative period [7, 8], suggesting there is unlikely to be an impact on timing of adjuvant therapy. In our own series of over 100 local perforator flaps, we have had no delays to adjuvant radiotherapy noted supporting the few studies which have not identified this as a problem. Other studies which have looked at the whole complement of oncoplastic BCS have also not found a significant difference in times to adjuvant therapy compared to standard BCS, although local flaps are not always represented prominently, if at all, in these studies [30–32].

Based on the available data, use of local perforator flaps for immediate partial breast reconstruction is unlikely to have a significant effect on delay to adjuvant radiotherapy, where indicated.

16.3.2 Local Flaps and Radiotherapy Planning

Knowledge about tumour bed localisation is crucial for radiotherapy planning, particularly if planning to deliver a boost to the tumour bed. Breast cancer provides additional challenges for radiotherapy planning as soft tissues undergo non-rigid deformations during surgery and the tumour itself no longer exists during planning [33]. Oncoplastic breast surgery moves tissue around to fill the defect following tumour excision and remote incisions are often used [30]. Therefore, traditional imaging and palpation assessment of the tumour bed is unreliable [34].

In a study of mini-LD flap-based partial breast reconstruction, using CT assessment, the location of the tumour bed was found to be completely outside of the original tumour quadrant location in 36% of cases [34]. This study found that accurate localisation of the tumour bed for delivery of boost radiotherapy was more likely if at least four marker clips were placed to the tumour bed at the time of surgery, prior to the oncoplastic reconstruction [34]. This finding has also been supported by Furet et al., who found that more than three clips were required for accurate tumour bed localisation after oncoplastic BCS compared to standard BCS [35]. The use of clips to mark the tumour bed in the setting of local flap-based reconstruction is shown in Fig. 16.4.

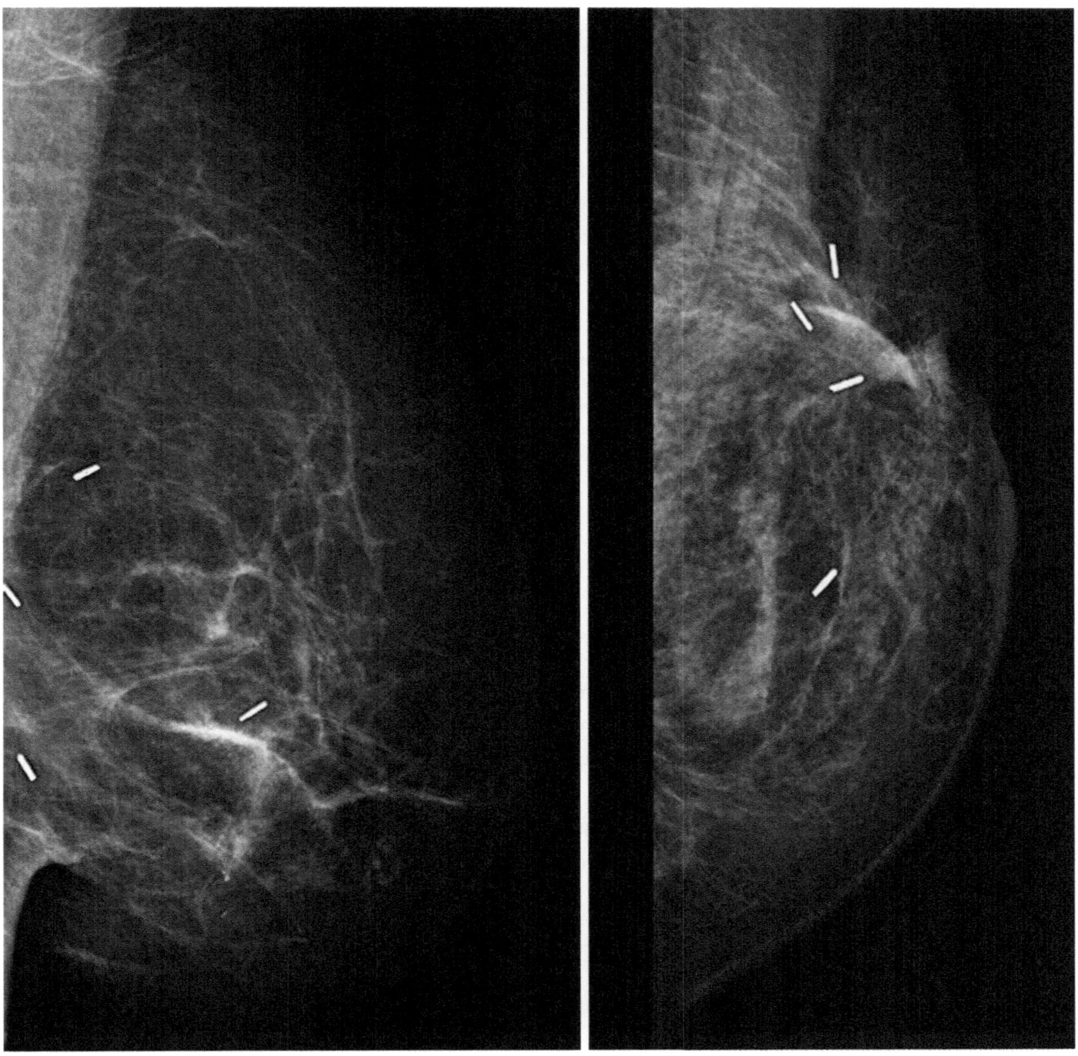

Fig. 16.4 Mammograms demonstrating use of four clips to localise the tumour bed in two patients who have undergone local flap-based reconstruction, demonstrating the extent of the tumour bed

When performing local flap-based reconstruction surgery, it is important to mark the site of the tumour bed intra-operatively prior to proceeding with the reconstruction, to facilitate radiotherapy planning. Based on the available evidence, at least four marker clips should be placed to delineate the edges of the tumour bed.

Key Points

The effect of local flaps on radiotherapy

- Immediate partial breast reconstruction using local perforator flaps is not significantly associated with a delay to adjuvant radiotherapy treatment.
- Marking the tumour bed intraoperatively with at least four marker clips prior to performing local flap reconstruction is important to enable accurate radiotherapy planning postoperatively.

16.4 Consideration 3: Previous Radiotherapy and Local Perforator Flaps

16.4.1 Indications for Local Flaps in Patients Who Have Had Previous Radiotherapy

Local flap reconstruction can also be used to fill defects left from prior BCS [6] or to correct deformities after previous mastectomy and reconstruction [36]. In many cases, these patients will have had prior radiotherapy, which must be taken into consideration when planning their surgery. An example of a prior irradiated field requiring local flap reconstruction is shown in Fig. 16.5. Prior radiotherapy may have effects on complications, timing of surgery and postoperative cosmesis.

16.4.2 Previous Radiotherapy and Early Complication Rates

The reported effects of previous radiotherapy in the setting of delayed autologous-tissue based reconstruction is variable [37]. There is very limited evidence available in relation to outcomes after delayed partial breast reconstruction, following BCS and prior radiotherapy. However, Youssif et al. showed a complication rate of 6% in 30 patients undergoing local flap reconstruction. Complications reported were one case of partial nipple areolar complex necrosis and one case of fat necrosis [6]. In the authors' own case series of 15 delayed local perforator flap reconstructions, where 80% of patients had received prior radiotherapy, a complication rate of 33% was seen—these were superficial surgical site infections or delayed wound healing problems at the donor sites assumed to be outside of the previous radiotherapy field (unpublished data). Therefore, it is impossible to determine the direct effect, if any, prior radiotherapy had on these complications in such small series. The authors recommend resecting any scar tissue at site of the defect in the delayed reconstruction setting, to "recreate" the original defect. Fresh, vascularised tissue in the form of the flap is then imported into this area which can help regenerate overlying skin and surrounding tissues, and reduce ischaemia-related complications.

Effects of radiotherapy on complications after autologous total breast reconstruction have been studied in more depth. One study has reported that vascular complications are more common (17.3% versus 9.6%) when flaps are placed into previously irradiated tissue compared to naïve tissue [38]. Overall complications have also been reported to be higher in those undergoing reconstruction following PMRT at 39% compared to 25% in non-irradiated patients [39]. On the other hand, other studies have shown no increase in major complications in those who have had prior radiotherapy compared to those who did not [18]. In a study of pedicled TRAM flap reconstruction

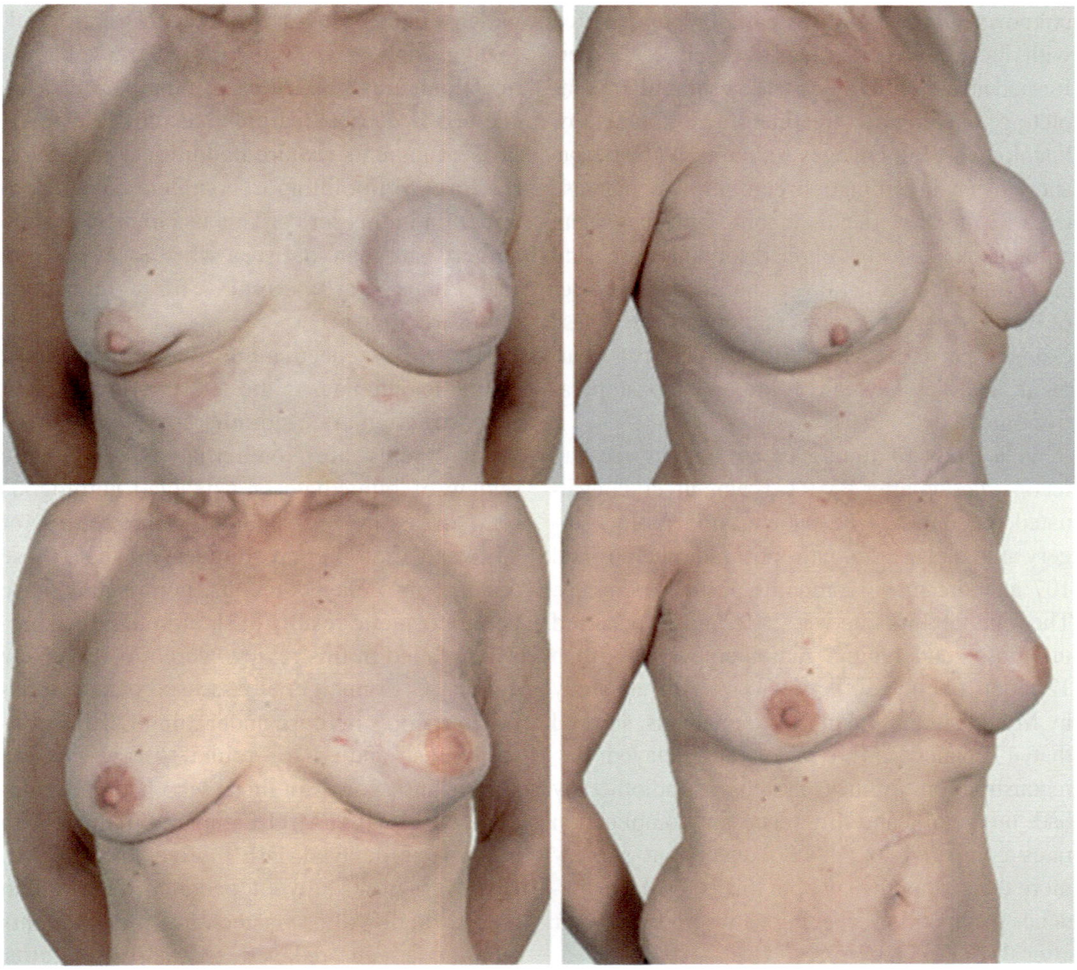

Fig. 16.5 Example of the use of a delayed local perforator flap to correct the deformity in the right breast following prior BCS and radiotherapy. This patient also underwent left breast capsulectomy and implant exchange to improve appearance after prior mastectomy and reconstruction

after mastectomy, the incidence of early complications and secondary surgery was no different between those who had radiotherapy pre- or post-reconstruction. In fact, there was a significant increase in flap contracture and a trend towards increased severity of fat necrosis in the group that underwent immediate reconstruction, followed by radiotherapy, compared to those who underwent delayed reconstruction after radiotherapy [13].

Strong evidence is lacking on the role prior radiotherapy plays in the early complication rate after delayed flap-based reconstruction. However, as radiotherapy has been linked to reduced vascular supply and delayed wound healing, it is prudent to warn patients of these possible complications when performing delayed local flap-based reconstruction in previously irradiated tissue.

16.4.3 Timing of Surgery After Prior Radiotherapy

It is generally accepted that further elective surgery should be deferred until the acute effects of radiotherapy have resolved to minimise the risk of complications, although the optimal timing is unknown. In their study of partial reconstruction with local perforator flaps, Youssif et al. performed all surgeries at least 12 months after completing oncological treatment [6]. Studies of histological skin changes following PMRT have shown that inflammation continues to increase over 12 months after treatment, with increasing amounts of elastin fibre disorganisation and clumping, and reduction in the average number of vessels per high powered field [40]. These changes persist, even at 12 months post treatment, and may have direct effects on postoperative outcomes.

In a study of timing of autologous fee-flap reconstruction after PMRT, Baumann et al. evaluated outcomes in 82 patients undergoing surgery at less than 12 months post radiotherapy and 107 at more than 12 months post-radiotherapy. The total fap loss rate was 2.6% and all occurred in those undergoing radiotherapy less than 12 months before surgery [41]. A separate study by Momoh et al. looking at 100 patients, showed that 17 patients who underwent delayed flap reconstruction within 6 months of radiotherapy had no significant difference in complication rates compared to 83 who underwent surgery more than 6 months later but this is low level evidence to support proceeding with surgery <1 year after PMRT [37].

Whilst the evidence is limited, it is common practice to wait between 6 and 12 months after radiotherapy before commencing delayed reconstruction. In our practice, we wait at least 6 months after completion of radiotherapy before proceeding to delayed local flap-based reconstruction.

16.4.4 Effects of Previous Radiotherapy on Cosmetic Appearance and Patient Reported Outcomes After Delayed Flap-Based Reconstruction

Data relating to patient-reported and cosmetic outcomes after delayed partial reconstruction with local flaps is lacking. In a single study of patients undergoing delayed reconstruction following previous BCS and radiotherapy, patient questionnaires at 3-, 6- or 12-months follow-up showed 94% satisfaction rates [6]. However, 26% of patients required additional surgery in the form of lipofilling to complete their reconstruction in this series. This is a higher revision surgery rate than that seen when local perforator flaps are used for immediate reconstruction.

There have been more studies looking at cosmetic outcomes in the setting of total breast reconstruction after radiotherapy. Results from these studies are conflicting. A systematic review of immediate and delayed autologous total breast reconstruction in the setting of adjuvant radiotherapy suggested that those undergoing delayed reconstruction may have better cosmetic results [42], although the studies included in this review were mostly of low quality. O'Connell et al. assessed patient satisfaction scores in those undergoing DIEP reconstructions and also found scores to be significantly lower in those who had an immediate DIEP with PMRT compared to those who underwent delayed DIEP after PMRT [43]. However, in a study of pedicled TRAM flap reconstruction after mastectomy, more patients who underwent delayed reconstruction after radiotherapy required revision surgery to the reconstructed breast, compared to patients who underwent immediate reconstruction followed by radiotherapy [13]. In this study, patients in both groups had similar aesthetic and psychological evaluations [13]. In O'Connell et al.'s study, those who underwent immediate DIEP with PMRT and those who underwent PMRT with delayed DIEP reconstruction had similar photography assessment scores [43]. Breast satisfaction scores have been shown to increase from baseline at 1 and 2 years after reconstruction both in patients who have had immediate reconstruction with PMRT and those who have had delayed reconstruction after PMRT [44]. This suggests it may be the reconstruction itself which plays a larger role in patient satisfaction, irrespective of the timing of radiotherapy.

Key Points

Previous radiotherapy and local perforator flaps

- Previous radiotherapy is associated with reduced vascular supply and delayed wound healing, which should be taken into account when planning delayed local flap reconstruction
- Local flap-based reconstruction should be delayed until 12 months after prior radiotherapy as this may be associated with a lower complication rate
- Patient satisfaction with cosmetic outcomes after delayed flap-based reconstruction in the setting of prior radiotherapy is generally high but revision surgeries may be required to complete their reconstruction

16.5 Future Considerations

16.5.1 Partial Breast Radiotherapy and Local Flaps

Partial breast radiotherapy has been shown in some trials to have similar outcomes in terms of recurrence-free survival at 5–10 years follow-up for invasive breast cancer compared to whole breast radiotherapy, with reductions in acute skin toxicity [4]. However, there is no reduction in fat necrosis rates at 3–5 years [4]. Partial breast radiotherapy can be considered in women aged 50 and over with tumours less than or equal to 3 cm, which are node negative [4].

These patients are less likely to require volume replacement reconstruction due to the smaller size of their tumours and partial breast radiotherapy is not currently routinely offered in most centres. Therefore, to date, there is no data relating to experience with partial breast radiotherapy and local flap reconstruction. Delivery of radiotherapy to the tumour bed would potentially result in differential effects to the flap compared to the residual normal breast tissue. Whether this would have significant effects on complications or cosmetic outcomes remains unknown at present.

16.6 Conclusions

The relationship between radiotherapy and local perforator flaps is important as most patients undergoing immediate or delayed partial breast reconstruction will undergo or have undergone radiotherapy treatment in their patient pathway. Local chest wall perforator flaps seem to tolerate radiotherapy well with no significant increase in complication rates seen after radiotherapy, although fat necrosis may be more commonly observed. Patient satisfaction with local perforator flap reconstruction remains high, even after delivery of adjuvant radiotherapy. Immediate reconstruction with local perforator flaps does not affect the ability to deliver appropriate radiotherapy regimens. Local perforator flaps are a good option for delayed partial breast reconstruction in patients who have received prior radiotherapy, with low complication rates and high patient satisfaction rates.

References

1. National Institute for Clinical Excellence. Early and locally advanced breast cancer: diagnosis and management. NICE Guideline NG101. London: NICE; 2018.
2. National Comprehensive Cancer Network. NCCN clinical practice guidelines in oncology (NCCN guidelines). Breast Cancer. Version 4.2020. Plymouth Meeting, PA: NCCN; 2020. p. 2020.
3. Carduso F, Kyriakides S, Ohno S, et al. Early breast cancer: ESMO clinical practice guidelines for diagnosis, treatment and follow-up. Ann Oncol. 2019;30:1194–220.
4. National Institute for Clinical Excellence. Early and locally advanced breast cancer: diagnosis and management. Evidence review for breast radiotherapy. NICE guideline NG101. London: NICE; 2018.
5. Hakakian CS, Lockhart RA, Kulber DA, Aronowitz JA. Lateral intercostal artery perforator flap in breast reconstruction: a simplified pedicle permits an expanded role. Ann Plast Surg. 2016;76(Suppl 3):S184–90.

6. Youssif S, Hassan Y, Tohamy A, et al. Pedicled local flaps: a reliable reconstructive tool for partial breast defects. Gland Surg. 2019;8(5):527–36.
7. Soumian S, Parmeshwar R, Chandarana M, Marla S, Narayanan S, Shetty G. Chest wall perforator flaps for partial breast reconstruction: surgical outcomes from a multicenter study. Arch Plast Surg. 2020;47(2):153–9.
8. Ho W, Stallard S, Doughty J, Mallon E, Romics L. Oncological outcomes and complications after volume replacement oncoplastic breast conservations – the Glasgow experience. Breast Cancer (Auckl). 2016;10:223–8.
9. Hillberg NS, Meesters-Caberg MAJ, Beugels J, Winkens B, Vissers YLJ, van Mulken YJM. Delay of adjuvant radiotherapy due to postoperative complications after oncoplastic breast conserving surgery. Breast. 2018;39:110–6.
10. Almasad JK, Slaah B. Breast reconstruction by local flaps after conserving surgery for breast cancer: an added asset to oncoplastic techniques. Breast J. 2008;14(4):340–4.
11. Martellani L, Manara M, Renzi N, Papa G, Ramella V, Arnez Z. Use of Licap and Ltap flaps for breast reconstruction. Acta Chir Plast. 2019;60(1):4–8.
12. Halyard MY, McCombs KE, Wong WW, et al. Acute and chronic results of adjuvant radiotherapy after mastectomy and Transverse Rectus Abdominis Myocutaneous (TRAM) flap reconstruction for breast cancer. Am J Clin Oncol. 2004;27(4):389–94.
13. He S, Yin J, Robb GL, et al. Considering the optimal timing of breast reconstruction with abdominal flaps with adjuvant irradiation in 370 consecutive pedicled transverse rectus abdominis myocutaneous flap and free deep inferior epigastric perforator flap performed in a Chinese Oncology Center. Ann Plast Surg. 2017;78(6):633–40.
14. Myung Y, Son Y, Nam T, et al. Objective assessment of flap volume changes and aesthetic results after adjuvant radiation therapy in patients undergoing immediate autologous breast reconstruction. PLoS One. 2018;13(5):e0197615.
15. Crisera CA, Chang EI, Da Lio AL, Festekjia JH, Mehrara BJ. Immediate free flap reconstruction for advanced-stage breast cancer: is it safe? Plast Reconstr Surg. 2011;128(1):32–41.
16. Cooke AL, Diaz-Abele J, Hayakawa T, Buchel E, Dalke K, Lambert P. Radiation therapy versus no radiation therapy to the neo-breast following skin-sparing mastectomy and immediate autologous free flap reconstruction for breast cancer: patient-reported and surgical outcomes at 1 year – a Mastectomy Reconstruction Outcomes Consortium (MROC) substudy. Int J Radiat Oncol Biol Phys. 2017;99(1):165–72.
17. Pont LP, Marcelli S, Robustillo M, et al. Immediate breast reconstruction with abdominal free flap and adjuvant radiotherapy: evaluation of quality of life and outcomes. Plast Reconstr Surg. 2017;140(4):681–90.
18. Berry T, Brooks S, Sydow N, et al. Complication rates of radiation on tissue expander and autologous tissue breast reconstruction. Ann Surg Oncol. 2010;17(Suppl 3):202–10.
19. Albino FP, Koltz PF, Ling MN, Langstein HN. Irradiated autologous breast reconstructions: effects of patient factors and treatment variable. Plast Recosntr Surg. 2010;126(1):12–6.
20. Roy PG, Tenovici AA. Staged approach to partial breast reconstruction to avoid mastectomy in women with breast cancer. Gland Surg. 2017;6(4):336–42.
21. Lee J, Bae Y, Audretsch W. Combination of two local flaps for large defects after breast conserving surgery. Breast. 2012;21:194–8.
22. Carrasco-Lopez C, Ibanez JFJ, Vila J, et al. Anterior intercostal artery perforator flap in immediate breast reconstruction: anatomical study and clinical application. Microsurgery. 2017;37:603–10.
23. Fujimoto H, Shiina N, Nagashima T, et al. Oncoplastic breast-conserving surgery using chest wall perforator flaps: three-dimensional quantitative analysis of the percentage of breast volume excised and changes over time in flap volume. J Surg Oncol. 2020;121:216.
24. Mericli F, Szpalski C, Schaverien MV, et al. The latissimus dorsi myocutaneous flap is a safe and effective method of partial breast reconstruction in the setting of breast-conserving therapy. Plast Reconstr Surg. 2019;143(5):927e–35e.
25. Lee S, Lee J, Lee S, Bae Y. Oncoplastic breast surgery with latissimus dorsi myocutaneous flap for large defect in patients with ptotic breasts: is it feasible when combined with local flaps? World J Surg Oncol. 2014;12:65.
26. Park TS, Seo JY, Razzokov AS, et al. Volumetric change of the latissimus dorsi muscle after postoperative radiotherapy in immediate breast reconstruction with an extended latissimus dorsi musculocutaneous flap. Arch Plast Surg. 2020;47(2):135–9.
27. Nam SB, Oh HC, Choi JY, et al. Volumetric change of the latissimus dorsi muscle after immediate breast reconstruction with an extended latissimus dorsi musculocutaneous flap. Arch Plast Surg. 2019;46:135–9.
28. Chatterjee JS, Lee A, Anderson W, et al. Effect of postoperative radiotherapy on autologous deep inferior epigastric perforator flap volume after immediate breast reconstruction. Br J Surg. 2009;96:1135–40.
29. Craig ES, Lentz R, Srinivasa D, et al. Three-dimensional analysis of how radiation affects Deep Inferior Epigastric Perforator (DIEP) flap volume, projection and position in breast cancer reconstruction. Ann Plast Surg. 2018;18:235–9.
30. Rose M, Svensson H, Handler J, Hoyer U, Ringberg A, Manjer J. Oncoplastic breast surgery compared to conventional breast-conserving surgery with regard to oncologic outcome. Clin Breast Cancer. 2019;19(6):423–32.
31. Kelemen P, Pukancsik D, Ujhelyi M, et al. Comparison of clinicopathologic, cosmetic and quality of life outcomes in 700 oncoplastic and conventional breast-conserving surgery cases: a single-centre retrospective study. Eur J Surg Oncol. 2019;45:118–24.

32. Dogan L, Gulcelik MA, Karaman N, Ozaslan C, Reis E. Oncoplastic surgery in surgical treatment of breast cancer: is the timing of adjuvant treatment affected? Clin Breast Cancer. 2012;139(3):202–5.
33. Wodzinski M, Skalski A, Ciepeila I, Kuszewski T, Kedzierawski P, Gajda J. Improving oncoplastic tumour bed localization for radiotherapy planning using image registration algorithms. Phys Med Biol. 2018;63(3):035024.
34. Alco G, Igdem A, Okkan S, et al. Replacement of the tumor bed following oncoplastic breast-conserving surgery with immediate latissimus dorsi mini-flap. Mol Clin Oncol. 2016;5(4):365–71.
35. Furet E, Peurien D, Fournier-Bidoz N, et al. Plastic surgery for breast conservation therapy: how to define the volume of the tumor bed for the boost? Eur J Surg Oncol. 2014;40(7):830–4.
36. Quinn EM, Highton L, Murphy J. Five year experience of oncoplastic volume replacement using local perforator flaps. 2020 Annual Meeting Official Proceedings, Volume XXI, Abstract 787329. Ann Surg Oncol. 2020;27:231–671.
37. Kronowitz SJ. Current status of autologous tissue-based breast reconstruction in patients receiving post-mastectomy radiation therapy. Plast Reconstr Surg. 2012;130(2):282–92.
38. Fosnot J, Fischer JP, Smartt JM Jr, et al. Does previous chest wall irradiation increase vascular complications in free autologous breast reconstruction? Plast Reconstr Surg. 2011;127(2):496–504.
39. Kroll SS, Schusterman MA, Reece GP, Miller MJ, Smith B. Breast reconstruction with myocutaneous flaps in previously irradiated patients. Plast Reconstr Surg. 1994;93(3):460–9.
40. Kung TA, Kidwell KM, Speth KA, et al. Radiation-induced skin changes after postmastectomy radiation therapy: a pilot study of indicators for timing of delayed breast reconstruction. J Reconstr Microsurg. 2019;35(3):209–15.
41. Baumann DP, Crosby MA, Selber JC, et al. Optimal timing of delayed free lower abdominal flap breast reconstruction after postmastectomy radiation therapy. Plast Reconstr Surg. 2011;127(3):1100–6.
42. Javaid M, Song F, Leinster S, Dickson MG, James NK. Radiation effects on the cosmetic outcomes of immediate and delayed autologous breast reconstruction: an argument about timing. J Plast Reconstr Aesthet Surg. 2006;59:16–26.
43. O'Connell R, Di Micco R, Khabra K, et al. Comparison of immediate versus delayed DIEP flap reconstruction in women who require postmastectomy radiotherapy. Plast Reconstr Surg. 2018;142(3):594–605.
44. Billig J, Jagsi R, Qi J, et al. Should immediate autologous breast reconstruction be considered in women who require postmastectomy radiation therapy? A prospective analysis of outcomes. Plast Reconstr Surg. 2017;139(6):1279–88.

Tumour Bed Boost Radiotherapy and Planning Following Partial Breast Reconstruction with Chest Wall Perforator Flaps

17

Emanuele Garreffa, Philip Poortmans, and Amit Agrawal

Contents

17.1 Background

The addition of a tumour bed (TB) boost radiation therapy (RT) to standard whole-breast irradiation (WBI) following breast conserving surgery (BCS) proportionally reduces ipsilateral breast tumour recurrence (IBTR) by about half [1]. As a constant proportional risk reduction depends on the initial recurrence risks, younger patients with higher-risk tumours (larger, triple-negative, or oestrogen receptor negative/human epidermal growth factor receptor 2-positive disease; and/or presence of lymphovascular invasion) derive the largest benefit in absolute terms [2].

Of the two types of oncoplastic breast surgery (OBS), displacement and replacement, this chapter is focussing on TB boost RT in replacement. Displacement type of OBS (such as mammaplasty) involves rearranging breast parenchyma to avoid volume defects following tumour excision, whilst replacement type of OBS involves filling in of tumour excision defect with tissue from beyond the breast, such as chest wall perforator flaps (CWPF). Patients receiving OBS

E. Garreffa
Breast Surgery, University Hospitals of Derby and Burton, Derby, UK
e-mail: emanuele.garreffa@nhs.net

P. Poortmans
Radiotherapy Department, Institut Curie, Paris, France
e-mail: philip.poortmans@gza.be

A. Agrawal (✉)
Oncoplastic Breast Surgery, Cambridge University Hospitals, Cambridge, UK
e-mail: amitagrawal@doctors.org.uk; amit.agrawal2@nhs.net

M. Hamdi et al. (eds.), *Pedicled Flaps in Partial Breast Reconstruction*,
https://doi.org/10.1007/978-3-031-08483-6_17

are usually younger and present with larger tumours; therefore, RT boost is particularly indicated. However, published studies on OBS do not provide RT regime details nor specify TB boost use. In a 2013 systematic review on volume displacement OBS and RT, TB boost was identified only in 11 out of 24 analysed studies [3]. Similarly, in a more recent systematic review in 2016, only 17 out of 37 studies on volume displacement OBS and 3 out of 11 studies on volume replacement OBS reported the use of boost RT [4]. This chapter focusses on the current evidence regarding the use of TB boost following partial breast reconstruction with CWPF.

17.2 Discussion

17.2.1 The Rationale of Tumour Bed Boost

Data from the European Organisation for Research and Treatment of Cancer (EORTC), "boost–no boost" trial, with a median follow-up of 18.2 years confirms that boost reduces the 20-year IBTR rate from 16.4% to 12.0%. However, the reduction was from 31% to 15% (HR, 0.37; 95% CI, 0.22–0.62; $p < 0.001$) in women aged 50 or less with high-grade cancers associated with high-grade Ductal Carcinoma in Situ (DCIS) [2]. Of note, it does not appear to translate into a significant overall survival benefit at 20 years (boost, 59.7%; no boost, 61.1%; $p = 0.323$) [1].

The joint Groupe European de Curietherapie (GEC) and the European Society for Radiotherapy & Oncology (ESTRO) Breast Cancer Working Group provided clinical guidance for the use of boost RT after WBI (either standard or hypo-fractioned) based on three stratified risk groups [5]. In the low-risk group (women aged 50 or more with unifocal, node negative cancers and clear surgical margins by at least 2 mm), the TB boost will only add little benefit and is therefore considered optional. In the intermediate-risk group (women aged 41–49, women aged 40 or less without risk factors or women aged 50 or more with risk factors), a TB boost of 10–16 Gy should be considered. Finally, in the high-risk group (women aged 40 or less with additional risk factors such as close margins, tumour size >3 cm, extensive associated DCIS, lymphovascular invasion, node positivity, multicentric or multifocal tumours, triple-negative phenotype, or residual tumour after neoadjuvant chemotherapy), an escalated boost ≥16 Gy is indicated.

17.2.2 Comparison Between Different TB Techniques

A study involving 2661 BCS patients who received 50 Gy whole breast radiation followed by 16 Gy of electrons, photons, or brachytherapy TB boost showed no differences in IBTR risk between these three variations at 5 years [6]. Another comparative study (2000–2005) in 1379 patients showed similar results between the three techniques at 8.8 years [7]. Limitations of both these studies were numerically disparate groups (dominated by electron TB) and a modest follow-up period.

17.2.3 Tumour Bed Boost After Volume Replacement Oncoplastic Breast Surgery with CWPF

At the time of writing of this chapter (March 2021), only four small studies on CWPF reported on the use of TB boost following BCS and partial breast reconstruction with CWPF [8–11], including 3 with patient outcomes [8, 10, 11]. A series [10] of 13 BCS patients who received fractionated WBI (45–50 Gy) and an additional TB boost (10 Gy) reported >95% overall patient satisfaction at 6 months (one reported fat necrosis needing surgical intervention). In another series [11] of two-stage CWPF surgery in 20 women, 19 patients had WBI with a 12 TB boost. Good aesthetic outcomes and high patients satisfaction rates within 6 months were observed with an anonymised patient survey. However, it is generally agreed that RT-related changes in shape and asymmetry often need a longer follow-up. A longer follow-up study (2 years) [8] analysed the change in flap volume over time in a cohort of 33 CWPF patients. All received 40–50 Gy WBI, and an additional 16 patients with close or positive margins received a 10 Gy TB boost [Personal Communication]. In the 26 patients with >2 years follow-up, the authors observed that most patients maintained at least 80% of the initial flap volume with only four patients (15.4%), with flap volume loss over 40%.

17.2.4 Challenges to Tumour Bed Contouring and Boost Delivery Planning in Volume Replacement Oncoplastic Breast Surgery

In volume displacement techniques with major parenchymal rearrangement, the possibility of TB site relocation with potential issues in accurate TB identification and planning of boost delivery was identified early in practice [3, 12]. However, in contrast, likely because volume replacement surgery became more popular recently, discussion over the accuracy of TB contouring after volume replacement surgery is more recent [9, 13].

17.2.4.1 Tumour Bed Displacement

A discordance between pre-operative gross tumour volume and post-surgical contoured TB was first identified after volume replacement OBS with LD mini-flap being performed for over two decades, discussion has gained ground more recently. In a study of 22 patients, there was a marked TB shift in 36.4% of the patients where the post-operative boost volume was identified in an entirely different quadrant to the pre-operative tumour site [13]. A common practice in UK [14] is to place markers (such as surgical clips) to help define the TB during computed tomography simulation images for planning boost localisation, size, and dose [15]. In Europe and Asia, this practice is increasing too [16–20].

In CWPF, despite the use of cavity clips, the accurate contouring of the TB can still be challenging. A recent study by the senior author's group reviewed the radiotherapy planning scans of 28 CWPF patients and compared the TB volume identified by an oncologist using cavity clips (oTB) with the surgical specimen volume (SPV) [9]. Data suggested that, if based solely on clips, TB contouring in CWPF can produce an underestimation of the boost target volume (average SPV-oTB—44.5 mL). On the other hand, TB identified by combining the clips with the flap delineated by a surgeon on planning CT scan (sTB) appeared to provide a closer correlation of target volume with the actual specimen volume (average SPV-sTB—1.02 mL), albeit with larger volumes. The volume, if it were to be estimated this way in actual practice, will represent the non-breast flap tissue filling the lumpectomy defect and could, in theory, be spared from TB and its adverse consequences [9, 15].

17.2.4.2 Larger Target Volume

Contrary to volume displacement techniques and simple BCS, where the lumpectomy defect is closed by opposing the cavity walls, in CWPF, the surgical defect is filled volume-for-volume by the flap, leaving the cavity walls separated. The breast tissue located within 1.5 cm of the perimeter of the excised tumour is at greater risk of true in-breast recurrence and is thereby defined as the "clinical target volume" (CTV) for the boost [21–23].

Even in the absence of adverse WBI effects, boost RT alone may result in varying degrees of focal retraction or indentation and asymmetry due to either local fibrosis or fat necrosis, resulting in parenchymal loss [15]. As the evidence of long-term effects of boost RT comes from patients from the pre-OBS era (though there may be some early unidentified OBS patients within these trials) [1, 24–26], the same adverse aesthetic effects in OBS might even be exacerbated [27, 28]. Before these reported adverse outcomes, seroma used to be surgically perceived as a natural filler of the uncorrected relatively larger WLE defect (BCS with 5+ mm margins) camouflaging as initial good postoperative outcome until after RT. Reported RT trial data, especially from long-term follow-up, will be from an era when OBS was an exception in very few surgical hands and hence may not strictly be comparable to current outcomes. Any fibrosis secondary to seroma (especially if complicated with bleeding/infection) [25] should be less common in the current surgical practice since now most breast surgeons should repair WLE defects.

However, in the setting of volume replacement OBS, where the oncoplastic excision volume is larger than in simple BCS [29, 30] and the replaced flap tissue is interposed between the cavity walls, a target boost volume including a rim of breast parenchyma adjacent to the TB would be larger. Such a larger boost volume may impair the long-term aesthetic outcome due to boost-related adverse effects [15, 31, 32]. As a potential solution, a ring-shaped boost, marked as a 5 mm rim of breast tissue around the TB and sparing the central flapped area, may be an option. Such a boost, although challenging to reproduce in treatment planning and delivery practice due to dose diffusion, may allow a substantial reduction of the target volume (−127.6% average target volume reduction) [9].

An alternative approach, and potentially a way around the problems of TB identification and unnecessary radiation to the replaced flap tissue, could be to change the sequence of treatment by delivering RT either preoperatively or intraoperatively. The use of preoperative RT has less negative impact on the aesthetic outcome [15, 33] and could potentially allow the delivery of a boost dose directly to the tumour and the surrounding penumbral tissue before surgery and therefore close to 100% accuracy. However, the evidence is scarce, until recently only from small [34] or retrospective studies [35], with a minimal representation of OBS patients. The preparatory prospective phase II PAPBI-1 multicentre study, that closed early due to poor accrual, investigated the impact of preoperative accelerated partial breast irradiation (PAPBI) on local control, breast fibrosis, and cosmetic outcome. The 5-year analysis of 133 women showed promising results, which are now being investigated in an ongoing randomised trial comparing pre- with postoperative PBI [36]. A combination of IMRT with an integrated boost followed by hormone treatment given before surgery is currently being tested in a UK feasibility trial which has not expressly included or excluded OBS patients [37].

The use of intraoperative RT (IORT) as an alternative to WBI has the potential advantages of improved accuracy in the delivery of RT, convenience for the patient, reduced skin toxicity and improved aesthetic outcomes [15]. Two randomised controlled trials have investigated this approach with discordant results [38, 39], and a wider introduction of this approach is currently being debated [40]. With electron-based IORT, as used in the ELIOT trial and in several other studies in PBI and in TB boost, much larger volumes can be treated compared to low-energy X-rays [41, 42]. The approach in which after lumpectomy, the CTV boost is administered preceding the OBS procedure is currently being discussed as a topic of prospective studies.

17.2.5 Is a Boost Necessary After Volume Replacement Surgery?

With decreasing local recurrence rates following improved diagnostic approaches as well as local and systemic treatments, the extent of RT of the breast after local tumour excision is put into discussion, even for high-risk patients [43]. De-escalation in breast cancer RT includes precise target volume definition and contouring [44], hypofractionation by reducing the number of fractions and the total dose [45], volume reduction with PBI for low-risk patients [46] and omission of the boost [47].

A weak point of most studies evaluating the TB boost is the definition of the CTV. Following the pivotal research findings of Holland [48], the presence of residual tumour cells decreases with the distance from the edge of the primary tumour. Based on that, the concept of the boost emerged, which was later fine-tuned to the definition of a CTV for the boost consisting of the 1.5 cm rim of tissue surrounding the primary tumour (2 cm for partial breast irradiation, which is indicated for low-risk patients instead of the boost that is indicated for high-risk patients) [21]. This 1.5 cm margin can be reduced by the tissue removed already with the lumpectomy, preferably anisocentric in six directions (provided that the pathology report describes this and in a reliable way). As the lumpectomy rarely removes the primary tumour in a geometrically perfectly centric position, the margins that are removed (and should be deduced from the 1.5 cm) are seldom, if ever equal in all directions [49]. Thereby, the lumpectomy cavity in general, poorly represents the anatomically correct boost CTV and, unfortunately, as previously stated in most of the studies that we described, the lumpectomy cavity, including a margin for potential microscopic spread, is erroneously expected to constitute the boost CTV. Moreover, the size of the margin varies depending on local experience and protocol, which should not be the case—in contrast, the margin between CTV and planning target volume should be made dependent on that. Many uncertainties in the definition of the clinical target volume are related to uncertainties in the localisation of the site of the original tumour within the breast after lumpectomy, more after OBS [50]. OBS is increasingly shown to have lower rates of margin positivity when compared to wide local excision or quadrantectomy [29, 30, 51–54], regardless of individual margin widths [55]. Oncoplastic resections also have a lower tumour-to-specimen ratio [29] with larger surgical margins, frequently well beyond 1 cm (particularly in volume displacement OBS) [30].

Suppose the purpose of the TB boost is to target the 1.5 cm of breast tissue surrounding the tumour. In that case, one could discuss whether this is still necessary for the setting of these oncoplastic escalated surgical margins. It is worth noting, however, that even though it could be easy to achieve >1 cm margins in volume displacement OBS (particularly for lower pole tumours in larger breasts), this might not be the case in volume replacement OBS which generally involves smaller surgical specimens [29] and is indicated in patients with higher tumour-to-breast ratios. Furthermore, the current trend in expanding the indications of OBS to larger tumours, often with satellite lesions identified pre-operatively, and even multifocal and multicentric cancers will reduce the chances of obtaining wide surgical margins [56]. The decision to include a boost in the RT treatment plan should consider not only the patient's age and tumour histology but also the surgical procedure performed and a three-dimensional assessment of the surgical specimen as well as 3D reconstruction of the CTV boost.

17.3 Conclusions

OBS is a recent innovation in breast surgery, led initially by displacement options and, more recently, replacement options. Undoubtedly, OBS leads to better surgical aesthetics, however, evidence on long-term outcomes following RT is limited. It is logical to extrapolate that it will be superior to traditional BCS with uncorrected tumour bed defect. However, OBS should remain a tool when indicated, and most women with small tumours might still have the best outcomes with procedures that involve minimal tissue damage. Furthermore, indications and planning for additional TB boost are generating discussions in the radiation oncology teams, given the recentness of these surgical innovations with early gains that need to be made more robust for long-term gains.

Ethical Statement

Funding No funding was provided by any source for this chapter.

Conflict of Interest We declare that there is no actual or potential conflict of interest in relation to this article. All the authors have no financial or personal relationship with other people or organizations that could inappropriately influence (bias) this work.

References

1. Bartelink H, Maingon P, Poortmans P, et al. Whole-breast irradiation with or without a boost for patients treated with breast-conserving surgery for early breast cancer: 20-year follow-up of a randomised phase 3 trial. Lancet Oncol. 2015;16(1):47–56.
2. Vrieling C, van Werkhoven E, Maingon P, et al. Prognostic factors for local control in breast cancer after long-term follow-up in the EORTC boost vs no boost trial: a randomized clinical trial. JAMA Oncol. 2017;3(1):42–8.
3. Schaverien MV, Stallard S, Dodwell D, Doughty JC. Use of boost radiotherapy in oncoplastic breast-conserving surgery - a systematic review. Eur J Surg Oncol. 2013;39(11):1179–85.
4. Yoon JJ, Green WR, Kim S, et al. Oncoplastic breast surgery in the setting of breast-conserving therapy: a systematic review. Adv Radiat Oncol. 2016;1(4):205–15.
5. Polo A, Polgár C, Hannoun-Levi JM, et al. Risk factors and state-of-the-art indications for boost irradiation in invasive breast carcinoma. Brachytherapy. 2017;16(3):552–64.
6. Poortmans P, Bartelink H, Horiot JC, Struikmans H, Van den Bogaert W, Fourquet A, Jager J, Hoogenraad W, Rodrigus P, Wárlám-Rodenhuis C, Collette L, Pierart M. EORTC Radiotherapy and Breast Cancer Groups. The influence of the boost technique on local control in breast conserving treatment in the EORTC 'boost versus no boost' randomised trial. Radiother Oncol. 2004;72(1):25–33.
7. Verhoeven K, Kindts I, Laenen A, et al. A comparison of three different radiotherapy boost techniques after breast conserving therapy for breast cancer. Breast. 2015;24(4):391–6.
8. Fujimoto H, Shiina N, Nagashima T, Sangai T, Sakakibara J, Takada M, Teranaka R, Takishima H, Kawasaki Y, Ohtsuka M. Oncoplastic breast-conserving surgery using chest wall perforator flaps: three-dimensional quantitative analysis of the percentage of breast volume excised and changes over time in flap volume. J Surg Oncol. 2020;121:216.
9. Garreffa E, Hughes-Davies L, Russell S, Lightowlers S, Agrawal A. Definition of tumor bed boost in oncoplastic breast surgery: an understanding and approach. Clin Breast Cancer. 2020;20(4):e510–5.
10. Munhoz AM, Montag E, Arruda E, Brasil JA, Aldrighi JM, Gemperli R, Filassi JR, Ferreira MC. Immediate conservative breast surgery reconstruction with perforator flaps: new challenges in the era of partial mastectomy reconstruction? Breast. 2011;20(3):233–40.
11. Roy PG, Tenovici AA. Staged approach to partial breast reconstruction to avoid mastectomy in women with breast cancer. Gland Surg. 2017;6(4):336–42.
12. Munhoz AM, Montag E, Arruda EG, et al. The role of the lateral thoracodorsal fasciocutaneous flap in immediate conservative breast surgery reconstruction. Plast Reconstr Surg. 2006;117(6):1699–710.
13. Alço G, Igdem S, Okkan S, et al. Replacement of the tumor bed following oncoplastic breast-conserving surgery with immediate latissimus dorsi mini-flap. Mol Clin Oncol. 2016;5(4):365–71. https://doi.org/10.3892/mco.2016.984.
14. Coles CE, Wilson CB, Cumming J, et al. Titanium clip placement to allow accurate tumour bed localisation following breast conserving surgery: audit on behalf of the IMPORT Trial Management Group. Eur J Surg Oncol. 2009;35(6):578–82.
15. Agrawal A. Oncoplastic breast surgery and radiotherapy-adverse aesthetic outcomes, proposed classification of aesthetic components, and causality attribution. Breast J. 2019;25(2):207–18.
16. Aznar MC, Meattini I, Poortmans P, Steyerova P, Wyld L. To clip or not to clip. That is no question! Eur J Surg Oncol. 2017;43(7):1145–7.
17. Borm KJ, Schönknecht C, Nestler A, et al. Outcomes of immediate oncoplastic surgery and adjuvant radiotherapy in breast cancer patients. BMC Cancer. 2019;19(1):907.
18. Kelemen P, Pukancsik D, Újhelyi M, et al. Comparison of clinicopathologic, cosmetic and quality of life outcomes in 700 oncoplastic and conventional breast-conserving surgery cases: a single-centre retrospective study. Eur J Surg Oncol. 2019;45(2):118–24.
19. Kim JB, Kim DK, Lee JW, et al. The usefulness of pedicled perforator flap in partial breast reconstruction after breast conserving surgery in Korean women. Arch Plast Surg. 2018;45(1):29–36.
20. Rose M, Svensson H, Handler J, Hoyer U, Ringberg A, Manjer J. Oncoplastic breast surgery compared to conventional breast-conserving surgery with regard to oncologic outcome. Clin Breast Cancer. 2019;19(6):423–432.e5.
21. Boersma LJ, Janssen T, Elkhuizen PH, et al. Reducing interobserver variation of boost-CTV delineation in breast conserving radiation therapy using a preoperative CT and delineation guidelines. Radiother Oncol. 2012;103:178–82.
22. Freedman GM, Anderson PR, Hanlon AL, Eisenberg DF, Nicolaou N. Pattern of local recurrence after conservative surgery and whole-breast irradiation. Int J Radiat Oncol Biol Phys. 2005;61(5):1328–36.
23. Lehman M, Hickey BE, Francis DP, See AM. Partial breast irradiation for early breast cancer. Cochrane Database Syst Rev. 2014;(6):CD007077.
24. Collette S, Collette L, Budiharto T, et al. Predictors of the risk of fibrosis at 10 years after breast conserving therapy for early breast cancer: a study based on the EORTC Trial 22881-10882 'boost versus no boost' [published correction appears in Eur J Cancer. 2009;45(11):2061]. Eur J Cancer. 2008;44(17):2587–99.
25. Mukesh MB, Barnett G, Cumming J, et al. Association of breast tumour bed seroma with post-operative complications and late normal tissue toxicity: results from the Cambridge Breast IMRT trial. Eur J Surg Oncol. 2012;38(10):918–24.

26. Vrieling C, Collette L, Fourquet A, et al. The influence of patient, tumor and treatment factors on the cosmetic results after breast-conserving therapy in the EORTC 'boost vs. no boost' trial. EORTC Radiotherapy and Breast Cancer Cooperative Groups. Radiother Oncol. 2000;55(3):219–32.
27. Brouwers PJAM, van Werkhoven E, Bartelink H, Fourquet A, Lemanski C, van Loon J, Maduro JH, Russell NS, Scheijmans LJEE, Schinagl DAX, Westenberg AH, Poortmans P, Boersma LJ. Young Boost Trial research group. Predictors for poor cosmetic outcome in patients with early stage breast cancer treated with breast conserving therapy: results of the young boost trial. Radiother Oncol. 2018;128(3):434–41.
28. Lansu JT, Essers M, Voogd AC, Luiten EJ, Buijs C, Groenendaal N, Poortmans PM. The influence of simultaneous integrated boost, hypofractionation and oncoplastic surgery on cosmetic outcome and PROMs after breast conserving therapy. Eur J Surg Oncol. 2015;41(10):1411–6.
29. Garreffa E, Kankam HKN, Bali R, et al. Achieving margin clearance following oncoplastic breast surgery in comparison with simple wide local excision: a three-dimensional specimen assessment. ANZ J Surg. 2020;90(11):2346–52.
30. Clough KB, Benyahi D, Nos C, Charles C, Sarfati I. Oncoplastic surgery: pushing the limits of breast-conserving surgery. Breast J. 2015;21(2):140–6.
31. Al Uwini S, Antonini N, Poortmans PM, Boersma L, Hurkmans C, Leer JW, Horiot JC, Struikmans H, Bartelink H. The influence of the use of CT-planning on the irradiated boost volume in breast conserving treatment. Radiother Oncol. 2009;93(1):87–93.
32. Borger JH, Kemperman H, Smitt HS, Hart A, van Dongen J, Lebesque J, Bartelink H. Dose and volume effects on fibrosis after breast conservation therapy. Int J Radiat Oncol Biol Phys. 1994;30(5):1073–81.
33. Lightowlers SV, Boersma LJ, Fourquet A, Kirova YM, Offersen BV, Poortmans P, Scholten AN, Somaiah N, Coles CE. Preoperative breast radiation therapy: indications and perspectives. Eur J Cancer. 2017;82:184–92.
34. Bollet MA, Kirova YM, Antoni G, et al. Responses to concurrent radiotherapy and hormone-therapy and outcome for large breast cancers in post-menopausal women. Radiother Oncol. 2007;85:336–45.
35. Poleszczuk J, Luddy K, Chen L, et al. Neoadjuvant radiotherapy of early-stage breast cancer and long-term disease-free survival. Breast Cancer Res. 2017;19:75.
36. Bosma SCJ, Leij F, Vreeswijk S, Maaker M, Wesseling J, Vijver MV, Scholten A, Rivera S, Bourgier C, Auzac G, Foukakis T, Lekberg T, Bongard D, Loo C, Rutgers E, Bartelink H, Elkhuizen PHM. Five-year results of the Preoperative Accelerated Partial Breast Irradiation (PAPBI) trial. Int J Radiat Oncol Biol Phys. 2020;106(5):958–67.
37. Clinicaltrials.gov. Neo-RT: a study investigating whether changing the sequence of treatments (starting radiotherapy followed by hormone therapy before surgery) is feasible (Neo-RT). n.d.. https://clinicaltrials.gov/ct2/show/NCT03818100. Accessed 26 Jul 2020.
38. Orecchia R, Veronesi U, Maisonneuve P, et al. Intraoperative irradiation for early breast cancer (ELIOT): long-term recurrence and survival outcomes from a single-centre, randomised, phase 3 equivalence trial. Lancet Oncol. 2021;22(5):597–608.
39. Vaidya JS, Bulsara M, Baum M, et al. Long term survival and local control outcomes from single dose targeted intraoperative radiotherapy during lumpectomy (TARGIT-IORT) for early breast cancer: TARGIT-A randomised clinical trial. BMJ. 2020;370:m2836.
40. Sasieni PD, Sawyer EJ. Intraoperative radiotherapy for early breast cancer - insufficient evidence to change practice. Nat Rev Clin Oncol. 2020;17(12):723–4.
41. Fastner G, Gaisberger C, Kaiser J, Scherer P, Ciabattoni A, Petoukhova A, Sperk E, Poortmans P, Calvo FA, Sedlmayer F, Leonardi MC. ESTRO IORT Task Force/ACROP recommendations for intraoperative radiation therapy with electrons (IOERT) in breast cancer. Radiother Oncol. 2020;149:150–7.
42. Kaidar-Person O, Meattini I, Zippel D, Poortmans P. Apples and oranges: comparing partial breast irradiation techniques. Rep Pract Oncol Radiother. 2020;25(5):780–2.
43. Poortmans PMP, Arenas M, Livi L. Over-irradiation. Breast. 2017;31:295–302.
44. Offersen BV, Boersma LJ, Kirkove C, Hol S, Aznar MC, Biete Sola A, Kirova YM, Pignol JP, Remouchamps V, Verhoeven K, Weltens C, Arenas M, Gabrys D, Kopek N, Krause M, Lundstedt D, Marinko T, Montero A, Yarnold J, Poortmans P. ESTRO consensus guideline on target volume delineation for elective radiation therapy of early stage breast cancer. Radiother Oncol. 2015;114(1):3–10.
45. Marta GN, Coles C, Kaidar-Person O, Meattini I, Hijal T, Zissiadis Y, Pignol JP, Ramiah D, Ho AY, Cheng SH, Sancho G, Offersen BV, Poortmans P. The use of moderately hypofractionated post-operative radiation therapy for breast cancer in clinical practice: a critical review. Crit Rev Oncol Hematol. 2020;156:103090.
46. Marta GN, Barrett J, Porfirio GJM, Martimbianco ALC, Bevilacqua JLB, Poortmans P, Riera R. Effectiveness of different accelerated partial breast irradiation techniques for the treatment of breast cancer patients: systematic review using indirect comparisons of randomized clinical trials. Rep Pract Oncol Radiother. 2019;24(2):165–74.
47. Kayali M, Jaoude JA, Ramia P, Assi H, Geara F, Poortmans P, Zeidan YH. Post-lumpectomy radiation therapy boost in breast cancer patients: evidence revisited. Ecancermedicalscience. 2021;15:1194.
48. Holland R, Veling SH, Mravunac M, Hendriks JH. Histologic multifocality of Tis, T1-2 breast carcinomas. Implications for clinical trials of breast-conserving surgery. Cancer. 1985;56(5):979–90.

49. Bartelink H, Bourgier C, Elkhuizen P. Has partial breast irradiation by IORT or brachytherapy been prematurely introduced into the clinic? Radiother Oncol. 2012;104(2):139–42.
50. Poortmans P, Aznar M, Bartelink H. Quality indicators for breast cancer: revisiting historical evidence in the context of technology changes. Semin Radiat Oncol. 2012;22(1):29–39.
51. Chakravorty A, Shrestha AK, Sanmugalingam N, et al. How safe is oncoplastic breast conservation? Comparative analysis with standard breast conserving surgery. Eur J Surg Oncol. 2012;38(5):395–8.
52. Clough KB, Lewis JS, Couturaud B, Fitoussi A, Nos C, Falcou MC. Oncoplastic techniques allow extensive resections for breast-conserving therapy of breast carcinomas. Ann Surg. 2003;237(1):26–34.
53. Giacalone PL, Roger P, Dubon O, et al. Comparative study of the accuracy of breast resection in oncoplastic surgery and quadrantectomy in breast cancer. Ann Surg Oncol. 2007;14(2):605–14.
54. Kaur N, Petit JY, Rietjens M, et al. Comparative study of surgical margins in oncoplastic surgery and quadrantectomy in breast cancer. Ann Surg Oncol. 2005;12(7):539–45.
55. Bali R, Kankam HKN, Borkar N, et al. Wide local excision versus oncoplastic breast surgery: differences in surgical outcome for an assumed margin (0, 1, or 2 mm) distance. Clin Breast Cancer. 2018;18(5):e1053–7.
56. Silverstein MJ, Savalia N, Khan S, Ryan J. Extreme oncoplasty: breast conservation for patients who need mastectomy. Breast J. 2015;21(1):52–9.

Quality of Outcomes

18

Leonardo Pires Novais Dias
and Moustapha Hamdi

Contents

18.1 Background

Breast cancer is the most commonly occurring cancer in women, and around one out of eight women will present the disease during their lifetime. According to GLOBOCAN 2020, female breast cancer recently surpassed lung cancer as the leading cause of cancer incidence worldwide. Besides that, breast cancer is only the fifth leading cause of cancer mortality (Fig. 18.1) [1]. Indeed, the proportion of mortality rates has been decreasing since the 1980s [2, 3]. Currently, the breast cancer death in a 5-year follow-up is around 5%, 5% and 10% for patients with 55 years, 65 years and 75 years at diagnosis, respectively [4].

Breast cancer care has changed dramatically over the last decades. The introduction of screening programs permitted early diagnosis that, combined with a better understanding of breast cancer behaviour, led to less aggressive local and systemic treatment protocols. Breast cancer surgery evolved from radical mastectomy to breast-conserving procedures followed by radiotherapy. Neoadjuvant chemotherapy consent tumour

L. P. N. Dias
Head of the Breast Surgery Department, Mater Dei Hospital, Salvador, Brazil
e-mail: leonardo.dias@materdei.com.br

M. Hamdi (✉)
Head of the Plastic Surgery Department, Brussels University Hospital, Vrije Universiteit Brussel, Brussels, Belgium
e-mail: moustapha.hamdi@uzbrussel.be

M. Hamdi et al. (eds.), *Pedicled Flaps in Partial Breast Reconstruction*,
https://doi.org/10.1007/978-3-031-08483-6_18

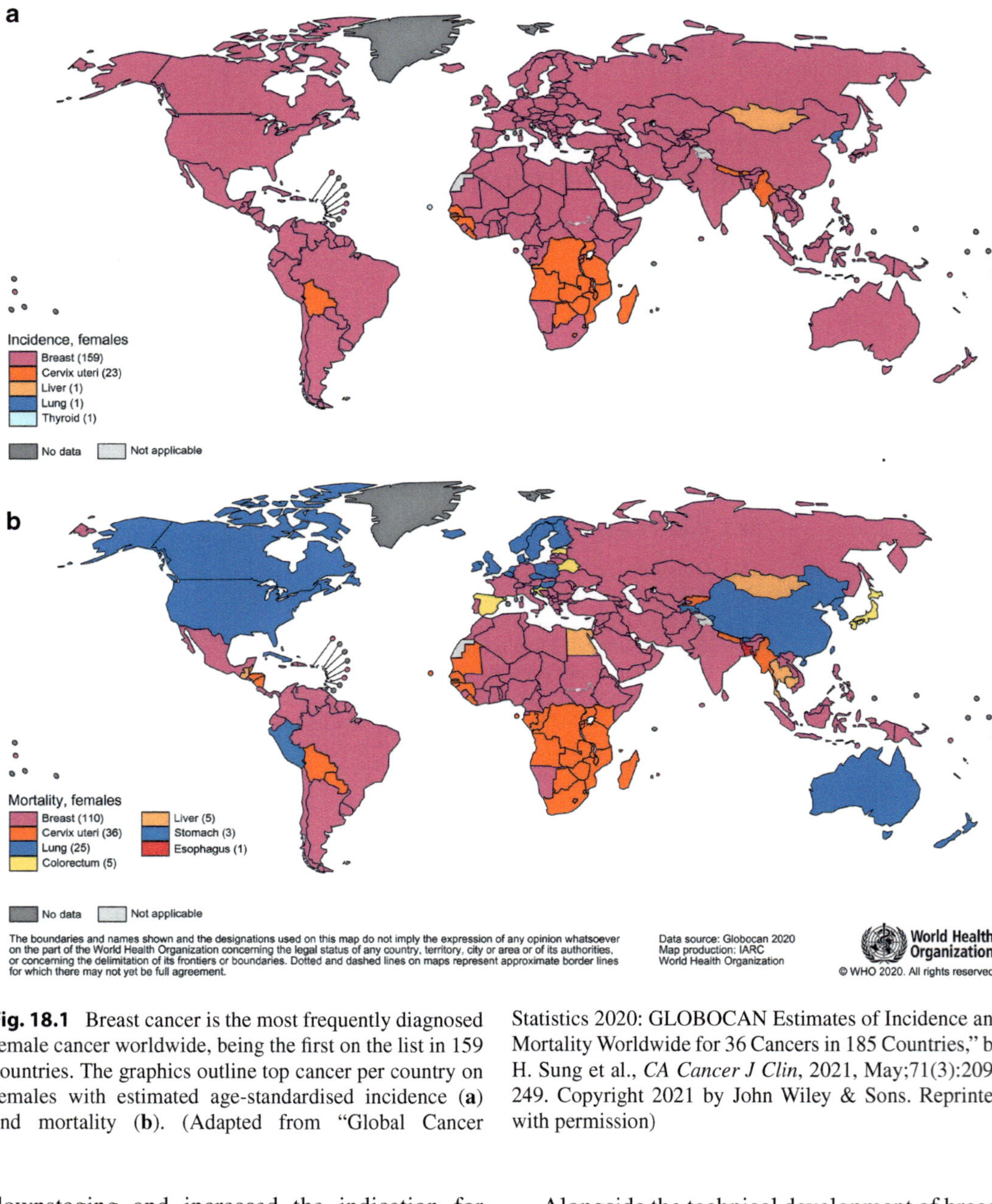

Fig. 18.1 Breast cancer is the most frequently diagnosed female cancer worldwide, being the first on the list in 159 countries. The graphics outline top cancer per country on females with estimated age-standardised incidence (**a**) and mortality (**b**). (Adapted from "Global Cancer Statistics 2020: GLOBOCAN Estimates of Incidence and Mortality Worldwide for 36 Cancers in 185 Countries," by H. Sung et al., *CA Cancer J Clin*, 2021, May;71(3):209–249. Copyright 2021 by John Wiley & Sons. Reprinted with permission)

downstaging and increased the indication for breast-conserving surgery. These were the first steps for the oncoplastic breast surgery, which combines extensive oncological resections with aesthetic techniques increasing the final cosmetic result. As a consequence, patients are living longer and better [5, 6].

Alongside the technical development of breast cancer treatment, the mentality over the disease changed remarkably. Back in the 1970s, the quality of outcomes for breast cancer treatment was evaluated mainly by the oncological safety, and aspects related to breast reconstruction or quality of life were considered secondary. Ahead oncologic safety, there were other motives why patients did not demand any restoration. The interval from primary cancer surgery to delayed reconstruction dwindled the patient's engagement in any additional operation. In addition, reimbursement was customarily not feasible since the aesthetic image of the breast was acknowledged as superficial self-indulgence. However, in the following decades, breast cancer awareness and advocacy reduced the stigma regarding the disease through education, which led to patient empowerment. New values in the breast cancer culture encouraged women to demand better quality of life after therapy, which became an essential part of treatment assessment. Today, shared decision-making puts the patient at the centre of the treatment plan, and all related clinical aspects must be discussed beforehand [7–11].

18.2 Breast Cancer Surgery

All advancements in breast cancer care increased long-term survival for most women with early breast cancer. Those survivors would live with their post-treatment issues for the rest of their days. In reply, strides in the surgical field were performed based on the fusion amid oncological safety and cosmetic techniques giving rise to oncoplastic breast surgery. This concept can be applied for both mastectomy and breast-conserving surgery [12].

One of the premature concerns regarding oncoplastic techniques for breast-conserving surgery was oncological safety. However, recurrence has decreased progressively over the years for several reasons. The advancement in imaging techniques to preoperatively localise the cancer area and the progress of adjuvant protocols are two examples. Oncoplastic breast-conserving surgery also can lower the percentage of close or positive margins while reconstructing the breast. Using therapeutic mammaplasty and flaps, the surgeon can excise the entire extent of cancer, including some residual non-affected breast tissue surrounding cancer, without compromising the cosmetic result [13, 14].

There have been numerous attempts to classify oncoplastic procedures. Ordinarily, they are separated by whether the strategy involves volume displacement or volume replacement. Volume displacement or reshaping procedures interchange dermo-glandular flaps from the breast area to the defect site. On the other hand, volume replacement techniques use autologous tissues to restore the volume loss that follows tumour resection [15].

Large tumours, high tumour/breast volume ratio and petite breasts in partial breast resections are frequently correlated with lacks that are challenging to reconstruct with volume displacement techniques. Indeed, in such cases, the patient may need reconstruction using autologous local or distant flaps. Furthermore, with the volume-replacement method, remodelling of the contralateral breast is usually not required to achieve symmetry. The use of pedicled and free fasciocutaneous and musculocutaneous flaps has been described for partial breast reconstruction. Among these, pedicled perforator flaps are the newest procedures available [15–17].

The pedicled perforator flap technique has an advantage over other methods of autologous breast reconstruction, as it uses well-vascularised tissues and spares the underlying muscles, which results in lower donor site morbidity in terms of muscle function and seroma formation. According to the pedicle length, perforator flaps can be used to manage defects in almost every quadrant. The main pedicled flaps from the chest wall area are nourished by intercostal, thoracodorsal and superior epigastric arteries perforators [16–18].

18.3 Outcomes

Breast cancer treatment aims to prolong survival providing the highest quality of life during and after treatment. Breast reconstruction is one factor that can adversely impact a survivor's capacity to deal with the physical and psychological features of the treatment. Quality outcomes for breast reconstruction rely on components, directly and indirectly, related to surgery, which are divided into objective and subjective elements. Oncological safety, surgical complications and physical function are some examples of objective factors. At the same time, quality of life and satisfaction are considered subjective elements. On the other hand, cosmetic assessment is a result of a combination of both objective and subjective factors. The synergy between these before-mentioned factors will determine the quality of outcomes for breast reconstruction.

18.3.1 General Aspects

Because of its benefits and flexibility, the use of oncoplastic breast-conserving surgery has become widely accepted and applied in routine clinical practice. For example, a recent study reported that from 2007 to 2014, the total percentage of oncoplastic breast-conserving surgery increased from 4% to 15% among all breast cancer surgeries and by the end of 2014 was making up to 33% of all breast-conserving surgeries (Fig. 18.2) [19].

Lately, researchers have created some new instruments to increase the accuracy of the quality of breast reconstruction assessment. The idea is to offer reliable objective and subjective data over the final physical result and patient's perception while being submitted to reconstruction. From the objective point of view, the investigators developed the BCCT.core (Fig. 18.3), a cosmetic evaluation instrument based on the symmetry and pre-established patterns of the breast mound [20]. This device seeks to turn the evaluation of the final surgical result into a standard process, capable of being compared with other patients. The scientists also developed questionnaires related to the patient's view of the disease, the treatment experience and the result. The development and validation of an instrument such as BREAST-Q helped bridge this knowledge gap (Fig. 18.4), as it established a relationship between pre and postoperative assessments based on patients' satisfaction with their breasts and their quality of life [21]. It is a fact that breast cancer treatment is a complex issue and a challenging experience for the patient. In this scenario, baseline subjective scores are essential as women undergoing breast reconstruction may start the process with different levels of satisfaction with their bodies and self-esteem.

As there are multiple techniques in breast reconstruction, a collaborative process between patients and clinicians can help patients navigate the process using evidence-based, patient-centred data combined with patient preferences. Thus, we can say that a high-quality outcome starts with a well-informed and assisted patient who will make good choices. Currently, most women undergoing breast-conserving surgery choose breast reconstruction and state that it offers a quality of life advantages and is an indispensable opportunity to enhance rehabilitation from breast

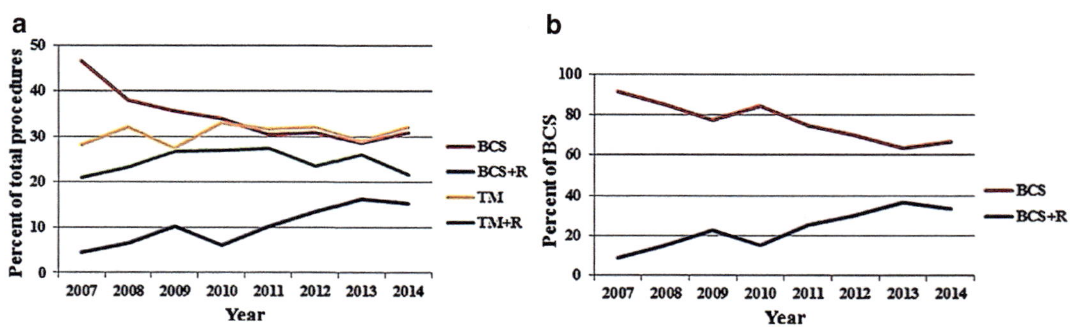

Fig. 18.2 (**a**) Graphic outlines the proportion of breast cancer procedures per year; (**b**) Proportion of breast-conserving surgery with or without reconstruction per year. *BCS* breast-conserving surgery, *BCS + R* breast-conserving surgery with reconstruction, *TM* total mastectomy, *TM + R* total mastectomy with reconstruction. (Adapted from "Operative and Oncologic Outcomes in 9861 Patients with Operable Breast Cancer: Single-Institution Analysis of Breast Conservation with Oncoplastic Reconstruction," by S. A. Carter et al., 2016, *Annals of surgical oncology*, *23*(10), 3190–3198. Copyright 2016 by Springer Nature. Reprinted with permission)

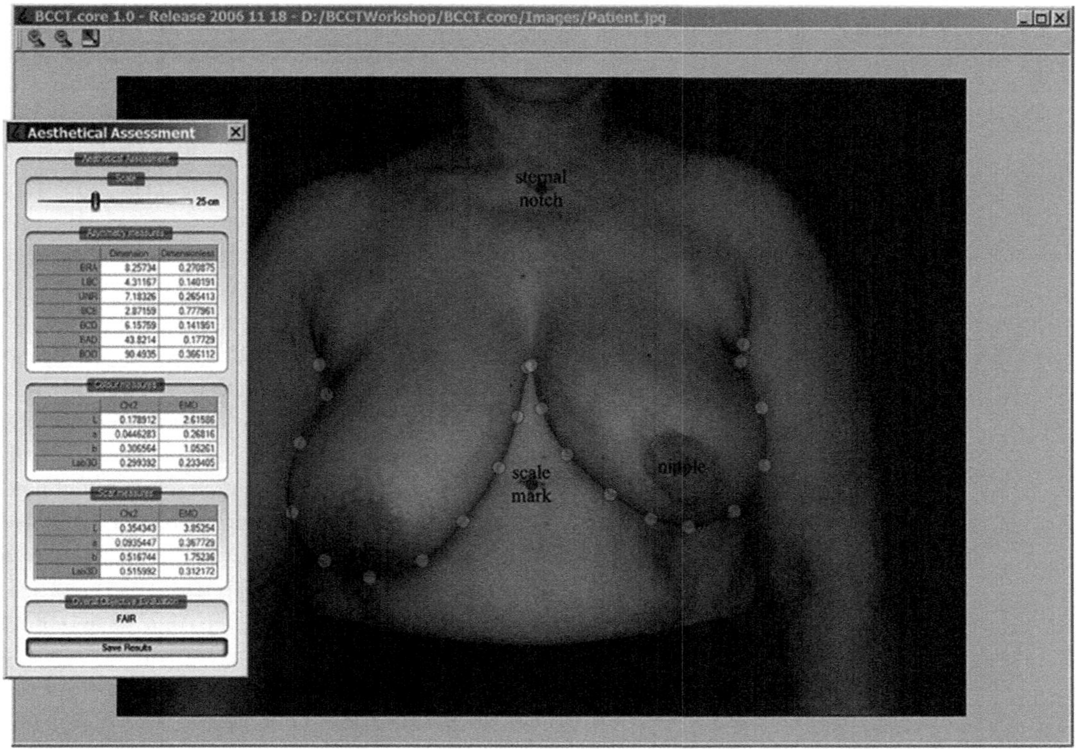

Fig. 18.3 BCCT.core software. Scale and reference points in the illustration. (Adapted from "Turning subjective into objective: the BCCT.core software for evaluation of cosmetic results in breast cancer conservative treatment," by M.J. Cardoso et al., 2007, *Breast*, 16(5):456–61. Copyright 2007 by Elsevier. Reprinted with permission)

cancer. Age alone should not discourage breast reconstruction. Older women who undergo breast reconstruction following breast-conserving surgery have similar outcomes and may have better quality of life-related results than those who do not [22].

18.3.2 Oncological Safety

Using chest wall perforator flaps for volume replacement following breast-conserving surgery was described initially in 2004 by Hamdi et al. and is a reliable procedure for patients with breast cancer [17]. During the following years, several subsequent papers described their use in clinical practice and reported outcomes. In 2013 Hamdi described that in a series with 93 patients submitted to partial breast reconstruction with perforators flaps, two cases needed surgical margin revision because these were compromised after final pathological assessment [16]. A systematic review by Pujji et al. published in 2021 with 432 patients submitted to partial breast reconstruction with pedicled perforator flaps reported a positive margin from 3% to 18%, with a pooled positive margin of 10.8%. Of these, 9.3% had re-excision of margins, and the rest was addressed to mastectomy. In addition, Pujji et al. reported a low local recurrence rate at 0–0.9%, and distal recurrence ranged from 0% to 10%, with a mean follow-up of 21 months (1–49) (Table 18.1) [23].

Quinn et al. reported in 2020 the most extensive series of cases of volume replacement oncoplastic breast-conserving surgery using local perforator flaps. The studied group was composed of 116 patients submitted to local perforator flaps from 2014 to 2020, and there were no local cancer

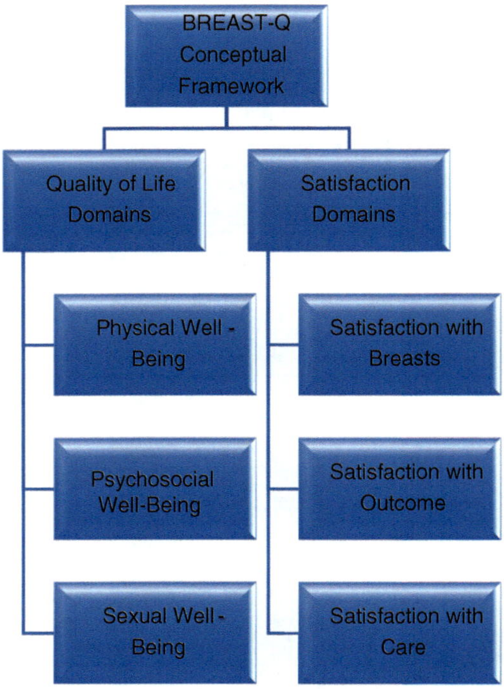

Fig. 18.4 BREAST-Q reported outcome framework for breast surgery. (Adapted from "Development of a new patient-reported outcome measure for breast surgery: the BREAST-Q," by A. L. Pusic et al., 2009, *Plastic and reconstructive surgery*, *124*(2), 345–353. Copyright 2009 by Wolters Kluwer Health. Reprinted with permission)

recurrences at a median follow-up of 37 months [31]. The second large case series was published by Soumian et al. in 2020 with 112 patients and presented a local recurrence index of 0.9% and distant recurrence of 0.9%. The Soumian et al. study was included in the systematic review of Pujji et al., which was discussed above [24].

A recent broader analysis of oncological safety for oncoplastic breast reconstruction was published by Raufdeen et al. in 2021. This systematic review compared oncoplastic breast-conserving surgery techniques, divided into volume replacement with latissimus dorsi (LD) flap, volume replacement non-LD flap and volume displacement. The volume replacement non-LD flap presented a lower probability of local recurrence (0.011 and 0.026) when compared to volume displacement (0.016 and 0.037) and volume replacement with LD flap (0.029 and 0.068). Even with a limited pool of data over breast reconstruction using chest wall perforator flaps, the results are positive [32].

Raufdeen et al. [32] study also reported a lower probability of mortality to volume replacement oncoplastic breast-conserving surgery non-LD flap compared to volume displacement and

Table 18.1 Oncological outcomes from the systematic review by Pujji et al. [23]

Oncological complications $n = x$ (%)						
Study	Positive margin	Re-excision	Completion mastectomy	Local recurrence	Distant recurrence	Death
Soumian et al. 2020 [24]	16 (14%)	15 (13%)	1 (0.9%)	1 (0.9%)	1 (0.9%)	0
Ojeda 2012 [25]	1 (4.6%)	NR	NR	NR	NR	NR
Roy 2016 [26]	4 (10%)	2 (5%)	2 (5%)	0	1 (2.5%)	0
Meybodi 2019 [27]	4 (18%)	4 (18%)	0	NR	NR	NR
Kim 2017 [28]	3 (7.5%)	3 (7.5%)	NR	NR	NR	NR
Hong 2019 [29]	1 (3%)	1 (3%)	0	0	0	0
Agrawal et al. 2020 [30]	5 (12.8%)	4 (10%)	1 (2.5%)	0	4 (10%)	1 (2.5%)
Total (range or mean)	34 (10.8%)	29 (9.3%)	4 (1.3%)	1 (0.45%)	6 (2.7%)	1 (0.45%)

NR not recorded

Adapted from "Systematic review of partial breast reconstruction with pedicled perforator artery flaps: Clinical, oncological and cosmetic outcomes," by O. Pujji et al., 2021, *European journal of surgical oncology: the journal of the European Society of Surgical Oncology and the British Association of Surgical Oncology*, *47*(8), 1883–1890. Copyright 2021 by Elsevier. Reprinted with permission volume replacement oncoplastic breast-conserving surgery LD flap (0.020 vs. 0.026 and 0.098). However, the oncological outcomes were worse in those patients who received volume replacement with LD flap. The LD flap is a technique established for decades and is frequently indicated after extensive resections of larger tumours since it provides a greater amount of tissue to restore the breast defect [32].

18.3.3 Surgical Complications

The before-mentioned study by Hamdi et al., published in 2013, listed only six seroma cases among thoracodorsal artery perforator (TDAP) flaps. There was no infection, haematoma or problem with the wound healing in this series [16]. On the other hand, Pujji et al. reported a complication rate of 12.3% and the haematoma was described in 1.9%, with half of these patients requiring a return to theatre for evacuation and wound wash out. In addition, 2.1% of patients developed a postoperative seroma. Flap necrosis was seen in 2.1%, with just one case of total flap necrosis. Sometimes, fat necrosis was described after radiotherapy treatment, and these patients underwent excision of the necrosed fat. Other complications included infection with 2.1%, wound dehiscence with 1.3% and venous congestion with 0.8% (Table 18.2) [23].

In Quinn et al. study, 101 repairs were performed as immediate partial breast reconstruction and 15 as delayed reconstructive procedures. The overall complication rate was 15%; most were minor surgical site infections, 1.7% required haematoma evacuation. Three patients who underwent delayed reconstruction required revision procedures, and one required a contralateral symmetrisation procedure. In addition, one patient in the immediate reconstruction group required additional lipofilling. Over time, the

Table 18.2 Clinical outcomes from the systematic review by Pujji et al. [23]

Clinical outcomes							
Clinical complications *n* = *x* (%)							
Study	Infection	Haematoma	Seroma	Flap necrosis (p = partial, t = total)	Fat necrosis	Wound dehiscence	Venous congestion
Munhoz 2011	0	0	0	0	1 (7.7%)	2 (15%)	0
McCulley 2015	0	0	0	0	0	0	1 (3.3%)
Soumian et al. 2020 [24]	0	4 (3.6%)	1 (0.9%)	0	1 (0.9%)	1 (0.9%)	0
Ojeda 2012 [25]	0	0	5 (23%)	0	0	1 (5%)	0
Roy 2016 [26]	0	2 (5%)	1 (2.5%)	1p (2.5%)	2 (5%)	0	0
Meybodi 2019 [27]	4 (18%)	0	1 (5%)	0	0	0	0
Kim 2017 [28]	0	0	0	4p (10%)	3 (7.5%)	0	2 (5%)
Abdelrahman et al. 2019 [33]	1 (4.8%)	1 (4.8%)	1 (4.8%)	2 (9.5%)	0	1 (4.8%)	0
Hong 2019 [29]	2 (6%)	0	0	0	2 (6%)	0	0
Carrasco-López et al. 2017 [34]	0	1 (7.1%)	0	1p (7.1%)	0	0	0
Agrawal et al. 2020 [30]	2 (5%)	0	0	1t (2.5%)	0	0	0
Total (range or mean)	9 (2.1%)	8 (1.9%)	9 (2.1%)	9 (2.1%)	9 (2.1%)	5 (1.2%)	3 (0.7%)

NR not recorded

Adapted from "Systematic review of partial breast reconstruction with pedicled perforator artery flaps: Clinical, oncological and cosmetic outcomes," by O. Pujji et al., 2021, *European journal of surgical oncology: the journal of the European Society of Surgical Oncology and the British Association of Surgical Oncology*, *47*(8), 1883–1890. Copyright 2021 by Elsevier. Reprinted with permission mean lesion size selected for immediate local flap reconstruction increased, operative times decreased, and the proportion of day case procedures expanded [31].

Another recent consecutive case series published by Schaverien in 2020 reported the outcomes of 21 patients submitted to volume replacement breast reconstruction and 16 of those who received the lateral intercostal artery perforator flap. No complication was registered in this group. However, four patients (19%) required a second intervention on the index breast, and one patient underwent contralateral symmetrisation [35].

18.3.4 Physical Function

Shoulder impairments are dramatically reduced with muscle-sparing LD flaps and other chest wall perforator flaps to restore the breast mound when compared to LD flaps. Amidst the chest wall perforator flaps, the TDAP flap harvesting is usually performed by splitting the muscle fibres without sacrificing the muscle itself. However, the harvesting technique combined with depriving the muscle of its primary blood supply may result in muscle atrophy and some decrease in function.

Bearing this in mind, Hamdi et al. reported in 2008 a prospective analysis of over shoulder function with 22 patients submitted to unilateral partial breast reconstruction with TDAP flap. Hamdi et al. used objective assessment to evaluate the discrepancy between sides shoulder mobility and found similar results. In addition, no statistically significant differences were observed in patients' groups submitted to axillary dissection or radiotherapy [36].

From the subjective point of view, a recent report published by Abdelrahman et al. described a comparative study with two equal groups of 21 patients submitted to immediate partial breast reconstruction, either with latissimus dorsi flap or TDAP flap. The study assessed the shoulder function using the Shoulder Pain and Disability Index at 3, 6 and 12 months during follow-up. Patients submitted to TDAP flap had a significantly lower motor disability of the shoulder when compared to the LD flap group at the same time intervals ($p < 0.001$) [33].

18.3.5 Cosmetic Outcomes

Pujji et al. [23] systematic review reported that 8 of 11 studies described cosmetic outcomes. The group of patients that rated the aesthetic result as good or excellent ranged from 76% to 100%. Besides the positive data showing that patients were satisfied with their breast reconstruction, most studies used different questionnaires, including self-generated ones. That limited the interpretation of the data even when using the same technique. In addition, only three studies used validated tools, though each one used a different assessment, which increased the confounding factor and reduced the accuracy of the analysis [23].

Fujimoto et al. published a study over long-term cosmetic outcomes after immediate partial breast reconstruction using chest wall perforators (33 patients) and breast-conserving surgery alone (167 patients). All patients were submitted to adjuvant radiotherapy, and 26 patients were followed for over 2 years. The aim analysis was performed using the BCCT.core. This software evaluates the latter aspect of the breast, including asymmetry, scar visibility and colour differences, then it produces a result of either poor, fair, good or excellent. The subjective analysis followed the four-category Harvard scale, using either poor, fair, good or excellent. Fujimoto et al. reported the relation between the extracted volume, the type of reconstruction and the ultimate aim and subjective assessments. When the resected volume exceeded 15%, the percentage of excellent or good outcomes was significantly higher in patients with flaps than in those with breast-conserving surgery alone (66% vs. 91% by aim assessment; $p < 0.05$; 48% vs. 96% by subjective assessment; $p < 0.01$, Fischer's exact test). More than half the patients submitted to chest wall perforator flap procedure maintained at least 80% of flap volume over 2 years after surgery (Figs. 18.5 and 18.6) [37].

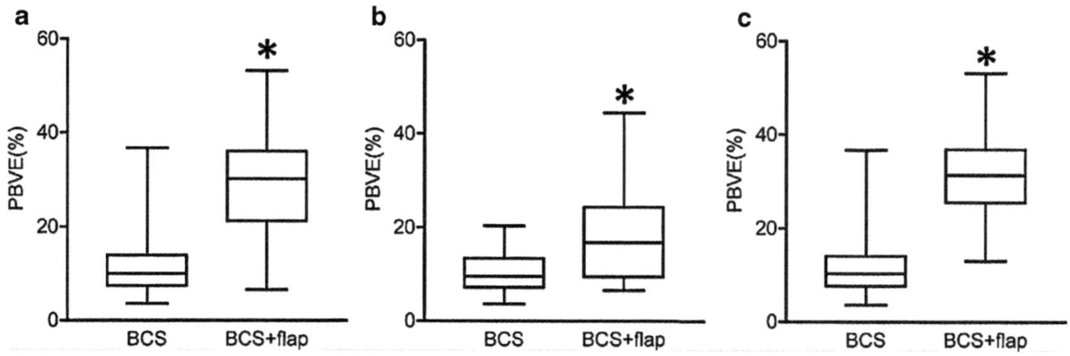

Fig. 18.5 Percentages of breast volume excised in patients who underwent breast-conserving surgery alone and breast-conserving surgery with flap. Tumours are located in all (**a**), inferior (**b**) and lateral (**c**) regions of the breast. *$p < 0.0001$. (Adapted from "Oncoplastic breast-conserving surgery using chest wall perforator flaps: Three-dimensional quantitative analysis of the percentage of breast volume excised and changes over time in flap volume," by H. Fujimoto, 2019, *Journal of surgical oncology*, https://doi.org/10.1002/jso.25809. Copyright 2019 by John Wiley & Sons. Reprinted with permission)

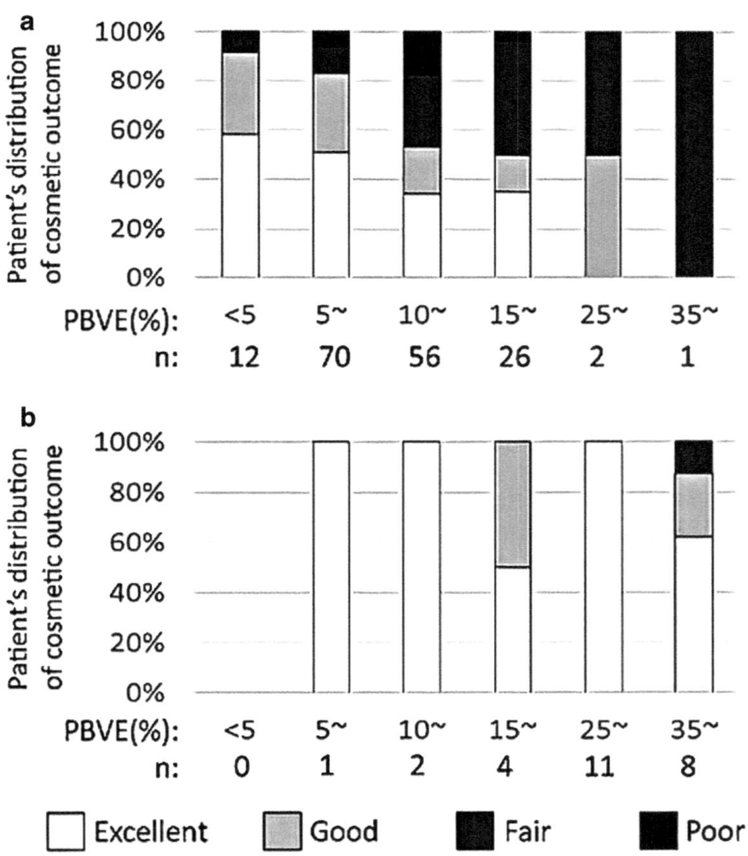

Fig. 18.6 Relationship between the volume excised from the breast and final cosmetic outcomes evaluated by the patients. Group (**a**) is related to patients submitted to breast-conserving surgery alone and group (**b**) to those submitted to breast-conserving surgery followed by reconstruction with chest wall flaps. (Adapted from "Oncoplastic breast-conserving surgery using chest wall perforator flaps: Three-dimensional quantitative analysis of the percentage of breast volume excised and changes over time in flap volume," by H. Fujimoto, 2019, *Journal of surgical oncology*, https://doi.org/10.1002/jso.25809. Copyright 2019 by John Wiley & Sons. Reprinted with permission)

18.3.6 Patient Satisfaction and Quality of Life

Agrawal et al. reported in 2016 results from research where the Breast-Q questionnaire was applied for eight patients submitted to partial breast reconstruction with chest wall perforator flaps. The Breast-Q score ranges between 0 and 100, the latter being the highest score. Mean results demonstrated satisfaction with breast around 90 points, physical well-being 82.9, psychosocial well-being 92.4, sexual well-being 77.7, back appearance 91.1 and shoulder and back function 82.9 [38].

Carrasco-López et al. also reported the results of the Breast-Q questionnaire of 14 patients submitted to breast reconstruction with anterior intercostal artery perforator flap. Scores were compared between baseline and post-local treatment. There was no difference between presurgical and postsurgical breast satisfaction scores with the breast, except for the patient who experienced a flap loss. Compared to pre-treatment scores, only four patients had a lower treatment outcome satisfaction score; in three cases, the patients reported changes in the overall breast consistency because of surgery and radiotherapy. In the fourth case, the dissatisfaction was because of the partial flap loss. No significant changes were observed in psychosocial and sexual well-being, except in the patient with partial flap loss (mean change 0 and 6.15). Curiously, there was a significant reduction in physical satisfaction after the breast reconstruction with a mean difference of 34.7% compared to baseline evaluation [34].

Agrawal et al. reported a prospective observational cohort study of 40 patients who had undergone breast conservation surgery plus chest wall perforator flaps reconstruction in a period of 3 years. Of these, 57.5% of patients had lateral intercostal artery perforator (LICAP) flap, 5% had lateral thoracic artery perforator (LTAP) flap, 27.5% had combined LICAP plus LTAP and 10% patients had anterior intercostal artery perforator flap. An informal questionnaire was developed and used to assess patient satisfaction at least 6 months after the completion of radiotherapy, using a 4-point Likert scale. Overall, 25 patients replied to the follow-up, 96% were satisfied with the scar and 88% were happy with the treated breast compared to the contralateral one. In addition, 92% declared to be well satisfied with their appearance in public and reaffirmed their confidence over the decision to undergo breast-conserving surgery (Table 18.3) [30].

18.4 Conclusions

Besides the lack of data, breast reconstruction using pedicled chest wall perforators flaps seems safe, with good cosmetic results and increased patients' quality of life. However, some aspects must be underscored for future discussion over the subject.

Objective factors related to breast reconstruction using chest wall perforators flaps are easily identified. The breast team has been gradually increasing the quality of assistance to avoid or reduce adverse outcomes related to these known

Table 18.3 Patient satisfaction after partial breast reconstruction with chest wall perforator flaps

Patient satisfaction	Highly unsatisfied	Unsatisfied	Satisfied	Highly Satisfied
How satisfied are you with your scar?	0 (0%)	1 (4%)	15 (60%)	9 (36%)
How happy are you with your treated breast in comparison to the opposite breast?	0 (0%)	3 (12%)	9 (36%)	13 (52%)
How comfortable are you going out in public?	0 (0%)	2 (8%)	12 (48%)	11 (44%)
Do you feel, in retrospect, that you should have opted for a mastectomy?	0 (0%)	2 (8%)	2 (8%)	19 (84%)

Adapted from "Chest wall perforator flaps in partial breast reconstruction after breast conservation surgery: an additional oncoplastic surgical option," by S. K. Agrawal et al., 2020, *Ecancermedicalscience*, *14*, 1073. CC BY 3.0

objective factors. On the other hand, assessment over the subjective factors is still in a grey zone area. Lack of reliable data and difficulties in standardising analysis are examples of the obstacles the breast team faces in current times. However, while these answers are not yet available, the take-home message of this chapter is that the patients' desires are supreme in determining the breast reconstruction plan. While some patients are considerably pleased with their breast shape, others have been expecting for an occasion to have an aesthetic procedure, reduction or augmentation. This concept means that patients have different baselines that need to be addressed differently while treating breast cancer. Therefore, personalised plans will definitely improve patient satisfaction and outcomes.

References

1. Sung H, Ferlay J, Siegel RL, Laversanne M, Soerjomataram I, Jemal A, Bray F. Global Cancer Statistics 2020: GLOBOCAN estimates of incidence and mortality worldwide for 36 cancers in 185 countries. CA Cancer J Clin. 2021;71(3):209–49. https://doi.org/10.3322/caac.21660.
2. Malvezzi M, Carioli G, Bertuccio P, Boffetta P, Levi F, La Vecchia C, Negri E. European cancer mortality predictions for the year 2019 with focus on breast cancer. Ann Oncol. 2019;30(5):781–7. https://doi.org/10.1093/annonc/mdz051.
3. Althuis MD, Dozier JM, Anderson WF, Devesa SS, Brinton LA. Global trends in breast cancer incidence and mortality 1973-1997. Int J Epidemiol. 2005;34(2):405–12. https://doi.org/10.1093/ije/dyh414.
4. Eloranta S, Smedby KE, Dickman PW, Andersson TM. Cancer survival statistics for patients and healthcare professionals - a tutorial of real-world data analysis. J Intern Med. 2021;289(1):12–28. https://doi.org/10.1111/joim.13139.
5. Waks AG, Winer EP. Breast cancer treatment: a review. JAMA. 2019;321(3):288–300. https://doi.org/10.1001/jama.2018.19323.
6. Strach MC, Prasanna T, Kirova YM, Alran S, O'Toole S, Beith JM, Poortmans P, McNeil CM, Carroll S. Optimise not compromise: the importance of a multidisciplinary breast cancer patient pathway in the era of oncoplastic and reconstructive surgery. Crit Rev Oncol Hematol. 2019;134:10–21. https://doi.org/10.1016/j.critrevonc.2018.11.007.
7. Sakorafas GH, Safioleas M. Breast cancer surgery: an historical narrative. Part III. From the sunset of the 19th to the dawn of the 21st century. Eur J Cancer Care. 2010;19(2):145–66. https://doi.org/10.1111/j.1365-2354.2008.01061.x.
8. Angarita FA, Elmi M, Zhang Y, Look Hong NJ. Patient-reported factors influencing the treatment decision-making process of older women with non-metastatic breast cancer: a systematic review of qualitative evidence. Breast Cancer Res Treat. 2018;171(3):545–64. https://doi.org/10.1007/s10549-018-4865-0.
9. Gu J, Groot G, Boden C, Busch A, Holtslander L, Lim H. Review of factors influencing women's choice of mastectomy versus breast conserving therapy in early stage breast cancer: a systematic review. Clin Breast Cancer. 2018;18(4):e539–54. https://doi.org/10.1016/j.clbc.2017.12.013.
10. O'Mahony M, Comber H, Fitzgerald T, Corrigan MA, Fitzgerald E, Grunfeld EA, Flynn MG, Hegarty J. Interventions for raising breast cancer awareness in women. Cochrane Database Syst Rev. 2017;2(2):CD011396. https://doi.org/10.1002/14651858.CD011396.pub2.
11. Katz SJ, Lantz PM, Janz NK, Fagerlin A, Schwartz K, Liu L, Deapen D, Salem B, Lakhani I, Morrow M. Patient involvement in surgery treatment decisions for breast cancer. J Clin Oncol. 2005;23(24):5526–33. https://doi.org/10.1200/JCO.2005.06.217.
12. Kaufman CS. Increasing role of oncoplastic surgery for breast cancer. Curr Oncol Rep. 2019;21(12):111. https://doi.org/10.1007/s11912-019-0860-9.
13. De La Cruz L, Blankenship SA, Chatterjee A, Geha R, Nocera N, Czerniecki BJ, Tchou J, Fisher CS. Outcomes after oncoplastic breast-conserving surgery in breast cancer patients: a systematic literature review. Ann Surg Oncol. 2016;23(10):3247–58. https://doi.org/10.1245/s10434-016-5313-1.
14. Kosasih S, Tayeh S, Mokbel K, Kasem A. Is oncoplastic breast conserving surgery oncologically safe? A meta-analysis of 18,103 patients. Am J Surg. 2020;220(2):385–92. https://doi.org/10.1016/j.amjsurg.2019.12.019.
15. Bertozzi N, Pesce M, Santi PL, Raposio E. Oncoplastic breast surgery: comprehensive review. Eur Rev Med Pharmacol Sci. 2017;21(11):2572–85.
16. Hamdi M. Oncoplastic and reconstructive surgery of the breast. Breast. 2013;22(Suppl 2):S100–5. https://doi.org/10.1016/j.breast.2013.07.019.
17. Hamdi M, Van Landuyt K, Monstrey S, Blondeel P. Pedicled perforator flaps in breast reconstruction: a new concept. Br J Plast Surg. 2004;57(6):531–9. https://doi.org/10.1016/j.bjps.2004.04.015.
18. Hamdi M, Van Landuyt K, de Frene B, Roche N, Blondeel P, Monstrey S. The versatility of the intercostal artery perforator (ICAP) flaps. J Plast Reconstr Aesthet Surg. 2006;59(6):644–52. https://doi.org/10.1016/j.bjps.2006.01.006.
19. Carter SA, Lyons GR, Kuerer HM, Bassett RL Jr, Oates S, Thompson A, Caudle AS, Mittendorf EA, Bedrosian I, Lucci A, DeSnyder SM, Babiera G, Yi M, Baumann DP, Clemens MW, Garvey PB, Hunt KK, Hwang RF. Operative and oncologic outcomes in 9861

patients with operable breast cancer: single-institution analysis of breast conservation with oncoplastic reconstruction. Ann Surg Oncol. 2016;23(10):3190–8. https://doi.org/10.1245/s10434-016-5407-9.
20. Cardoso MJ, Cardoso J, Amaral N, Azevedo I, Barreau L, Bernardo M, Christie D, Costa S, Fitzal F, Fougo JL, Johansen J, Macmillan D, Mano MP, Regolo L, Rosa J, Teixeira L, Vrieling C. Turning subjective into objective: the BCCT.core software for evaluation of cosmetic results in breast cancer conservative treatment. Breast. 2007;16(5):456–61. https://doi.org/10.1016/j.breast.2007.05.002.
21. Pusic AL, Klassen AF, Scott AM, Klok JA, Cordeiro PG, Cano SJ. Development of a new patient-reported outcome measure for breast surgery: the BREAST-Q. Plast Reconstr Surg. 2009;124(2):345–53. https://doi.org/10.1097/PRS.0b013e3181aee807.
22. Quemener J, Wallet J, Boulanger L, Hannebicque K, Chauvet MP, Régis C. Decision-making determinants for breast reconstruction in women over 65 years old. Breast J. 2019;25(6):1235–40. https://doi.org/10.1111/tbj.13438.
23. Pujji O, Blackhall V, Romics L, Vidya R. Systematic review of partial breast reconstruction with pedicled perforator artery flaps: clinical, oncological and cosmetic outcomes. Eur J Surg Oncol. 2021;47(8):1883–90. https://doi.org/10.1016/j.ejso.2021.03.249.
24. Soumian S, Parmeshwar R, Chandarana M, Marla S, Narayanan S, Shetty G. Chest wall perforator flaps for partial breast reconstruction: surgical outcomes from a multicenter study. Arch Plast Surg. 2020;47(2):153–9. https://doi.org/10.5999/aps.2019.01186.
25. Lopez Ojeda AB, Lopez CC, Rodrigues TAG, et al.Thoracodorsal artery perforator (TDAP) flap in immediate breast reconstruction and the role of preoperative mapping: a clinical experience. Eur J Plast Surg. 2013;36:165–170.
26. Roy PG. One-stage vs. two-stage approach for partial breast reconstruction with lateral chest wall perforator flaps. Canc Treat Res Commun, 2016;92016:56–61.
27. Meybodi F, Cocco AM, Messer D, et al.The modified lateral intercostal artery perforator flap. Plast Reconstr Surg Glob Open. 2019;7(2). Article e2066.
28. Kim JB, Eom JR, Lee JW, Lee J, Park HY, Yang JD. Utility of two surgical techniques using a lateral intercostal artery perforator flap after breast-conserving surgery: a single-center retrospective study. Plast Reconstr Surg. 2019;143(3):477e–487e.
29. Hong S, Wang S, Liu J, Qiang Z, Zheng X, Chen G . Usefulness of lateral thoracic adipofascial flaps after breast-conserving surgery in small-to moderate-sized breasts. Clin Breast Canc. 2019;19(5):370–376.
30. Agrawal SK, Shakya SR, Nigam S, Sharma A, Datta SS, Ahmed R. Chest wall perforator flaps in partial breast reconstruction after breast conservation surgery: an additional oncoplastic surgical option. Ecancermedicalscience. 2020;14:1073. https://doi.org/10.3332/ecancer.2020.1073.
31. Quinn EM, Burrah R, O'Ceallaigh S, Highton L, Murphy J. Six-year experience of oncoplastic volume replacement using local perforator flaps. J Plast Reconstr Aesthet Surg. 2021;74(9):2184–93. https://doi.org/10.1016/j.bjps.2020.12.083.
32. Raufdeen F, Murphy J, Ahluwalia M, Coroneos CJ, Thoma A. Outcomes in volume replacement and volume displacement techniques in oncoplastic breast conserving surgery: a systematic review. J Plast Reconstr Aesthet Surg. 2021;74:2846. https://doi.org/10.1016/j.bjps.2021.06.004.
33. Abdelrahman EM, Nawar AM, Balbaa MA, Shoulah AA, Shora AA, Kharoub MS. Oncoplastic volume replacement for breast cancer: latissimus dorsi flap versus thoracodorsal artery perforator flap. Plastic Reconstr Surg. 2019;7(10):e2476. https://doi.org/10.1097/GOX.0000000000002476.
34. Carrasco-López C, Julian Ibañez JF, Vilà J, Luna Tomás MA, Navinés López J, Pascual Miguel I, Fernandez-Llamazares-Rodriguez J, Higueras-Suñe C. Anterior intercostal artery perforator flap in immediate breast reconstruction: anatomical study and clinical application. Microsurgery. 2017;37(6):603–10. https://doi.org/10.1002/micr.30171.
35. Schaverien MV, Kuerer HM, Caudle AS, Smith BD, Hwang RF, Robb GL. Outcomes of volume replacement oncoplastic breast-conserving surgery using chest wall perforator flaps: comparison with volume displacement oncoplastic surgery and total breast reconstruction. Plast Reconstr Surg. 2020;146(1):14–27. https://doi.org/10.1097/PRS.0000000000006911.
36. Hamdi M, Salgarello M, Barone-Adesi L, Van Landuyt K. Use of the thoracodorsal artery perforator (TDAP) flap with implant in breast reconstruction. Ann Plast Surg. 2008;61(2):143–6. https://doi.org/10.1097/SAP.0b013e318158fd7b.
37. Fujimoto H, Shiina N, Nagashima T, Sangai T, Sakakibara J, Takada M, Teranaka R, Takishima H, Kawasaki Y, Ohtsuka M. Oncoplastic breast-conserving surgery using chest wall perforator flaps: three-dimensional quantitative analysis of the percentage of breast volume excised and changes over time in flap volume. J Surg Oncol. 2020;121:216. https://doi.org/10.1002/jso.25809.
38. Agrawal A, Mirshekar-Syahkal B. Use of combination of modules of BREAST-Q in partial breast reconstruction with lateral chest wall perforator flap. Eur J Surg Oncol. 2016;42(5):S39.

A Systematic Review of Partial Breast Reconstruction with Pedicled Perforator Artery Flaps: Clinical, Oncological and Cosmetic Outcomes

19

Ojas Pujji, Vivienne Blackhall, Laszlo Romics, and Raghavan Vidya

Content

With breast cancer becoming the most common cancer worldwide in women [1], significant strides are being made in its management to ensure a balance between ontologically safe resection and adequate cosmesis without compromising short- and long-term clinical outcomes.

Chest wall perforator flaps (CWPFs) provide a useful solution for those women undergoing breast conservation surgery (BCS) who would otherwise have to undergo mastectomy due to poor cosmetic outcome of the residual breast tissue. There is limited evidence studying CWPFs [2–5].

A systematic review was conducted which included eight case series, two prospective cohort studies and one randomised controlled trial (RCT) evaluating the clinical, oncological and cosmetic outcomes of pedicled perforator flaps for partial breast reconstruction following excision of primary breast cancer between 1990 and July 2020 [6].

Baseline characteristics of patients and tumour are presented in Table 19.1.

Oncological and clinical outcomes are shown in Tables 19.2 and 19.3.

Our review demonstrated a positive margin rate at 3–18% and a low local recurrence rate at 0–0.9%, which is in line with the outcomes reported following BCS (7–22% incomplete excisions and 0–7% local recurrence rate) [7]. Our results are also in line with other reviews evaluating a range of oncoplastic techniques including volume replacement and displacement [8–10].

Disclaimer: This chapter is partially based on 'Pujji OJS, Blackhall V, Romics L, Vidya R. Systematic review of partial breast reconstruction with pedicled perforator artery flaps: Clinical, oncological and cosmetic outcomes. Eur J Surg Oncol. 2021 Aug;47(8):1883–1890'.

O. Pujji · R. Vidya (✉)
Department of Breast Surgery, The Royal Wolverhampton NHS Trust, Wolverhampton, UK
e-mail: Ojas.pujji@nhs.net; Raghavan.Vidya@nhs.net

V. Blackhall
Registrar in General Surgery, The Queen Elizabeth University Hospital, Glasgow, Scotland, UK

L. Romics
Gartnavel General Hospital, Glasgow, Scotland, UK
e-mail: Laszlo.romics@nhs.net

M. Hamdi et al. (eds.), *Pedicled Flaps in Partial Breast Reconstruction*,
https://doi.org/10.1007/978-3-031-08483-6_19

A total of 52 clinical complications were seen across the 432 cases (12.3%). Haematoma was described in eight cases (1.9%), with four of these patients requiring a return to theatre [11–14]. Nine patients developed a postoperative seroma (2.1%) [14, 15]. Flap necrosis was seen in nine patients (2.1%), eight of which were partial [12, 13, 16]. Fat necrosis was described in a total of nine cases (2.1%) [12, 14, 17–19]. Other complications included infection (9; 2.1%) [13–16], wound dehiscence (5; 1.3%) and venous congestion (3; 0.8%).

Table 19.1 Cohort baseline characteristics

Characteristic	Value	Reference
Age	28–83 years	[20]
BMI	18–32	[16, 17, 21]
Breast size	A-D cup	[6, 21, 22]
T stage		[6, 11, 12, 22]
T1	18–69.2%	
T2	30.7–71%	
T3	0–12.5%	
N stage		[6, 21, 22]
N0	50–52%	
N1	22.5–38%	
N2	10–20%	
N3	0–5%	
Indication for surgery		[6, 9, 14]
Invasive cancer	53.8–92.5%	
DCIS	7.7–14.3%	
Most common tumour location-UOQ	23.1–72.7%	[6, 11, 14]
Mean specimen weight	62.5–164.7 g	[6, 11, 14]
Mean hospital stay	1–10 days	[11, 14, 21]

Eight studies reported on cosmetic outcomes as rated by the patient. Most patients had a positive opinion regarding the cosmetic appearance of their reconstructed breast. The majority of patients were satisfied with the appearance of the breast or rated the cosmetic outcome as either good or excellent (range 76.2–100%).

The use of CWPFs is expanding for partial breast reconstruction following BCS for breast cancer. However, larger RCTs or prospective studies with long-term follow-up are required to demonstrate the safety and acceptability of CWPFs with well-defined outcome measures and qualitative assessment of patient experience and perceptions of the technique.

Table 19.2 Oncological outcomes from the systematic review by Pujji et al. [6]

Oncological outcomes $n = x$ (%)						
Study	Positive margin	Re-excision	Completion mastectomy	Local recurrence	Distant recurrence	Death
Soumian [14]	16 (14%)	15 (13%)	1 (0.9%)	1 (0.9%)	1 (0.9%)	0
Lopez Ojeda [23]	1 (4.6%)	NR	NR	NR	NR	NR
Roy [11]	4 (10%)	2 (5%)	2 (5%)	0	1 (2.5%)	0
Meybodi [15]	4 (18%)	4 (18%)	0	NR	NR	NR
Kim [16]	3 (7.5%)	3 (7.5%)	NR	NR	NR	NR
Hong [18]	1 (3%)	1 (3%)	0	0	0	0
Agrawal [24]	5 (12.8%)	4 (10%)	1 (2.5%)	0	4 (10%)	1 (2.5%)
Total (range or mean)	34 (10.8%)	29 (9.3%)	4 (1.3%)	1 (0.45%)	6 (2.7%)	1 (0.45%)

Note: *NR* not recorded. Adapted from 'Systematic review of partial breast reconstruction with pedicled perforator artery flaps: Clinical, oncological and cosmetic outcomes', by O. Pujji et al., 2021, *European journal of surgical oncology: the journal of the European Society of Surgical Oncology and the British Association of Surgical Oncology*, *47*(8), 1883–1890. Copyright 2021 by Elsevier. Reprinted with permission

Table 19.3 Clinical outcomes from the systematic review by Pujji et al. [6]

Clinical outcomes							
Clinical complications $n = x$ (%)							
Study	Infection	Haematoma	Seroma	Flap necrosis (p = partial, t = total)	Fat necrosis	Wound dehiscence	Venous congestion
Munhoz [17]	0	0	0	0	1 (7.7%)	2 (15%)	0
McCulley [25]	0	0	0	0	0	0	1 (3.3%)
Soumian [14]	0	4 (3.6%)	1 (0.9%)	0	1 (0.9%)	1 (0.9%)	0
Lopez Ojeda [23]	0	0	5 (23%)	0	0	1 (5%)	0
Roy [11]	0	2 (5%)	1 (2.5%)	1p (2.5%)	2 (5%)	0	0
Meybodi [15]	4 (18%)	0	1 (5%)	0	0	0	0
Kim [16]	0	0	0	4p (10%)	3 (7.5%)	0	2 (5%)
Abdelrahman [12]	1 (4.8%)	1 (4.8%)	1 (4.8%)	2 (9.5%)	0	1 (4.8%)	0
Hong [18]	2 (6%)	0	0	0	2 (6%)	0	0
Carrasco-Lopez [13]	0	1 (7.1%)	0	1p (7.1%)	0	0	0
Agrawal [24]	2 (5%)	0	0	1t (2.5%)	0	0	0
Total (range or mean)	9 (2.1%)	8 (1.9%)	9 (2.1%)	9 (2.1%)	9 (2.1%)	5 (1.2%)	3 (0.7%)

Note: *NR* not recorded. Adapted from 'Systematic review of partial breast reconstruction with pedicled perforator artery flaps: Clinical, oncological and cosmetic outcomes', by O. Pujji et al., 2021, *European journal of surgical oncology : the journal of the European Society of Surgical Oncology and the British Association of Surgical Oncology*, *47*(8), 1883–1890. Copyright 2021 by Elsevier. Reprinted with permission

References

1. Cancer incidence for common cancers. https://www.cancerresearchuk.org/health-professional/cancer-statistics/incidence/common-cancers-compared#heading-Two:%202020. Accessed 17 Mar 2020.
2. Haloua MH, Krekel NM, Winters HA, et al. A systematic review of oncoplastic breast-conserving surgery: current weaknesses and future prospects. Ann Surg. 2013;257:609–20.
3. Yiannakopoulou EC, Mathelin C. Oncoplastic breast conserving surgery and oncological outcome: systematic review. Eur J Surg Oncol. 2016;42:625–30.
4. Campbell EJ, Romics L. Oncological safety and cosmetic outcomes in oncoplastic conservation surgery, a review of the best level of evidence literature. Breast Cancer. 2017;9:521–30.
5. Youssif S, Hassan Y, Tohamy A, et al. Pedicled local flaps: a reliable reconstructive tool for partial breast defects. Gland Surg. 2019;8(5):527–36.
6. Pujji OJS, Blackhall V, Romics L, Vidya R. Systematic review of partial breast reconstruction with pedicled perforator artery flaps: clinical, oncological and cosmetic outcomes. Eur J Surg Oncol. 2021;47(8):1883–90. https://doi.org/10.1016/j.ejso.2021.03.249. Epub 2021 Apr 13. PMID: 33895022.
7. Haloua MH, Krekel NM, Winters HA, Rietveld DH, Meijer S, Bloemers FW, et al. A systematic review of oncoplastic breast-conserving surgery: current weaknesses and future prospects. Ann Surg. 2013;257(4):609–20. https://doi.org/10.1097/SLA.0b013e3182888782. PMID: 2347050.
8. Moher D, Liberati A, Tetzlaff J, Altman DG, The PRISMA Group. Preferred reporting items for systematic reviews and meta-analyses: the PRISMA statement. PLoS Med. 2009;6(7):e1000097. https://doi.org/10.1371/journal.pmed.1000097.
9. Yoon JJ, Green WR, Kim S, et al. Oncoplastic breast surgery in the setting of breast-conserving therapy: a systematic review. Adv Radiat Oncol. 2016;1(4):205–15.
10. Romics L, Macaskill EJ, Fernandez T, Simpson L, Morrow E, Pitsinis V, et al. A population-based audit of surgical practice and outcomes of oncoplastic breast conservations in Scotland—an analysis of 589 patients. Eur J Surg Oncol. 2018;44(7):939–44. https://doi.org/10.1016/j.ejso.2018.04.004. Epub 2018 Apr 13. PMID: 29705287.
11. Roy PG. One-stage vs two-stage approach for partial breast reconstruction with lateral chest wall perforator flaps. Cancer Treat Res Commun. 2016;9:56–61.
12. Abdelrahman EM, Nawar AM, Balbaa MA, Shoulah AA, Shora AA, Kharoub MS. Oncoplastic volume replacement for breast cancer: latissimus dorsi flap versus thoracodorsal artery perforator flap. Plast Reconstr Surg Glob Open. 2019;7(10):e2476.
13. Carrasco-Lopez C, Julian Ibanez JF, Vila J, Luna Tomas MA, Navines Lopez J, Pascual Miguel I, et al.

Anterior intercostal artery perforator flap in immediate breast reconstruction: anatomical study and clinical application. Microsurgery. 2017;37(6):603–10. https://doi.org/10.1002/micr.30171. Epub 2017 Mar 28. PMID: 28370199.
14. Soumian S, Parmeshwar R, Chandarana M, Marla S, Narayanan S, Shetty G. Chest wall perforator flaps for partial breast reconstruction: surgical outcomes from a multicenter study. Arch Plast Surg. 2020;47(2):153–9.
15. Meybodi F, Cocco AM, Messer D, et al. The modified lateral intercostal artery perforator flap. Plast Reconstr Surg Glob Open. 2019;7(2):e2066.
16. Kim JB, Eom JR, Lee JW, Lee J, Park HY, Yang JD. Utility of two surgical techniques using a lateral intercostal artery perforator flap after breast-conserving surgery: a single-centre retrospective study. Plast Reconstr Surg. 2019;143(3):477e–87e.
17. Munhoz AM, Montag E, Arruda E, et al. Immediate conservative breast surgery reconstruction with perforator flaps: new challenges in the era of partial mastectomy reconstruction? Breast. 2011;20(3):233–40.
18. Hong S, Wang S, Liu J, Qiang Z, Zheng X, Chen G. Usefulness of lateral thoracic adipofascial flaps after breast-conserving surgery in small-to moderate-sized breasts. Clin Breast Cancer. 2019;19(5):370–6.
19. Ayman A, Mohamed R, Farahat A, Hashem T. The role of thoracodorsal artery perforator flap in oncoplastic breast surgery. J Egypt Natl Canc Inst. 2017;29(2):83–7.
20. Martin RC, et al. Quality of complication reporting in the surgical literature. Ann Surg. 2002;235:803.
21. Hamdi M, Van Landuyt K, Monstrey S, Blondeel P. Pedicled perforator flaps in breast reconstruction: a new concept. Br J Plast Surg. 2004;57(6):531–9.
22. Institute of Health Economics (IHE). Quality appraisal of case series studies checklist. Edmonton, AB: Institute of Health Economics; 2014. http://www.ihe.ca/research-programs/rmd/cssqac/cssqac-about.
23. Lopez Ojeda AB, Lopez CC, Rodrigues TAG, et al. Thoracodorsal artery perforator (TDAP) flap in immediate breast reconstruction and the role of preoperative mapping: a clinical experience. Eur J Plast Surg 2013;36:165e70.
24. Agrawal SK, Shakya SR, Nigam S, Sharma A, Datta SS, Ahmed R. Chest wall perforator flaps in partial breast reconstruction after breast conservation surgery: an additional oncoplastic surgical option. Ecanc Med Sci 2020;14:1073. https://doi.org/10.3332/ecancer.2020.1073. Published 2020 Jul 17.
25. McCulley SJ, Schaverien MV, Tan VK, Macmillan RD. Lateral thoracic artery perforator (LTAP) flap in partial breast reconstruction. J Plast Reconstr Aesthetic Surg 2015;68(5):686e91.

GPSR Compliance

The European Union's (EU) General Product Safety Regulation (GPSR) is a set of rules that requires consumer products to be safe and our obligations to ensure this.

If you have any concerns about our products, you can contact us on ProductSafety@springernature.com

In case Publisher is established outside the EU, the EU authorized representative is:

Springer Nature Customer Service Center GmbH
Europaplatz 3
69115 Heidelberg, Germany

Batch number: 10732801

Printed by Printforce, the Netherlands